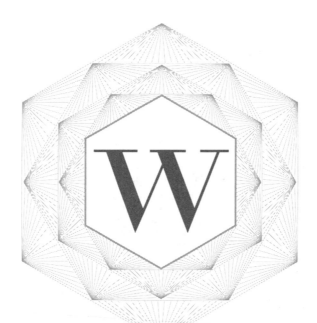

SUPER
WOMAN R~X~

Discover the Secrets to Lasting Health, Your Perfect Weight, Energy, and Passion with Dr. Taz's Power Type Plans

TASNEEM BHATIA, MD

RODALE.

RODALE *wellness*

Live happy. Be healthy. Get inspired.

Sign up today to get exclusive access to our authors, exclusive bonuses,
and the most authoritative, useful, and cutting-edge information
on health, wellness, fitness, and living your life to the fullest.

Visit us online at RodaleWellness.com
Join us at RodaleWellness.com/Join

© 2017 by Tasneem Bhatia, MD

All rights reserved. No part of this publication may be reproduced or transmitted in any form
or by any means, electronic or mechanical, including photocopying, recording, or any other
information storage and retrieval system, without the written permission of the publisher.

Rodale books may be purchased for business or promotional use or for special sales.
For information, please e-mail BookMarketing@Rodale.com.

Printed in the United States of America

Photo credits: Mitch Mandel/Rodale Images (pages 260 *bottom* and 272 *bottom*);
Thom MacDonald/Rodale Images (page 272 *top*); Matt Rainey/Rodale Images
(page 273 *bottom*); Photodisk (page 307); and Beth Bischoff (all remaining image)

Illustration credits: 123RF (page 41) and Peter Hermes Furian/123RF (page 43)

Book design by Christina Gaugler

Library of Congress Cataloging-in-Publication Data is on file with the publisher.

ISBN 978–1–62336–858–6 hardcover

Distributed to the trade by Macmillan

2   4   6   8   10   9   7   5   3   1   hardcover

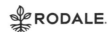

We inspire health, healing, happiness, and love in the world.
Starting with you.

To the original Super Woman—
my mom—and a super woman to be—my daughter, Rania.
Thank you, Mom; you have created a legacy that you may not
still understand. Rania, I cannot wait to see what you will do—
you picked the title of this book and you make me laugh
and feel so very proud every day.

Contents

Introduction

BEEP...BEEP...BEEP!

That cannot be my alarm. I swear I just went to bed.

The clock says 5 a.m., so that's a yes, and once I've opened my eyes, the race is on.

Remember the first Superman movie starring Christopher Reeve? In one scene, Superman flies around the earth so fast that he is able to reverse its orbit and turn back time to save Lois Lane. My mornings have a similar race-around-the-earth feel to them. Thankfully, what looks like a complete flurry is really a finely tuned morning routine that meets my needs and sends my family—and me—out the door energized and happy. Here's how it goes.

I carefully crawl out of bed and navigate the obstacle course that is my bedroom (often, I have nighttime visitors: my 8-year-old son Kubby and my daughter, Rania, 9, plus the stuffed animal family that comes with them). Once I'm safely in the hallway, I stumble downstairs (this takes 30 seconds) and boil water in the kettle for my must-have morning tea (2 to 3 minutes). While that's happening, I decide if it's a food prep or a workout day (I alternate). Based on my decision, I either throw on my workout clothes or pull out the cutting board, knife, veggies, and fruit and do some extra-healthy-food prep work to keep my family—and myself—stocked for easy grab-and-go noshing (5 minutes)—but first, my precious tea. It's my own concoction made from a regular Lipton black tea bag steeped with cinnamon sticks, raw ginger, and cardamom (the additions help my digestive system). I'd love to sip my morning drink luxuriously with my feet propped up—ha!—but on a work and school day that's just a fantasy. Instead, I guzzle tea from the hot mug and head to our exercise room for 30 to 40 minutes. My workouts consist of a variety of exercises—from cardio on our elliptical or spin bike to strength training, Pilates, and/or yoga. I switch it up according to my energy levels, with 10 minutes or so of meditation tacked on at the end. If it's a food prep day, I'll spend my time washing and cutting fruits and veggies, packing lunches and snacks for all of us, and prepping for dinner. If there's any time left, I'll get in a few yoga poses, or at least seek a few minutes of peace by reading a page from one of my favorite inspirational books, meditating, journaling, or praying.

By six o'clock, the second alarm goes off (this one's in my head). It's time to wake the kids, get breakfast on the table, shower, dress, check homework, sign sports or field-trip forms, resolve Girl Scout issues, leave lists for the after-school nanny, deal with my daughter's hair drama, find any missing clothing and/or shoes, get the kids out the door for school, and send a very grumpy non-morning-person husband off to work.

By now it is around seven. I eat my breakfast, usually a green power smoothie with added protein (see recipes on page 194), and take my supplements—omega-3s, a B-complex, collagen, evening primrose oil, and a small dose of thyroid hormone. I check my calendar for the day, answer work e-mails, make a to-do list, jump in the car and fight Atlanta traffic for 20 to 30 minutes, and make it to work to see *you*. My days are filled with many women just like you and me who strive to manage and balance all the moving pieces of our lives like plate-spinning Chinese acrobats.

Phew.

And that's just the first couple hours of the day.

Here's the thing: While my morning routine might sound like a recipe for boiling over, a formula for a meltdown, or an invitation to a nervous breakdown—it's anything but.

I wake up energized and happy, I arrive at work full of passion and excitement, and I come home at night feeling content and fulfilled. I love my life, and I thrive each and every day!

I'm often asked how I do it all—with two young children, a husband who works full time, my own full-time practice, my work teaching residents at Emory University, and a host of other roles. I've been told on more than one occasion that I must be some sort of super woman, but I know that I'm no different than any other woman. So how do I do it? I've discovered and harnessed an amazing source of super powers inside myself—super powers available to you, too. All of us have caches of dormant powers just waiting for the right mixture of activating practices, strategies, and ingredients—all tailored to us!

YOUR MISSING SUPER POWERS

So why haven't you heard of these real-life super powers?

Modern society demands that we be super women but doesn't bother to show us how to tap the necessary super human powers we need to meet all of life's obligations and responsibilities. We're expected to simultaneously juggle careers, children, and family; to have a social life and maintain our households, budget, and cars; to handle schoolwork and arrange for after-school activities; to cook healthy meals, pack nutritious lunches (remember, no peanut butter), and have sparkling clean refrigerators full of healthy food; to find time to exercise; and to be slim, beautiful, stress free, and smiling at all times. Did I mention that we're also supposed to look like we're 25 even when we're more than a few years north of that?

> Research shows that women have more stress in their daily lives than men; our health suffers more under the burden of stress.

And yet, we're surprised when we break down, blow up, freak out, fall into a fog or a funk, suffer from back and neck pain, gain weight, can't get pregnant, or get diagnosed with diabetes, heart disease, or cancer. When things get bad enough, we march off to the doctor, where we're poked and prodded and prescribed medications to manage and control—but not to truly solve and heal—our health woes. Some of us will try herbal therapies we've read about, go on a yoga retreat, or commit to sitting on a cushion and saying "om" for 30 minutes a day. Or maybe we'll try yet another diet—vegan or vegetarian, a juice fast, or the next trendy paleo plan—or sign up for a gym membership, only to fail to use it within weeks of swearing "this time is going to be different!"

> Compared to men, women are twice as likely to suffer from anxiety and three times as likely to be diagnosed with depression.

The reason that the majority of health solutions fail is that they are given as a blanket prescription (take drug X for your high blood pressure, a paleo diet is best to lose weight, and so on). Plus, these methods just aim to manage your symptoms or your disease without getting to the root of what is causing the high blood pressure or the weight gain in you personally, with all your individual traits, genetics, quirks, and strengths. Nope, it's just "follow this diet and lose weight," "follow that exercise plan and get fit," "take this medication to sleep better," and so on. These solutions assume that we are all alike, and that we just need to manage our symptoms or conditions. Most health professionals offer remedies without ever stopping to inquire, "Who are you?" and "What's the actual source of the root cause of the problems here?"

Most diets, health plans, fitness programs, beauty regimens, and mood makeovers—even the best out there—offer one answer, one plan, one diet, and one workout. Even those that claim to look at diet from your unique hormonal, genetic, or personality type usually end up offering only one plan. And the rare book that does offer individualized plans such as blood type diets only takes into account one factor— blood type—instead of all the valuable indicators from a wide variety of medical disciplines from around the world and across the span of thousands of years. I learned the hard way that following a standard plan, designed for the average woman, just won't cut it. I know from many years of experience with countless women that each and every one of you is as unique as your fingerprint, as distinct as your DNA, and as complex as Egyptian hieroglyphics. For you, me, and all women looking for a better way, the status quo just won't cut it.

WHAT THIS BOOK IS ABOUT

Enter *Super Woman Rx*: This is *the* definitive guide to health and wellbeing for women specifically because it's a design for living that is anything but one-size-fits-all. It is personalized, tailored and created for you—it is the ultimate biohack of your health. (*Biohack* is a term first coined to describe the do-it-yourself biology increasingly taking place among small groups to explore and study life and living organisms.) We will use the term to describe your own small but powerful do-it-yourself study of *you*.

In the chapters to come, you'll investigate and identify (biohack) your own unique chemistry, energy drains, and imbalances, and you'll use your findings to discover your individual Power Type. You'll continue to biohack your own chemistry and characteristics by using a specific prescriptive and predictive plan based on *you*. You'll pinpoint exactly what needs addressing and you'll transform your health and your life so that you'll wake up enthusiastic, invigorated, and inspired to live. By the end of this book you'll be jumping out of bed and into your day. Biohacking your own health is how you tap into your source of power, energy, and spark!

Mainstream solutions don't work, because you are about as mainstream as your closet—or shoes. While I would love to be 6 feet tall, that's never going to be a reality. Instead, I focus on and embrace the uniqueness that is me, and because I do, I thrive in my life. You will too!

WHAT MAKES THE SUPER WOMAN RX SPECIAL?

I've discovered a Power, or rather, Powers—the Five Power Types, to be exact. The beauty of the diverse background and training I've been fortunate enough to obtain is that I know and can share a reliable way to predict a plan for your health and your life that is truly healing and empowering. I'm a medical doctor, a certified nutritionist, acupuncturist, yoga teacher, Traditional Chinese Medicine practitioner, functional medicine doctor, and an integrative and holistic physician. Whether you are in your early twenties or settled into retirement, by taking the time to dig down deep to discover your core, your roots, your unique Power Type, *Super Woman Rx* provides a method that will dictate and guide you through every health and life decision, so you will thrive in your life. When you follow the steps in this book you will connect all the dots in your health history that will then show you the exact sort of intervention, nutritional changes, herbal support, exercises, mental and spiritual practices, and household habits you need to unlock your own super powers.

And yes, all of this has taught me how to restore balance in myself, my family, and friends, but even more importantly, this knowledge allows me to fulfill my lifetime dream of helping my patients and all of you realize and be your highest, most *POWERFUL* selves. This is a vantage point from which you can contribute to your relationships, your work, and your families. All this by identifying *your* ONE Power Type to start unleashing your super powers! This is the recipe for creating super women out of all of us!

Today, I'm happy, healthy, energetic, and full of inspiration and enthusiasm. I have clear skin, luxurious hair, and I'm a healthy and fit weight. The biggest difference is that I now wake up ready and excited to take on the day—I feel like Super Woman!

MY JOURNEY FROM SUPER DRAINED TO SUPER CHARGED

It wasn't always that way.

In 2001, I had arrived—or so I thought. I'd accomplished my lifelong dream of becoming a doctor. After completing medical school and my residency, I had become a pediatrician and then an emergency medicine physician. I was still unsure of my footing, still trying financially to establish myself, and I was still single and navigating the world of relationships and dating, but I was also at the beginning of my dream career and my future looked bright. I should have been walking on air. Instead, I felt like I was stuck in deep mud. I was 28 years old.

While I loved treating patients, I was chronically stressed, overwhelmed, and exhausted. I'd gained 10 extra pounds that wouldn't budge despite long, intense, and frequent exercise sessions. My PMS was fierce and my periods were irregular. My face was covered in cystic acne, my joints were always achy, and my once long and thick hair was coming out in clumps. I'd open my eyes in the morning and immediately squeeze them shut again. I dreaded the day ahead. I'd shuffle to the bathroom and shower in the dark to avoid looking at myself. I was miserable. To get through the demands of the day, I gulped down multiple cups of coffee, even though they never seemed to clear up my foggy head.

I wanted my mojo back. I mean, who wants to feel hormonally imbalanced and be bald and overweight at *any* age, let alone 28?

Since I was an emergency room doctor who believed in the medical system, I started trying to solve my issues by going to doctor after doctor to figure out how to get back to feeling like my younger, more energetic, healthy self. But after countless visits with general practitioners, as well as specialists, I still didn't get the answers I was looking for; instead, I'd be sent off for yet more lab work or another appointment, or prescribed an ever-growing list of medications to help manage my symptoms. Each physician suggested more tests and then invariably offered more drugs to manage and control the myriad of symptoms I was struggling with—and nothing worked.

My turning point came the day I crashed my car.

I had just started another new prescription, this time prescribed by a world-renowned specialist who told me that it was my only chance of avoiding total baldness by the time I turned 30! The side effects caused by the drug included dizziness and a drop in blood pressure (I naturally run low BP numbers to begin with), but I was so frazzled and desperate to fix my unresolved health issues that I didn't read the side effect label on the medicine—I just blindly trusted this doctor and his reputation. The next day I was driving to work when I got really dizzy and almost passed out. I swerved, briefly lost control of my car, and hit the sidewalk. Thankfully, only my car was hurt, but that was my wake-up call. In that moment, I realized I had to figure out a better way to get healthy. There had to be a different way—I was *done*!

That was my moment of clarity. I was entirely fed up and frustrated. I knew that the conventional medicine in which I'd been trained had failed me. I realized that the mainstream medical paradigm needed a makeover, and so did I. So I went back to my roots.

I started digging deeper into alternative options for health and healing. I studied, harder than ever before, looking into nutrition and the relationships between food as medicine, Traditional Chinese Medicine, acupuncture, Ayurveda, and more. My mother had always been a believer in the healing power of nutrition, and so I started there. I went back to several traditional Ayurvedic (Indian health) recipes from my childhood. I continued my own personal nutritional investigation and developed my diet as I went. I was so energized by my new eating plan that I took it to the next level and studied and became a certified nutrition specialist, decided to go gluten free, and then to remove dairy from my diet. My face started to clear up. I researched supplements and matched them to my nutritional deficiencies and symptoms—a link I only became aware of after studying holistic medicine. I started taking B vitamins and omega-3s. After a month, my hair stopped falling out. I started investigating how stress affects health; I learned to meditate and started doing yoga again. I stopped feeling miserable, my energy soared, and I slept soundly. From then on, I was on fire. I had healed myself and I wanted more!

At this point, I was a certified nutritionist. I registered for training in Traditional Chinese Medicine (TCM) and acupuncture and became a licensed acupuncturist and TCM practitioner. I studied Ayurvedic practices and learned more about this ancient system of medicine. Finally, I became certified as an integrative and holistic medicine doctor, after completing a fellowship with Dr. Andrew Weil, and opened my own practice. Along the way I authored two highly successful books, *The 21-Day Belly Fix* and *What Doctors Eat*, and now I'm excited to expand my scope with this comprehensive prescriptive plan for women's health.

Today, I'm a physician and a woman who has found superior health, happiness, and vitality for myself and for my family, friends, and more than 10,000 patients because I stepped outside of the conventional medical box. I expanded my medical training and viewpoint to include the best from the entire world's health and healing disciplines—conventional, complementary, alternative, and holistic—including nutrition, Chinese medicine, acupuncture, Ayurvedic treatments, and more.

At 45, I'm far busier than I used to be. I continue to run my own practice, CentreSpring MD—formerly the Atlanta Center for Holistic and Integrative Medicine—where I see more than 160 patients a month. The center has grown from a two-person/two-room operation (when I started it was just my sister-in-law and me) to a practice with 14 patient rooms, four doctors and four nurse practitioners, and two locations, not to mention a large staff and a jam-packed schedule. We're expanding the practice again as this book goes to press because we can't keep up with the hundreds of new patients who keep coming through the door each month looking for better options for their health, and because we know that our approach to medicine yields lasting results. I'm also an associate professor at Emory University School of Medicine, I travel and speak all over the world several times a year, I appear on television once or twice a month as a health expert, and I have a beautiful family (Kubby, Rania, and my husband, Vik).

As I said, I'm no different than any other woman. I can get tired, I can overdo it, and I can still get sick—I'm not super human. But because I know how to use the powerful clues my body gives me, I do have access to potent super powers that help me to accomplish more while staying balanced, healthy, and happy. Thankfully, that means that I usually sidestep the pitfalls of fatigue, stress, depression, illness, and more while keeping up with an incredibly busy life. This power is available to you, too. My own path has taught me a lot about moving through the different stages of life as a woman—through my free and single twenties; my family-starting, career-solidifying thirties; and now my forties, where I'm the healthiest and happiest I've ever been. I've seen the power of the Super Woman Rx transform countless women from all different decades and phases of life, from late teens to late eighties and every age in between.

HOW TO USE THIS BOOK

You won't find a one-size-fits-all plan here. You will discover that you fit into one of five distinct and individualized Power Types.

Hold on.

Five Types?

I realize that I just finished telling you how unique you are, and I still hold to that, but at the same time, I have found that there are five key patterns or types of women who benefit from unique recommendations. When you determine your Power Type (in Chapter 3), you'll choose the one 3-Week Power Plan that is tailored to your unique blueprint. Your plan will guide you as to how to eat, exercise, socialize, meditate, and care for your body to achieve the results you seek. You will understand how your chemistry is connected to your life and the decisions you make along the way. These plans are based on the five general types of women I meet in my practice again and again—the five amazing kinds of super women I meet every day.

As you follow your 3-Week Power Plan, you'll see and feel your unique super powers awakening. You'll slim down and tone up effortlessly, look and feel younger and be full of energy, and feel happier and more relaxed than ever before. Regardless of your age and wellness status, you will learn how to consider and evaluate every nuance and aspect of your health, personality, and body type to determine the best plan for your Power Type.

The *Super Woman Rx* is the ultimate women's resource guide for health and well-being—the ultimate biohack of your health. You are your own best healer and keeper of your own unique super powers. This book is designed to show you a better way to connect the dots to find the best diet, the best exercise and mind and body tools, and the best beauty regimen for you.

Here's a quick look at how the book is organized.

Part I: I'll start off in Chapter 1 by covering the background you need to know to understand the situation most women find themselves stuck in—overwhelmed and burned out. In Chapter 2, you'll dive right in with the Mojo Meter, a test that will show you where you are out of balance in your life right now. In Chapter 3, you'll determine which Super Woman Power Type you are—what makes you uniquely *you*. Chapter 4 will educate you on the tools every super woman needs to thrive in our super demanding world. Here you'll learn all about the background, healing practices, and transformative power of the many tools and disciplines we will be blending. This is your reference guide, a place you can return to as you move through the *Super Woman Rx* for your basic explanation of the principles and philosophies from which we will pull.

Part II: Here is where we get into the meat of your 3-Week Power Plan. In these next five chapters, you'll find detailed information about your unique Power Type, and you will begin an individualized 3-Week Power Plan customized to meet your needs.

Part III: In this section, I'll take you to the next level and provide all the extra ingredients—recipes, exercises, mind-body strategies, and your super beauty regimen—to round out your Power Plan and reclaim your super powers.

Throughout the book you'll see testimonies from *real* super women who have followed the 3-Week Power Plans and have felt the results of fantastically superior super powers in their lives!

I guard my health like the precious and rare jewel it is. I've learned the hard way that when I let *me* slip from top priority, this super woman quickly finds herself feeling as drained as Superman when exposed to kryptonite, and all my super powers disappear in a flash. I'm here to show you how to find and activate your super powers, to get your mojo back, and to live the super woman life you were meant to live.

Your health is rightfully yours. Are you ready to take it back?

Let's do this!

PART

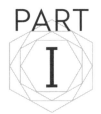

I

ACTIVATE YOUR INNER SUPER POWERS

ARE YOU A Gypsy Girl, a Boss Lady, a Savvy Chick, an Earth Mama, or a Nightingale? In the next four chapters, you will identify your unique Power Type.

Think back for a moment to a time when you felt and looked alive. Picture your life—before long workdays, jam-packed schedules, kiddie or teen craziness, family drama, husbands or boyfriends or partners, pets, noisy neighbors, needy parents—go beyond all that to a time when you felt invincible—on top of the world—*alive*! Maybe it's that moment where you put on your favorite dress and it fit perfectly (go get 'em), or when a "good hair day" was a frequent occurrence, and you were actually happy with your selfies or your Polaroids or your Canon 360s. Or maybe it was when you could go to the gym without feeling self-conscious about your body, or any time you felt truly free and happy—think back to when *you* were your own *super hero*.

Too long ago to remember? Not sure what I am talking about? We cannot let that happen. You will feel this way again, and this book will give you the recipes, the secrets, and the formula to live an empowered and impassioned life. But that starts by learning more about *you*, by finding your *type*—your *Power Type*—a blend of your medical needs, personality, and unique values.

Read on for the formula that will give you energy, vitality, beauty, and inner peace—leading you to your natural and divinely inspired inner, given gifts.

Chapter 1 starts you off by explaining the problem plaguing today's super women (that's all of us!). Chapter 2 introduces a self-assessment test that will help you establish a baseline for where you're at in regard to energy and balance. In Chapter 3 you'll get down to work by identifying your Power Type, and in Chapters 4 and 5, we'll go in-depth into the nuances and healing practices that identify, heal, and amplify *your* Power Type.

CHAPTER 1

THE SUPER WOMAN SYNDROME

WE ARE SUPPOSED to do it all—and do it well—or so we think.

Modern womanhood means maintaining the demands of multiple roles: businesswoman, employee, mother, spouse, daughter, sister, homemaker, breadwinner, caretaker, chore and homework supervisor, family taxi driver, meal planner, or some mixture of these and more. And whatever roles we fill, we're supposed to perform them looking eternally youthful, serene, and happy. We are expected to be super women, and we manage, but it comes at a cost. Women today show increased rates of anxiety, depression, chronic stress and fatigue, migraines, heart disease, strokes, and infertility. Consider these findings.

- Women experience twice the rate of depression that men do, regardless of race or ethnic background. Researchers suspect that many factors unique to women's lives play a role in developing depression, including genetics, hormones, abuse and oppression, and interpersonal, psychological, and personality characteristics.

- From their teen years until around age 50, women are twice as likely to suffer from anxiety as men, according to the Anxiety and Depression Association of America.

- While men and women report similar levels of stress, women are more likely to report that their stress levels are increasing and much more likely than men to report negative emotional and physical symptoms of stress, such as headaches, feeling like crying, and having indigestion, according to a 2010 survey of more than 1,600 men and women.

◆ Women are two to four times more likely to be diagnosed with chronic fatigue syndrome than men. Women are also more likely to experience difficulty falling and staying asleep (63 percent versus 54 percent of men), to experience pain at night (58 percent versus 48 percent), and to experience fatigue during the day, according to a National Sleep Foundation poll.

◆ According to the Migraine Research Foundation, women make up 28 million of the more than 38 million reported sufferers of this severe health condition. Women's migraines also occur more often, last longer, and are more severe than men's.

◆ Heart disease is the number one killer of women, with 90 percent of women having one or more heart disease risk factors.

◆ Each year 55,000 more US women than men have a stroke, according to the National Stroke Association, and women's recovery rates after stroke lag those of men.

◆ Nearly 11 percent of women in the United States (more than six million) experience infertility issues, according to the National Survey of Family Health (data are for 2006 to 2010).

◆ Polycystic ovary syndrome (PCOS), also known as Stein-Leventhal syndrome, is one of the most common hormonal endocrine disorders in women. Five to 10 percent of women of childbearing age are affected by PCOS. But this statistic is grossly underestimated, with many more going undiagnosed.

Juggling all these different roles lends itself to a unique array of health problems that we didn't face before in our history as women. Given the multitasking demands and multiple challenges of modern life—e-mails, cell phone calls and texts, lists, more lists, housework—something has got to give. All of this results in sacrifices in other areas of our lives—it creates dis-ease on many fronts, psychologically, spiritually, emotionally, and physically.

Think back to what you know of your own family history. My grandmother didn't work outside the home and did not have much of an education, my mother-in-law gave up her career as a physician in India to raise her family, and my mother—the first super woman I knew—was determined to finish her education despite being married off at 19. She worked 18-hour days, 7 days a week to see her three daughters turn into their own versions of her super woman self. The bottom line is this: Women have many more choices and options today, but we also have to meet multiple demands and handle more responsibilities. As amazing as our opportunities are, we often forget one very important variable—our health!

MULTIPLE ROLES EQUAL BIG TROUBLE

A UK study in 2013 made headlines globally, with its evidence that women were better multitaskers than men. What the research didn't cover was that taking on the multiple roles of mother, career woman, wife, etc., takes a toll—not to mention stressing over meeting the ridiculous, unrealistic demands of feminine perfection, of being "beautiful." Women have to work twice as hard to get half as much, and all the duties and demands drain our energy, health, and happiness. According to a 2013 Mayo Clinic survey, women are more likely to suffer from skin disorders, osteoarthritis and joint issues, back problems, lung diseases, anxiety and depression, headaches and migraines, asthma, thyroid issues, and anemia than their male counterparts. The average American woman today weighs 166.2 pounds and is 5 feet 4 inches tall, which gives her a BMI of 28.5 (25 to 29 is considered overweight, while a BMI of 30 or higher is considered obese). Finally, consider that it used to be men who were more likely to suffer from heart disease; today women have taken the lead in deadly heart attacks.

I hear similar stories from hundreds of women every month who come to me complaining of all of the above mentioned ailments and more—all of it boiling down to feeling overwhelmed but with no place to cut back. Woman after woman tells me how she's failed to find solutions to her health even after numerous appointments with multiple doctors and specialists, trials on prescription medications that come with too many side effects, and dozens of tests that yielded no answers at all. The fact is that we women are in trouble. We want and deserve it all, but our health and our relationships are suffering. Most of us want or need to have both a career and a family life, but even for those who decide or need to do one thing at a time (stay home or focus on career), today's pressures are just as overwhelming.

Let's take moms. Have you called a stay-at-home mom lately? If you have, I'm willing to wager that she *wasn't* at home when she answered. It's more likely that she was taxiing kids to or from after-school activities, assisting in the classroom, coaching soccer or leading a Girl Scout troop, and on and on. And if she *was* home, it's a sure bet that she was busy doing some sort of work: cooking, cleaning, doing laundry, putting away groceries, supervising homework, putting a bandage on a boo-boo, and/or paying the bills. She sure wasn't lounging around the pool, popping bonbons into her mouth. Mom-ing is a full-time job all on its own.

Alternatively, the women who are the CEOs, stockbrokers, and business owners—a different set of pressure points—are usually either the breadwinners for their families or have sacrificed the pursuit of a family as they pursued a career. Many of my CEO friends feel anxiety and urgency to keep up with their male counterparts at the table and put in as many or more hours to prove themselves. They hop on planes, manage meetings, build teams, and watch the bottom line, afraid of—almost panicked at—the idea of taking a moment to slow down to nurture their energy and their spirits.

And then there are the women who do both—they have children and/or parents to care for *and* they run companies, lobby for world peace, and sign up as room mom, troop leader, or PTA president year after year.

It's too much, and we don't have the powers to keep it all up all the time. I know I didn't. It's trying to juggle too many different roles and please too many people that burns us out, fries our brains, and destroys our health. Yes, you might bring home the bacon, but you also are probably getting fried to a crisp.

WHAT'S NEXT: ACTIVATING YOUR SUPER POWERS

I found my super powers, I restored my health and well-being, and I found my purpose and my gifts. I've helped countless women do the same and understand that it is all related—that by learning your chemistry and finding your type, you will also find your own super powers. You cannot broker world peace, run a business, or look amazing without understanding this formula. In this book, I make sure these super powers are available to *you* too!

Most diets, weight loss plans, even health regimens tend to be one-size-fits-all, but you are a unique individual who requires a customized plan to fit your specific Power Type. Nowhere is this one-size-fits-all mentality more obvious than when looking at the popular diets on the market. Most weight loss plans are generic—trying to appeal to the "average" woman and making claims that they will work for all women. Sure, a lot of diet programs tweak the amount of calories allowed based on your height, age, and weight goal—but they don't go far enough. You and I are far from average—you are amazing and capable, and you also have a unique makeup that deserves an equally individualized plan to improve your health and happiness. That's what you're about to learn. There are a few diet books out there that recognize and address the need for different plans for different types of individuals. *Eat Right 4 Your Type*, *The GenoType Diet*, and *The Diet Cure*, for example, attempt to offer a somewhat customized program for different individuals, but these diets still only focus on one sort of "typing," such as blood type, genetic history, or common hormones while ignoring so many other factors, including Eastern medicine typing, body clues, laboratory values, and emotional makeup.

Conventional Western medicine focuses on the management and control of symptoms and disease, not on finding a true solution to the underlying problem. There is value in conventional mainstream medicine—but alone, it is a broken system. I don't want you to have the same frustrating experience I had 15 years ago. There is a better way! The best health care is a blend of several of the best and most valuable healing practices from around the globe, ancient and modern, from the East and the West—and it's all truly within your reach. You've already started by reading this book!

READY?
Turn the page to begin reclaiming your super powers.

CHAPTER 2

YOUR MOJO METER: TAKING YOUR PULSE

HAVE YOU LOST IT? Has your mojo gone missing or your spark gone dark?

I know you can get IT—your mojo—back. You will go back to lighting up a room, warming a space, and spreading your vibrancy through everything you touch. I see it all the time. In fact, my favorite moments in practice are when I get to see the light come back on in a woman's eyes, when her face glows and she transforms from dim and dull to bright and full. I could not have asked for a better job. It's my purpose and my passion—getting you back to you.

When I first meet a new patient at my practice, CentreSpring MD, I spend a few hours on her care. That might seem like a lot, especially since the average doctor's visit runs all of 10 minutes, but I think getting to know you is crucial. I want you to think in the same way. This chapter is your new-patient appointment in print form. Don't worry—it won't take you as long as it takes me since you already know you!

WHAT EXACTLY IS THE MOJO METER?

Your mojo is your spark or your energy, verve, joyfulness, vigor, inspiration, enthusiasm, passion, inner light, divine goddess. Whatever you want to call IT, you want IT working in tip-top shape. Think back again to a day you felt truly happy and beautiful. Well, that was just a mini dose of mojo—I'm going to show you how to turn that fleeting feeling into Super Energy and make it last every moment of every day!

The sort of mojo I'm talking about tapping into is your source of a true zest for life, or the get-up-and-go type of energy that gets you excited to experience all the blessings and opportunities in the hours ahead. That energy begins with your health and with the realization that you have to periodically check in with yourself to understand where you are on the spectrum of health and happiness. A mantra here or there can help, a vitamin B_{12} shot may get you through the week, but to get and keep all of your inner super powers fully and optimally charged at all times, you have to be able to put all the pieces of *you* together. That means knowing how to do an inner self-analysis of where you are right at this very moment. That's just what the Mojo Meter does: It's your check-in, checkup, and your way to check out where you are at this period of time in your life. Instead of searching on Dr. Google, you can use your knowledge of yourself (you are the expert) to take the following test to get a balanced and objective picture of you (this is how you begin to *biohack* your health). By checking everything from your energy levels to the quality of your mood, the condition of your hair and skin, and even your periods (yes, we're going to talk about that and more), you'll be able to see where you need a little help, a stronger nudge, or a full-on intervention. This test will help you to know whether you need a rest, a boost, or a complete overhaul.

The Test

It's time to dive in and take your pulse. Answer the following questions True or False based on how you'd rate the last few months of your life. Don't overthink it; just go with the first instinctive response that pops up. Go with the answer that comes to you within the first 10 seconds after reading the question. Answering this way will give you a vivid snapshot of your energy level and health right now. You'll use this baseline to know where to go next. And you'll return and retake this test as you move through your 3-Week Power Plan and beyond.

The Mojo Meter

Part A

1. I look forward to waking up every morning.		T | F
2. I get dressed easily in the morning.		T | F
3. I have clothes that I love and feel confident wearing.		T | F
4. I eat breakfast at home, before checking e-mails.		T | F

5. I assemble and plan my food for the day.	T | F
6. I have shiny, healthy hair.	T | F
7. I have clear, smooth skin.	T | F
8. I am within 5 pounds in either direction of my ideal weight.	T | F
9. I have strong nails.	T | F
10. I am content with my figure and appearance.	T | F
11. I have boundless energy throughout the day.	T | F
12. I have good focus and concentration.	T | F
13. I feel mentally sharp.	T | F
14. I don't lose my words or forget things.	T | F
15. I look forward to going to work.	T | F
16. I look forward to coming home.	T | F
17. I am free of pain.	T | F
18. I have regular and consistent menstrual cycles.	T | F
19. I am actively in an intimate relationship.	T | F
20. I have found my life partner.	T | F
21. I have a strong, supportive family.	T | F
22. I am surrounded by community.	T | F
23. I have found a way to connect to my spirit.	T | F
24. I love where I live.	T | F

Part B

25. I suffer from frequent headaches.	T | F
26. I have interrupted sleep more than three nights per week.	T | F
27. I am battling hair loss.	T | F
28. I have acne and/or eczema.	T | F
29. I have unexplained weight gain.	T | F
30. I am unhappy with my weight.	T | F
31. I am unhappy with my figure.	T | F
32. I dread having to dress or enter my closet.	T | F
33. I hesitate to turn on lights in the bathroom.	T | F
34. I hesitate to get on the scale.	T | F
35. I have frequent indigestion.	T | F
36. I have irregular periods.	T | F

37.	I have had a chronic illness or disease in the last 5 years.	T | F
38.	I have terrible PMS or perimenopausal/menopausal symptoms.	T | F
39.	I have chronic pain.	T | F
40.	I have joint swelling or joint pain.	T | F
41.	I am in a difficult or disjointed relationship.	T | F
42.	I am estranged from family or lack family.	T | F
43.	I do not have a companion.	T | F
44.	I hate my job.	T | F
45.	I detest the career I have chosen.	T | F
46.	I am seeking a life change and not sure how to get there.	T | F
47.	I crash through the day and it is difficult to sustain my energy.	T | F
48.	I have crying episodes.	T | F
49.	I have poor motivation.	T | F
50.	I find it difficult to concentrate.	T | F
51.	I suffer from overthinking/mind racing.	T | F
52.	I do not maintain connection to my spirit.	T | F

Scoring

Add up the True answers as follows:

For questions in Part A, numbers 1 to 24, every True answer = 1. Add them all up (you will have a positive number). Write your number here: _____.

For questions in Part B, numbers 25 to 52, each True answer = -1. Add them all up (you will have a negative number). Write your number here: _____.

Now add Part A and Part B together. The equation will look like this: A + (-B) or A−B (since B will be a negative number).

If you scored:

19 to 24: Congratulations! Your mojo is at a max right now, so go for it. Find that dream job, start your family, or launch a fund for world peace. Whatever your vision, you are in a good place to embrace it. Just don't get overconfident. Appreciate where you are now, and use the Super Woman Rx to reinforce and stabilize your already healthy and happy life. This is a reference book for your entire life, and you can still take it to the next level. Plus, life will still happen. Chances are, you will hit speed bumps when you are not at your peak, challenges that will require you to ramp up your defenses, or transitions that need addressing. Continue on with the next chapters to help you reinforce your motivation to keep on doing the right things for you, and to shed some light to how you can do even better. Plan on retaking the Mojo Meter every 4 months.

7 to 18: Caution, slippery slopes ahead. It's time to do a bit of digging. You are starting to lose your edge and could use some leveling and balancing out. Your score indicates that you are seeing early warning signs that the life you are living and the way you're taking care of yourself may not really maximize your energy and your super powers. It's time to get started. Over the next chapters, you'll learn how to pinpoint exactly what your unique Super Woman needs to thrive. While your mojo shows many strong areas, there are regions that need improvement. In the next chapter you'll be able to pinpoint your unique type and know how to specifically address the energy areas that need a boost.

1 to 6: Repairs and restoration required. Proceed with caution. Your score indicates that you're out of touch with your super powers and need a tune-up. You need to stop and check in, or you will soon be checked out. Your health is drained on more than one front; let's work to get you back on track. The Super Woman Rx will empower you to get on the right eating, exercise, and mental health plan to get back into balance and operating at your optimal level of health and happiness. Read on.

-27 to 0: Major overhauling needed! Halt! Stop what you are doing and read this book! Your mojo is in trouble. You are checked out, disconnected, and divided from yourself. It's time to get started on some major rehab work. You are obviously in the middle of some spiritual, physical, mental, or emotional crisis. In the next chapter you'll learn how to begin assembling your team of health interventionists and supporters: your family members, friends, doctors, counselors, and so on.

IT'S TIME TO TAKE action. You now know where you stand. This will help you to move forward clearly and consciously, with the motivation, desire, and hunger you need to tap into your super powers. There is no happy without healthy, and no passion without chemistry, so let's get your mojo back—claim IT and own IT. How? First you have to find your unique fingerprint—your Power Type and the formula that will super charge your mojo.

Ready to find your Power Type? Turn the page!

CHAPTER 3

MEET YOUR POWER TYPE: TAKE THE POWER TYPE TEST

GYPSY? BOSS LADY? SAVVY CHICK? EARTH MAMA? OR NIGHT-INGALE? Which one are you? Are you just one of these types, or a blend of a few? What exactly is a Power Type?

Welcome to the Power Type Test. This assessment will help you determine your unique characteristics, personality, strengths, and weaknesses and will help you to establish the type of Super Woman Rx plan you'll benefit from most.

Paleo, gluten or lactose free, vegan or vegetarian? Pre- or postmenopausal? Sedentary, active, or athletic? Underweight, normal, or overweight?—who are you?

Some of these labels are choices, some are not. Regardless, they recognize that individuals vary and that any given person will thrive with one diet or activity over another.

Still, there are so many other factors and layers to take into consideration above and beyond just a person's diet or quantity of exercise. Narrowing down health and well-being into so few categories would be like trying to build a house by just looking at the best paint colors and plumbing—what about the foundation, electric wiring, lighting, insulation, and so on?

I am fortunate to meet countless women every week in my practice. I see some similarities among my patients, and many differences. Each woman has a story, a unique fingerprint and mission. Let's take a look.

Mary is 40 years old. She is tall and slender, with brown eyes and long, dark brown hair. Her hair started to get dry recently and she noticed the same dryness in her skin. While she has always been anxious, her anxiety has worsened lately, with frequent episodes of heart palpitations, middle-of-the-night waking, and restlessness. A part of this anxiety may be due to elevated stress and frustration with ongoing infertility issues—she finally met the love of her life and now wants to start a family.

Janice is 28 years old. With short blonde hair and moist, thick skin, Janice is a medium to heavily built woman who has struggled with weight her whole life. She has battled excess weight and been self-conscious and uncomfortable in her body since she was a child. After years of yo-yo dieting and days in and out of weight management programs, her self-esteem is deeply affected—she has never dated. To make matters worse, her doctor recently told her that she is prediabetic and that she may be a full-blown diabetic by the time she turns 30 if she continues at this rate.

Denise is 56 years old. Her hair is a beautiful ebony color and she has a rich olive skin complexion. Her eyes are gorgeous, with long eyelashes and thick eyebrows. She has lived an amazing life so far, running a company, raising children, and being happily married. While she appears to have everything, she has recently noticed an underlying unhappiness starting to brew—she battles bouts of depression, a new issue for her, and is frustrated with teenagelike acne now popping up on her face. Her doctor recommended an antidepressant, but she is reluctant, not having taken any medications for many years. She breaks down frequently but isn't sure where the surge of emotions and frustrations is coming from.

Three women—all very different—all with unique issues.

None of them knows the others; they are different in terms of age, body type, height, hair, skin, digestive issues, and health concerns. Interestingly, these three women came to me after trying out extremely similar diets and exercise programs from the same health book that suggested the same magic-bullet fix to their health and well-being issues. Silly, right? But this is what happens in most situations. Go into any Jenny Craig, Nutrisystem, or Weight Watchers building and you'll see a wide variety of women of various heights, ages, and weights who are all prescribed pretty similar food and exercise plans. Sure, the amount of calories may be tweaked a little, but that's about as far as it goes for most plans. Ditto for patients at a doctor's or nutritionist's office: different patients, same general exercise and food recommendations. That's the main reason most diets, exercise plans, and health regimens fail—they rely on the one-size-fits-all paradigm. Each of us has different nutritional, physical, mental, and spiritual needs. But most health experts, doctors, nutritionists, books, plans, and programs only offer one sort of solution.

That's not what I do. At my practice, CentreSpring MD, my team spends a lot of time trying to understand each woman's unique challenges and issues, and then develops a customized plan she uses to successfully move forward and see long-term results. I opened my doors back in 2009 with just one little office and one receptionist. I actually shared office space with my dentist husband—him in the front, and me in the back. At the time, my vision was to stay small and to still have plenty of time at home with my children. I was excited to offer people an alternative to the regular rushed doctor's visit and the dismal and frustrating reality of running around from appointment to appointment that I'd experienced. The bank didn't want to give me a loan for a holistic and integrative medical practice because they didn't understand what I was doing. I remember overhearing one loan officer saying, "What's she doing, swinging chickens in the air and waving herbs around?" I certainly did offer a different sort of experience. I'd do a long history to get to know a patient, and then I'd use a blend of acupuncture, nutritional counseling, general medical care and tests, Chinese medicine (herbs and supplements), and so on. Even though this was just 8 years ago, at the time, people in Atlanta (where I am based) didn't understand exactly what I was doing, and insurance sure didn't cover (and still doesn't) most patient appointments—so folks had to pay cash. Business was slow at first, but my patients loved the results and improvements in health. Word of mouth about my practice spread. By 2010, I needed to hire more clerical help and a nurse. I began to have trouble keeping up with the demand—at one point our office was overflowing so I used Vik's (my husband) dental chairs to do acupuncture on patients. I will never forget the look on his face the day he walked in to see his entire dental space taken over by my patients! By 2011, I was invited to appear on radio and television shows to discuss my practice and my philosophy of health and well-being; first we gained national, and then global, recognition! I began doing regular appearances on local and national television stations and was invited to be a regular columnist in a major magazine publication.

From 2011 to today, we have seen more than 10,000 women in my practice and we're still growing. We're up to multiple locations and we're bursting at the seams yet again—as this book goes to press we continue to evolve to meet the ever-growing demands of women around the world in the most effective and personal way possible. This book is my practice in print to help all women who aren't able to come and see me personally.

WHAT MAKES *SUPER WOMAN RX* UNIQUE?

Very few doctors and practices today take the time to put it *all* together or use multiple systems of medicine to arrive at that point. I have education and experience as an emergency medicine doctor, a pediatrician, and an integrative medical physician. I've been trained and educated in Chinese medicine, acupuncture, Ayurveda (a holistic system of medicine developed in India), nutrition, and anti-aging and regenerative medicine. *These different systems of medicine stress the importance of discovering the power that comes when you respect and learn about the distinctiveness and uniqueness of each and every person.* Looking at each woman from multiple perspectives and healing disciplines allows for a more complete picture of the challenges and issues facing each woman. Most importantly, I help hundreds of women each and every month to uncover their own unique blueprint; to understand deeply their characteristics, personality, and unique issues; and I teach them how to use that knowledge to access their inner super powers and to heal themselves. The treatment plans that we offer differ from patient to patient. We do *NOT* practice a one-size-fits-all philosophy at CentreSpring MD. I have also built and trained a team of amazing providers to do the same. At CentreSpring MD, each patient has access to a team of physicians, nurse practitioners, acupuncturists, nutritionists, and other health specialists in Ayurveda, craniosacral therapy, counseling, and hypnosis. This book provides that same team approach.

FIND YOUR POWER TYPE, FIND YOUR PERFECT PLAN

Let's face it, successfully finding and sticking to a healthy lifestyle (one that really works for you) is challenging to say the least. Every year new plans, books, methods, health gurus, media messages, and podcasts tell us about the next quick fix to become healthier, happier, younger, slimmer, fitter—or just better. But which is right for you? How do *you* stop feeling overwhelmed and burned out? How do *you* improve *your* energy, reduce *your* anxiety, and overcome *your* funk? How do *you* lose the weight and shed the fat? Should *you* be gluten free, dairy free, vegan, or vegetarian? Should *you* cut out all carbs and go sugar free? Should *you* run marathons or just do yoga? What about strength training? Is it okay if *your* bedtime is midnight as long as *you* sleep in? How much sleep do *you* really need? Why did *you* get cancer, diabetes, arthritis, or an auto-immune disease?

Here's the answer to all of the above: It depends.

I'm not trying to be vague, glib, or difficult. The reality is that each of us is truly different and your answers depend on who you are. I learned this through my own health discoveries and transformations, and through working on the health and life metamorphoses of thousands of women.

Access to successful healing and maximized super powers depends specifically on who you are, what your energy level and metabolism are like, your body type, your unique chemical composition, family history, nutritional needs, genetics, and more. Some of you do better with vigorous exercise, while others do better with yoga and tai chi. Some of you have a proclivity for high blood pressure or stress, while others of you are not easily flustered. You might have sensitivities to dairy or gluten, or you may need more or less protein in your diet. The test you'll complete on the following pages provides an organized series of questions that work to biohack your Power Type and will unlock the mystery of who you are and how to awaken the inner super powers that are dormant inside you right this very moment.

You can predict the formula for your best health! The golden nuggets of information to super charge your health are not elusive. Not only are super human health powers possible, but it's easier to access them than you might think.

Ready to begin biohacking your health and finding your Power Type?

Determining Your Personal Power Type

Who are you? The Power Type Test is a self-assessment questionnaire that will help you categorize yourself into one of these five distinct Power Types.

+ Gypsy Girl
+ Boss Lady
+ Savvy Chick
+ Earth Mama
+ Nightingale

By the end of this chapter you will have a clear snapshot of YOU as you are right now, which will give you strong clues as to how you'll proceed to improve your health, happiness, and life. Your Power Type is simply the classification that you belong to at this point in time. No one Power Type is better than another, there are pros and cons to each, and there's a high probability that you'll be making use of more than one Power Type as you move through your own personal journey.

The reality is that most of us exhibit some components from all five of the Power Types, but there will be one that dominates. This is your starting point, but this is also a test that you'll repeat. That's because your Power Type often changes and fluctuates depending on your life stage or the circumstances surrounding you. You may be a Gypsy Girl today, but a Nightingale a few months—or a decade—from now. Some changes happen with hormonal fluctuations, health issues, seasonal variations, or even new stressors.

I'm being vague about Power Types on purpose because I don't want to bias your responses.

This test consists of eight categories and 51 total questions. It's a good idea to retake the test every couple months since your Power Type can change—just as your life changes.

The Power Type Test

Important Instructions! Circle the answer that best describes you. For some of the questions you may find it difficult to choose, but don't overthink it—go with what feels like the most likely answer, or imagine what a friend would say about you. *One caveat: Make answer f—None of the above or not applicable—a rare choice. If you choose more than a couple of these, it can throw off the test.* The scoring directions come after you've finished all the questions. Once again, remember that you are only allowed to choose one answer per question, so choose what resonates with you the most. Have fun!

I. PHYSICAL APPEARANCE

Hair

1. My hair is best described as:
   a. Thin and sparse
   b. Thin but of average volume
   c. Medium volume
   d. Falling out; I am losing hair
   e. Full and abundant volume
   f. None of the above or not applicable

2. My hair is typically:
   a. Dry
   b. Dry with areas of oiliness (such as the central scalp)
   c. Slightly oily (I need to wash daily)
   d. Oily on the scalp with dry, brittle ends overall
   e. Luxuriant and shiny (I can wash every 3 or 4 days)
   f. None of the above or not applicable

3. My hair strands are:
   a. Thin and break easily
   b. Thin but strong (when I pull one from the scalp it is tough to break it)
   c. Thick
   d. Mixed, with areas of thicker and thinner strands that break easily
   e. Thick and coarse
   f. None of the above or not applicable

Skin

4. My skin is usually:
   a. Dry and quick to wrinkle
   b. Oily with areas of dryness
   c. Oily
   d. Dry with patches of oiliness
   e. Moist and firm
   f. None of the above or not applicable

5. My skin:
    a. Wrinkles easily
    b. Is subject to occasional breakouts, especially of eczema or contact dermatitis
    c. Is prone to acne on my jaw and chin
    d. Wrinkles easily and is prone to acne or blemishes on my forehead and chin
    e. Is clear, with few blemishes, and slow to wrinkle
    f. None of the above or not applicable

6. When I touch or pull on my skin:
    a. It feels dry and rough.
    b. There are areas of roughness.
    c. It is moist and oily, with breakouts.
    d. It is dry and irritated or inflamed.
    e. It is moist and responds to pressure easily.
    f. None of the above or not applicable

Body

7. My body build is best described as:
    a. Slender and/or thin
    b. Thin with some muscle
    c. Medium with good muscle tone
    d. Thin to medium with some muscle loss
    e. Medium to large, with areas of fat deposition
    f. None of the above or not applicable

8. My weight:
    a. Remains consistently low (I am lean and have trouble gaining weight)
    b. Fluctuates (I gain or lose easily)
    c. Is fairly consistent as long as I work out
    d. Decreases when I'm stressed or overworked
    e. Is stubborn (I gain easily and tend to be overweight)
    f. None of the above or not applicable

II. SYMPTOMS
Energy

9. My energy is:
   a. Irregular—I alternate between high highs and low lows
   b. Consistent, but I occasionally crash or become overwhelmed
   c. Consistently positive (I feel on top of the world!)
   d. Low—I have trouble getting going, or I crash in the afternoons
   e. Just okay—I have more days of feeling low energy than high
   f. None of the above or not applicable

10. In terms of sleep patterns:
   a. I am up all night—I do my best work at night.
   b. I am up super early in the morning, before others—I hear the birds!
   c. I am awake as the day breaks, usually the same time every morning.
   d. I need more sleep than I did in the past and am often in bed before everyone else.
   e. I always oversleep—it's tough getting out of bed, even though I sleep through the night.
   f. None of the above or not applicable

11. My energy is:
   a. Lowest in the afternoon
   b. Low in the morning and afternoon
   c. Low in the morning only (I gain energy and feel better through the day)
   d. Low all day
   e. Lowest in the evening
   f. None of the above or not applicable

Sleep

Note: If you take a sleep-aid medication, either over the counter or prescription, please consider the following questions about your sleep patterns as they are when you are medication free.

12. I typically go to sleep:
   a. Past midnight
   b. Between 11 p.m. and midnight
   c. Between 10 p.m. and 11 p.m.
   d. No later than 10 p.m., and sometimes earlier
   e. By 10 p.m.
   f. None of the above or not applicable

13. I find my sleep:
   a. Difficult; I cannot fall asleep or stay asleep
   b. Difficult; I fall asleep but wake up frequently between three and four o'clock in the morning
   c. Good; I have more trouble falling asleep than staying asleep
   d. Okay; I often have trouble falling asleep, and will then sleep in
   e. Excessive; I can both fall asleep and stay asleep, often oversleeping
   f. None of the above or not applicable

14. When I do have trouble with sleep, it is most often because:
   a. My mind is restless and anxious.
   b. I worry about my to-do list and that my tasks won't get done.
   c. I stay up too late trying to get too much done before bedtime.
   d. I don't feel rested in the morning. I feel drained and can't get caught up because I'm too tired.
   e. I wake up wanting to stay in bed all day. I either procrastinate or lack motivation.
   f. None of the above or not applicable

Pain Issues

15. My pain can best be described as:
   a. Diffuse; I have a lot of joint pain
   b. Localized; I often have muscle aches and pains
   c. Minimal; I get sore occasionally
   d. Severe—especially abdominal and joint pain
   e. Moderate, mainly presenting as abdominal pain
   f. None of the above or not applicable

16. I experience pain:
   a. Often. I ache and hurt easily.
   b. Sometimes. I hurt a few days out of the month.
   c. Rarely. I rarely have or experience pain.
   d. Almost always. I am in pain most days of every week.
   e. Frequently, but not daily. I do experience pain a few days of the week.
   f. None of the above or not applicable

Mind/Thinking

17. My thinking patterns are:
    a. Erratic. I have trouble focusing and sustaining thoughts.
    b. Sharply unfocused. I can do many tasks at once but have to train my brain to stay on task.
    c. Razor sharp. I am usually on point and able to finish my to-do list.
    d. Densely hazy. I often feel brain fog or overly burdened.
    e. Periodically foggy. I can forget things occasionally.
    f. None of the above or not applicable

18. My thought process can be best described as:
    a. Scattered. My thoughts buzz around like hummingbirds in my head.
    b. Imaginative. I love to daydream.
    c. Linear. I think from point A to B without difficulty.
    d. Elliptical. Often, I'll follow one thought but then my mind will take detours and I'll end up with a different version of the same thought.
    e. Circular. My thoughts are often circular or cyclical—after a number of thoughts, I end up at the same thought.
    f. None of the above or not applicable

Digestive Issues

19. My belly issue is:
    a. Bloating, gas, and diarrhea
    b. Occasional discomfort
    c. Abdominal pain or constipation
    d. Occasional constipation or diarrhea
    e. Abdominal weight gain, indigestion, bloating
    f. None of the above or not applicable

20. My biggest digestive issue is:
   a. Irritable bowel syndrome (IBS), diarrhea dominant. I cycle between episodes of abdominal pain and diarrhea.
   b. Reflux. Food feels like it is coming back up into my throat or I have heartburn.
   c. Constipation. I have trouble having at least one bowel movement a day.
   d. Gastroparesis (delayed gastric emptying—food stays in stomach longer than it should). I have abdominal bloating, with extended feelings of fullness or nausea.
   e. IBS, constipation dominant. I cycle between episodes of abdominal pain and constipation.
   f. None of the above or not applicable

Temperature

21. I am:
   a. Frequently cold or easily chilled
   b. Occasionally cold or chilled
   c. Usually comfortable, but sometimes warm
   d. Someone who fluctuates between being cold and hot
   e. Easily overheated
   f. None of the above or not applicable

III. HORMONE BALANCE

22. My cycles are:
   a. Irregular
   b. Regular but light
   c. Regular
   d. Irregular but heavy
   e. Very heavy—I sometimes see clots
   f. None of the above or not applicable

23. During a cycle, I will use on average:
   a. Zero to two pads daily. I don't get a cycle or my cycle is very light.
   b. Two to four pads or tampons daily
   c. Four to six pads or tampons daily
   d. One to six pads or tampons daily—it varies
   e. More than six pads or tampons daily
   f. None of the above or not applicable

24. I experience:
    a. Irregular ovulation
    b. Ovulation but trouble getting pregnant
    c. Ovulation followed by cystic acne and hair loss
    d. Poor ovulation or no ovulation
    e. Ovulation with fibroids or uterine polyps
    f. None of the above or not applicable

25. In regards to my menstrual cycle, I feel worst:
    a. After ovulation
    b. The week before my cycle
    c. Just a few days prior to my cycle
    d. I feel bad all month and my cycle is irregular or nonexistent.
    e. Midcycle and the week before my cycle
    f. None of the above or not applicable

26. As my cycle approaches, I typically crave:
    a. Salt
    b. Salt and sugar
    c. Sugar
    d. Fat
    e. Sugar and fat
    f. None of the above or not applicable

27. My breasts are:
    a. Small, with minimal volume (an A cup or smaller)
    b. Small to medium (A to B cup)
    c. Medium (B cup)
    d. Changing—they were large and are now smaller, or they were small and are now larger
    e. Large to extra large (D cup or greater)
    f. None of the above or not applicable

28. My libido is:
    a. What is that? Nonexistent.
    b. Variable, but usually low. Once a week is enough.
    c. Average. I feel best when having sex one to three times a week.
    d. Variable, depending on how I feel.
    e. Great. Bring it on. I crave it and need it.
    f. None of the above or not applicable

29. My cycle:
    a. Makes me anxious or depressed
    b. Lowers my energy, and I get a little anxious and more sensitive
    c. Makes me irritable and angry
    d. Wipes me out—I just have no energy
    e. Is incapacitating; I have to take a day or more off of work
    f. None of the above or not applicable

IV. MOOD

Please answer the questions in the following category as if you were medication free.

30. I can best describe my overall mood as the following:
    a. I am usually anxious and nervous.
    b. I am prone to anxiety, but only when stressed.
    c. I can be irritable and very angry when stressed—yes, that is me yelling.
    d. I can have waves of depression and anxiety.
    e. I do get depressed often.
    f. None of the above or not applicable

31. I tend to wake up feeling:
    a. Nervous or anxious about the day ahead
    b. Hopeful that I'll have some time for reflection
    c. Ready to charge forward and take hold of the day
    d. Sluggish, dragging my feet because I don't feel good physically
    e. Dread about my to-do list
    f. None of the above or not applicable

32. I can best describe myself as:
    a. A bit flighty. I might flip-flop moods on you.
    b. Fairly even tempered. I get angry occasionally.
    c. Warm to hot tempered
    d. Calm and compassionate
    e. Even-steven. You can't usually ruffle my feathers.

V. DISEASES

33. I have been diagnosed with:
    a. Anxiety, ADHD, bipolar disorder, or schizophrenia
    b. Irritable bowel syndrome (IBS), colon cancer, or osteoporosis
    c. Inflammatory bowel disease, colon cancer, or a digestive disease
    d. Autoimmune disease, cancer, or immune deficiency
    e. Diabetes, breast cancer, or uterine cancer
    f. None of the above or not applicable

34. I battle:
    a. Infertility
    b. Migraine headaches
    c. Polycystic ovary syndrome (PCOS), endometriosis
    d. Chronic sinus infections
    e. Hypertension, high cholesterol and triglycerides
    f. None of the above or not applicable

35. I often get:
    a. Palpitations
    b. TMJ (temporomandibular joint) issues, pain in the jaw joint and muscles that control jaw movement, often including neck and shoulder pain
    c. Acne
    d. Allergies, frequent illnesses—I am sick every month
    e. Yeast infections
    f. None of the above or not applicable

VI. EMOTIONS

36. I cry:
    a. Easily
    b. Only when fatigued
    c. Rarely
    d. Hardly ever or never
    e. Often

37. I am happiest:
    a. Drawing, painting, or writing
    b. Strategizing or inventing
    c. Leading a team or being in charge
    d. Volunteering
    e. Serving or caring for others
    f. None of the above or not applicable

38. I get angry:
    a. Rarely
    b. Sometimes
    c. Often; I have to work to control my temper.
    d. Occasionally
    e. Hardly ever or never

39. I feel most loved when I am with:
    a. Animals
    b. Friends
    c. My community
    d. My church or spiritual community
    e. Children or a significant other

VII. RELATIONSHIPS

40. I have had:
    a. Many brief romantic relationships
    b. A few significant relationships. I don't mind being alone at times.
    c. One or two longer relationships. I don't have patience for someone who does not feel right.
    d. Three to five longer relationships.
    e. I am always in a relationship. I have trouble being alone.
    f. None of the above or not applicable

41. In a relationship, I crave:
    a. Romance—bring on the flowers, cards, and passion
    b. Some romance, some intellectual stimulation, and some solitary time to recharge
    c. A mental equivalent
    d. A nurturing partner who sees the world as I do
    e. Warmth and reassurance

42. Although I love my children, I often feel:
    a. Irritable or snappy around them
    b. That I enjoy them but need some time away
    c. That I enjoy them but anger easily
    d. Happy and content
    e. Protective and possessive—only I can best do this job
    f. None of the above or not applicable

VIII. WORK

43. I seek and enjoy:
    a. Creative work
    b. The opportunity to build teams, companies, and projects
    c. The opportunity to lead a team, company, or project
    d. Meaningful work that gives back to society or impacts the world in a lasting way
    e. Service-based work—caring for the sick, elderly, or children, as an example
    f. None of the above or not applicable

44. I'd describe myself as:
    a. An erratic worker—I get bursts of energy
    b. A consistently high-energy worker
    c. A steady and consistent worker
    d. A high-energy worker, but more recently having issues getting through the day
    e. A lower-energy, more methodical worker with only enough stamina to work part time

45. My favorite season is:
    a. Summer
    b. Spring
    c. Fall
    d. Fall and summer
    e. Winter

46. Of the colors below, my favorite is:
    a. Blue
    b. Purple
    c. Red or orange
    d. White
    e. Brown, beige, or cream

47. In my previous lab work, my total cholesterol readings have usually been:
    a. Low—less than 130
    b. Low normal—130 to 150
    c. High normal—150 to 170
    d. Normal—170 to 190
    e. Very high—I need medications (greater than 190)
    f. None of the above or not applicable

48. I am prone to having:
    a. A pallid skin tone or complexion
    b. Under-eye circles
    c. A thick, yellow-coated tongue
    d. Swollen joints
    e. A white-coated tongue

49. Of the animals below, the best to describe me is a:
    a. Hummingbird. I am always moving and humming along.
    b. Dolphin. I alternate between smooth sailing and jumping to new heights.
    c. Lion. I rule the jungle.
    d. Horse. I am happy to serve.
    e. Bear. I am comforting.

50. My favorite comfort foods are:
    a. Salty—potato chips
    b. Both salty and sweet—potato chips and chocolate
    c. Spicy foods
    d. Fried foods
    e. Sweets—ice cream and chocolate

51. My blood pressure runs:
    a. Low, <110/80
    b. Low normal, 110/80 to 120/80
    c. Normal, 120/80 to 130/80
    d. Occasionally low or high, 130/80 to 140/80
    e. Consistently high, >140/80

How to Score

Please use the instructions for determining your dominant Power Type as follows:

1. Count up your number of each answer.

   Total a's = _____

   Total b's = _____

   Total c's = _____

   Total d's = _____

   Total e's = _____

   Total f's = _____

2. Next, multiply each answer by the corresponding points below.

   A. Multiply total a answers by 1 = _____.

   B. Multiply total b answers by 2 = _____.

   C. Multiply total c answers by 3 = _____.

   D. Multiply total d answers by 4 = _____.

   E. Multiply total e answers by 5 = _____.

   F. Multiply total f answers by 0 = _____.

3. Final step: Add up all totals from above and write your answer here_____. Use this number to find your Power Type below.

   A. 50–95: You are a Gypsy Girl (see Chapter 5).

   B. 96–135: You are a Savvy Chick (see Chapter 7).

   C. 136–180: You are a Boss Lady (see Chapter 6).

   D. 181–225; You are a Nightingale (see Chapter 9).

   E. 226–270: You are an Earth Mama (see Chapter 8).

NOW YOU KNOW YOUR POWER TYPE: Congratulations! The questions you just answered have uncovered the path you need to take to activate your super powers. Just one more stop before you get started on your 3-Week Rx.

It's important to familiarize yourself with the tools and healing practices you'll be incorporating and how they all relate to each other to creat the most effective plan for your health. It's all laid out in the next chapter.

CHAPTER 4

SUPER TOOLS FOR SUPER WOMEN

YOU HAVE FOUND your Power Type and you're eager to get started. I know. I can feel you fidgeting impatiently in your seat, mentally yelling, "Give me my super powers ALREADY!" I understand, really I do—and we are getting close—but before we jump into the medical meat of your particular Power Type and your plan for rebalance and super powered living, I want to make sure you understand the language, philosophies, principles, practices, and tools we'll be using.

Formulating and creating the Super Woman Rx is the culmination of my more than 25 years of education in multiple systems of medicine and experience in treating over 10,000 patients. During this time, I've merged and integrated the BEST ideas from multiple healing practices, teachings, and systems of medicine and wisdom to create effective treatment and healthy lifestyle plans. The five easy-to-follow, highly successful Super Woman Rx Power Type plans at the heart of this book are the outcome of this incredible journey. But to fully understand where we are headed, you need a quick crash course on just what you'll be applying to your life. I want us all speaking the same language, and to provide you with the information that will fuel your commitment and motivation to make permanent changes for improved health, happiness, and well-being.

There are many different ways that medicine is defined, and the terminology can be confusing. For years after I started my practice, people (including other doctors) would ask my husband, "What exactly does your wife do?" and "Just what is integrative medicine?" Today, integrative medicine, which simply means the utilization of all appropriate, evidence-based medical practices and healing methods to achieve optimal health and happiness, is better known. Still, it's not what the majority of people experience when they go to the doctor. In 2015, the National Center for Health Statistics (part of the Centers for Disease Control and Prevention) and the National Institutes of Health released evidence showing that more than 33 percent of American adults, about 3 in 10, used some form of complementary and alternative medicine in 2012.

The typical scenario between patient and doctor goes something like this: You feel sick or are in pain, tired, stressed, or depressed. You make an appointment and go to the doctor. Your vitals are checked, sometimes blood is drawn, and usually you get a prescription for a medication, and sometimes a referral to another specialist, and off you go—with a follow-up appointment scheduled in 2 to 6 weeks. To boil this down even further, you go into the doctor's office with an existing issue or problem and the doctor quickly tries to assess what's going on, then gives you something to manage or control your symptoms. Sound familiar? Most doctor office visits last a little over 10 minutes, even less of that time is spent face-to-face with your actual doctor, and often the majority of that time your physician is typing into a computer rather than looking at you. It's perfunctory and impersonal, and definitely not enough time or attention to do a full analysis of the complex individual you are, to record a complete history, or to figure out what's going on currently with you—how could it be? It doesn't have to be this way.

There is so much more to be had from medicine and health in general. The one-dimensional Western or conventional view of sickness and health just described is entirely too limiting. I am here to share a new way of thinking about your health—one that is inclusive and holistic. This chapter will be your reference point.

On the following pages you'll find explanations and definitions for the healing practices you'll be incorporating in Super Woman Rx. These are the tools you'll be pulling from, which will change you from so-so or just okay to super powered. These practices may seem diverse—they are—and some may be far from your conventional understanding of and experience with medicine, disease, and healing—they are—but truly, all of these healing disciplines are vital components to creating a more powerful health toolbox than you've ever had access to before, and to creating the ultimate *you*.

THE ULTIMATE BIOHACK: SUPER WOMAN MEDICINE

Everything included in this book and in my medical philosophy and personal beliefs—all the Super Woman Rx recommendations, the 3-Week Power Plans, the exercises, the nutritional suggestions, the supplements, meditations, remedies, methods, and strategies—is based on scientifically tested medical and healing practices that have provided effective and impressive results either in clinical studies or in my own clinical practice. The approach you'll find here in *Super Woman Rx* is my practice in print form—your guidebook to evaluating the whole *you*—so you can become a powerful advocate for your health! This is your personal guide to biohacking yourself, or figuring out how to link your chemistry with the rest of your life. (For a review of what *biohacking* means, see page x.)

The purpose of this chapter is to break it all down—to explain to you all the components of what I know to be the best tools to use to find your center—your core—to empower you to spring forth into super health! This is what I believe medicine should be. What follows on these next pages are the main components that make up my practice, my beliefs, and the Super Woman Rx. The results will speak for themselves, but knowing why you are doing certain things can strengthen your motivation and commitment to your health, especially in the long term.

DEFINING MEDICINE

First let's take a look at how the main medical and healing practices we'll be using are generally defined. This chapter is not exhaustive, and there are other valuable medical disciplines, but the following are the ones most relevant to the Super Woman Rx.

Integrative Medicine

This formal term is probably closest to my definition of super woman medicine or biohacking, since integrative medicine involves bringing together the best of all systems of medicine—blending conventional medicine with scientifically sound alternative medical approaches in a coordinated and effective way. In the Super Woman Rx, we will integrate multiple systems of all the best medicines to create the best plan for you.

Conventional Medicine

Conventional medicine is also referred to as mainstream, standard, Western, orthodox, or allopathic medicine or biomedicine. It refers most often to a system in which doctors of medicine (MDs) or doctors of osteopathic medicine (DOs) and other health professionals including registered nurses, pharmacists, and therapists identify, diagnose, and treat symptoms and diseases using drugs, radiation, or surgery. This is the medicine you probably grew up with and what I described in the opening of this chapter. The scientific progress of this system of medicine is immense and focused on identifying diseases and conditions, many of which we will touch upon! Research is a great strength of this field, leading to a better understanding of genetics, the microbiome (see "Understanding Your Gut Microbiome" on page 000), and many other concepts.

Complementary Medicine

Complementary medicine combines a nonmainstream and a mainstream medical practice. What is important to note is that complementary medicine can simply mean adding an alternative remedy to a conventional one. Originally, complementary medicine didn't need to be based on any scientific evidence or clinical expertise. This meant that anyone could hang out a sign and say that using alternative treatment X (think snake oil), along with doing whatever your regular doctor said, would heal you—and could call it "complementary medicine."

Today, complementary medicine encompasses such things as having a cancer patient drink ginger tea to relieve nausea (an alternative treatment) while undergoing chemotherapy (mainstream medicine). Many practitioners utilize complementary medicine without realizing it when they recommend home remedies, food, or mind-body advice in conjunction with conventional medical care.

Holistic Medicine

According to the American Holistic Health Association, holistic medicine is "the art and science of healing that addresses the whole person—

UNDERSTANDING YOUR GUT MICROBIOME

Our understanding of the microbiome has exploded and continues to expand. The delicate balance of bacteria that begins in your mouth and inhabits your colon (aka your gut) and beyond is responsible for your digestive health, your mood, hormones, and more! How can your intestines affect your mind? It's all centered in the gut-brain axis, the connection between the brain in your head and the one in your gastrointestinal (GI) tract, or your gut. While your gut doesn't have the same physically concentrated gray matter as the brain inside your skull, it does act like a sort of second brain in that it is triggered by the fight-or-flight response just like the limbic system of your brain.

Picture a million different tiny living organisms in your mouth, esophagus, small intestine, and large intestine (all part of your gut). Those bugs have to live in harmony and are fed and watered by your diet and impacted by your stress and lifestyle. Understanding and balancing your individual microbiome is one of the keys to your super powers! When the bugs in your gut are out of balance, even the best food and lifestyle changes can yield minimal results. Your Power Type plan will help you rebalance your unique microbiome and reharness your super powers, so you can welcome in new energy!

body, mind, and spirit." Holistic medicine can include complementary and alternative medical practices, with a central focus on the blending and balancing of the mind, the body, spiritual health, and the connection between all of them.

Traditional Chinese Medicine (TCM)

While the goals of Western medicine and Traditional Chinese Medicine (TCM) are the same—healthy patients, pain reduction, disease management and treatment—their methods and philosophies vary widely. TCM focuses on the prevention of disease before it manifests or occurs rather than the control, management, and/or treatment of already existing disease. TCM is holistic. This means that it views all of you—your body, your emotional makeup, and your needs—as unique and individual. As a comparison, consider that Western medicine is reductionist, meaning that it reduces everything—from body parts and body systems to the mind and heart—to science, chemistry, and technology. In the Western reductionist model, decisions and treatments are based in the world of scientific studies that follows the rule of common averages—meaning if the average person has X, then she needs drug Y.

Let's look at an example. You go to your doctor complaining of frequent headaches. Your doctor diagnoses you with a migraine and writes a prescription for a migraine-blocking drug. This drug was found to work on a certain percentage of the population who complain of migraines. You take your prescription and go on your way. Hopefully you fall into the percentage of people the drug worked on, and not the percentage that had horrible side effects.

Now, let's say you go to your Chinese medicine physician. You complain of headaches. She will typically look closely at your face, tongue, and pulse and then determine where your energy, or *qi*, is blocked (more on this in a bit). If she determines that you have a digestive issue (that's the area where your qi is blocked), you will get a formula for nutrients, herbs, and acupuncture that targets the opening up of the energy flow of digestion. If your issue is stress or anxiety, then your prescription will target stress management and emotional balance with different nutrition recommendations, herbs, and acupuncture.

Chinese medicine is made up of several components. Here are the ones I've incorporated into the Super Woman Rx.

MERIDIANS

The theory of meridians in TCM is the belief that channels (aka meridians) of energy (aka qi, see page 38) govern the body and different body functions. The meridian system is the highway system of your body, and your meridians connect circulation to your organs to your tissues. Acupuncture pinpoints (literally) these meridians, or channels, to encourage a healthy and balanced movement of energy (qi).

There are 12 main meridians throughout your body. Each meridian is made up of a yin-yang pair (see page 38). Meridians can be healed and balanced with food, herbs, and acupuncture. An acupuncturist must completely understand the meridian system to provide effective treatment. For the purposes of the Super Woman Rx, you need to keep in mind only the following:

◆ **Kidney meridian:** considered the "life force," this meridian determines our energy, hormone balance, and the rate at which we age. We are gifted with this energy at birth.

◆ **Spleen meridian:** the master digestive meridian—the commander, so to speak, of your digestive system

◆ **Lung meridian:** responsible for detoxification and lung function

◆ **Heart meridian:** the seat of anxiety and depression; imbalances linked to chronic stress to the heart meridian result in heart disease

◆ **Pericardium meridian:** another meridian that influences anxiety and depression

◆ **Liver meridian:** also known as the laundromat, this is the major detoxification meridian of the body and where we clean out environmental toxins. Stagnation here can affect hormone balance.

◆ **Stomach meridian:** responsible for digestion and metabolism of our food

◆ **Gallbladder meridian:** governs fat metabolism—a weakness here can result in issues with dairy and meat

QI

Your life energy, believed to be gifted at birth, is dependent on the energy, or qi, of your parents. You can replenish or deplete your qi throughout your life continuum. If you are out of balance your qi is blocked, and blockages of qi create disease. Cancer, for example, is seen as a blockage of qi over time. Your qi runs through your body in an electrical circuit—almost like highways that traverse the body. Circulation, emotions, and food can all affect this flow of energy.

YIN AND YANG

The quality of your qi, or life energy, is determined by the Chinese philosophy of yin-yang balance. This is the belief that harmonious yet opposing forces make up the universe and balance each other out to create universal harmony. Yin is believed to be the nurturing female energy, while yang is the more aggressive male energy, and perfect balance between the two is the ultimate goal. In other words, balance for the mind, body, and life in general is a delicate dance of yin and yang. Too much stress, overwork, and aggression is an indication of yang excess, which affects your chemistry and physiology all the way down to your cellular functions. On the other hand, too much yin energy can sometimes lead to a deep depression.

The TCM Perspective on Hormones

The key to preserving and nourishing healthy hormones from a Chinese medicine perspective is striving for yin-yang balance by focusing on the right diet, digestive health, and strategies that promote stress

THE EAST/WEST GUIDE TO HORMONES

In conventional medicine, hormones are the chemical messengers secreted in your blood that tell your body what to do and how to feel. Most doctors treat hormonal imbalances with drugs, and not much else. We can master our hormones and reclaim our sanity by simply taking a walk back in medical history to almost 2,000 years ago, to another region of the world, where the delicate balance of our hormones was believed to be determined by our qi, or overall energy. Finding and sustaining that qi was paramount to preserving a woman's fertility and to helping her transition between the stages of her life.

Here, in *Super Woman Rx*, I'm going to teach you a way to shift your perspective about your hormones, literally to biohack your hormones. In addition to using conventional tools and other natural remedies to understand hormones, you are going to learn the Traditional Chinese Medicine (TCM) approach to your body's chemical messengers and how to use their diagnostic principles to change your life. TCM teaches that hormones are not just lab values but also a manifestation of the orchestra at work in your body—a reflection, in a sense, of your diet, sleep, lifestyle, and passions. Your hormones are your life energy, your qi, and to solve or balance any hormonal issue, you must balance your qi.

management (see "The East/West Guide to Hormones on page 39"). While Western medicine is just coming to terms with the link between diet and hormones, TCM has understood this relationship for more than 5,000 years! For the majority of super women I meet, a high-stress lifestyle results in yang excess (high stress hormones and too much masculine energy) and too little yin (low female hormones and too little female power), which can leave these women—*and you*—panicked, sleepless, and vulnerable to diseases. By adopting approaches that enhance yin energy, you can help your body naturally build and balance estrogen and progesterone. The number one tool used to balance hormones in TCM is food and nutrition.

TCM TECHNIQUES, METHODS, AND MODALITIES

The way you answered the questions in the Power Type test addressed the methods and modalities in this and later sections. Chinese medicine practitioners most often use the following procedures.

Face mapping

TCM practitioners link the color, condition, and texture of specific areas of your face to the health status of various organ systems in your body. Here's an overview of how face mapping works.

- **Face color/skin tint:** Red, pale, blue, yellow, or gray skin can indicate various issues. For example, gray and dull skin are linked to anemia, a reddish complexion can indicate congestion and an excess of heat, while a blue or purplish hue can hint at stagnation (a lack of circulation).

- **Breakouts/acne:** On your forehead, breakouts and acne are believed to indicate gallbladder congestion, which is often an issue for Boss Ladies and indicates that your body is not processing fats effectively. If the problem is between your eyebrows, it means your liver is weakening or becoming clogged. If your chin has pimples and/or blackheads it is often a digestive issue, and acne on your jaw is often hormonal.

- **Dark circles:** If you have dark circles under your eyes, it's a clue that you have a kidney meridian imbalance, common among Gypsy Girls and Savvy Chicks.

Tongue diagnosis

This is a primary diagnostic tool used in TCM, and these practitioners go far beyond the command to stick out your tongue and say ahhh. If you've been to see an acupuncturist, then you've probably experienced this. Looking at the tongue can offer hints about where a body is out of balance. Different areas are associated with specific meridians.

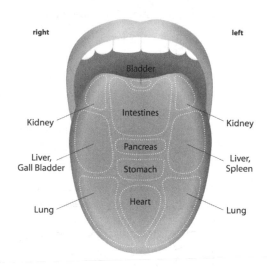

Tongue Reflexology Chart

right — left
Bladder
Kidney — Intestines — Kidney
Pancreas
Liver, Gall Bladder — Stomach — Liver, Spleen
Lung — Heart — Lung

Acupuncture

Acupuncture points are like traffic cops who work to regulate your qi by either blocking it or enhancing its flow. Needles, lasers, and magnets have all been used to unleash these blocked areas. The aim is always to achieve optimal balance between yin and yang in your body, where qi flows freely, preventing and treating disease.

Moxibustion

This is a TCM technique where the burning of herbs over acupuncture points is used to garner and collect energy and literally warm up a cold, undernourished body. It is often used when acupuncture may be too aggressive for a patient.

Cupping

Small suction cups are used to move energy through the body and detoxify the body. Many athletes have used cupping to heal sprains and strains.

Ayurvedic Medicine

The word *Ayurveda* means "the science of life," and it refers to a 5,000-year-old holistic system of medicine developed in India. This healing practice is a valuable diagnostic tool that helps to explain how your unique

WHERE EASTERN PHILOSOPHIES OVERLAP

TCM and Ayurvedic ideas and methodologies share certain concepts of elements or energies.

The Chinese believe in five seasons: autumn, winter, spring, summer, and late summer. Behind each season are elemental energies (the five elements): metal, water, wood, fire, and earth. You can see these energies in the world around us and in our own energies. In Ayurvedic philosophy, practitioners believe that each dosha is associated with an element that symbolizes the main energy of that dosha. Depending on your type, you will have one or two dominant energies or elements that reflect certain characteristics. In the chapters on specific Power Types, you'll learn which elements are key for you and how awareness of these energies can help you navigate your world.

- **Air/Wind/Metal:** associated with vata's flow and creativity and TCM's windy and transitional autumn
- **Fire:** associated with pitta's passion and TCM's fiery and hot summer
- **Earth/Wood:** associated with kapha's groundedness and TCM's late summer, when fire burns down and energy mellows, balanced with the strong, healthy growth cycle of spring
- **Air/Fire/Water:** associated with vata-pitta's visionary power and TCM's seasons of winter and summer, which are in turn associated with stillness, concentration, and passion that contains great power
- **Earth/Air/Wood:** associated with vata-kapha, kapha-pitta, or a blend of all types and all characteristics and seasons

personality traits, health risks, and body type are helpful signposts that point toward and guide your Power Type. Read on for a list of terminology, practices, and strategies used in this ancient wisdom and healing practice.

DOSHAS

In Ayurveda there are three main energies or personality types, called *doshas*, that govern and guide your inner and outer movements, transformations, and structure: *vata, pitta,* and *kapha,* and also combination types of vata-pitta, kapha-vata, and pitta-kapha. We all carry a unique proportion of these three main forces, with one or two types dominating at any given time. Understanding your dominant or combination dosha will help you to recognize your strengths, weaknesses, health risks, and personality traits. Using this as a guide will help you to know, without lab work or x-rays, why you might be deficient in fatty acids, if you are at risk for osteoporosis or anxiety, and so on. I also find it valuable to use doshas as a guide to diets—there are pitta-pacifying recipes or vata-balancing regimens that are helpful and part of the Power Plans to come. In the Super Woman Rx, we have used these doshas as one tool to identify your Power Type. Here is a quick primer on doshas to get you oriented.

Vata: Often described as thin, wiry, or lanky, the vata types are dominated by the air element and prone to dry skin or hair.

Pitta: Of medium build and athletic, pittas are associated with fire and have a tendency to generate and create heat, often resulting in digestive imbalance issues.

Kapha: More largely built and sometimes more heavyset, kaphas have slower metabolisms and thick hair and skin but a tendency to gain weight.

CHAKRAS

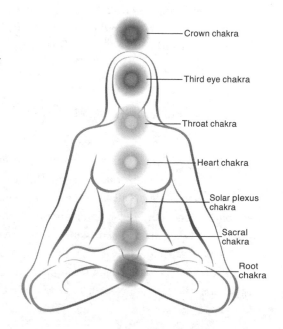

Crown chakra

Third eye chakra

Throat chakra

Heart chakra

Solar plexus chakra

Sacral chakra

Root chakra

Imagine a swirling wheel of energy where matter and consciousness meet: This is known as a *chakra,* and you have seven of them, according to Ayurveda. They are considered centers of spiritual power or wheels of energy that run throughout your body, starting from the base of your spine on up to the crown of your head. The energy in each chakra is known as *prana,* or life energy. The seven chakras represent different pranas: The Crown represents spirituality; the Third Eye represents mental focus, clarity, and intelligence; the Throat represents communication; the Heart represents love; the Solar Plexus represents confidence and control; the Sacral represents connection and acceptance; and the Root represents foundation and being grounded.

The goal with each is to keep them open and flowing. Chakras are thought to be connected to your psychological, emotional, and spiritual well-being. If a chakra gets blocked, then energy (prana) cannot flow, and you will experience health issues.

AYURVEDIC THERAPIES

Typing: In Ayurveda, a practitioner would take the time to identify your dosha by studying your face, tongue, and pulse, similar to the method in Chinese medicine. A lifestyle evaluation is also commonly performed.

Shirodhara: This is a technique where heated oil is poured over the forehead for an extended period of time, accessing the third eye chakra to calm your inner nerves, ease anxiety, and improve overall tranquility and vitality.

Abhyanga: This Sanskrit word can be translated as both "oil" and "love," and is a 15- to 20-minute self-massage technique that can ease anxiety, calm nerves, and enhance sleep. It is also beneficial to help hair grow luxuriantly, soften and soothe skin, and reduce wrinkles.

WHAT IS pH AND WHY DOES IT MATTER?

The abbreviation pH, which stands for "power of hydrogen," is a measure of the hydrogen concentration in your body. The pH scale ranges from 1 to 14, with 1 being completely acidic, 7 being neutral, and 14 being all alkaline. Our ideal pH is 7.3 to 7.45 and can be determined through either a saliva or urine test. If you are too acidic, you are more likely to suffer from digestive problems, heart disease, infertility, joint and muscular pain, and acne, and a weak immune system. Each of the Five Power Plans addresses your unique pH tendencies with diet, exercise, supplements, and mind-body tips that bring you back into balance.

SUPER-SIZED RECOMMENDATIONS

At my practice, CentreSpring MD, we combine all systems of the best medicine from around the world. I find that there are key nutrients, lab markers, and hormones that are often overlooked or minimized in the conventional setting. Here's a rundown of the vitamins, supplements, lab work, and hormone checks that I recommend.

Vitamins and Supplements You Need to Know

While each Power Type comes with her own set of customized vitamins and supplements, the short list below includes those that work on issues common to many super women of all types. If you see something here that you don't see in your 3-Week Power Plan—for example, you have digestive issues but don't see a digestive enzyme specified in your plan—it's okay to include it.

◆ **B vitamins** play a powerful yet often underestimated role in women's health. They are the key micronutrients involved in regulating hormone pathways and neurotransmitters, meaning that these miracle micronutrients can play a role in mood, sleep, energy, and beauty! The B-complex supplement you choose should include the following types and amounts of B vitamins. If you can't find a B vitamin supplement that has these amounts, buy them separately. I find that B vitamins that are methylated (more biologically available) often work best, especially for those who have MTHFR (a gene that prevents them from using a standard B vitamin supplement correctly). For more information, see Resources, page 316. Here's the rundown.

  - **B_1 (thiamin), 25 milligrams:** converts food into fuel, helps your body metabolize fats and proteins

  - **B_2 (riboflavin), 25 milligrams:** helps you convert food into fuel

  - **B_5 (pantothenic acid), 50 milligrams:** helps your body convert food into fuel and use fats and proteins as energy

  - **B_6 (pyridoxine), 25 milligrams:** helps your body make neurotransmitters for normal brain development and function, stabilizes mood

  - **B_{12} (cobalamin), 1,000 micrograms:** works to improve energy

(continued on page 48)

ANTI-INFLAMMATORY EATING—FOODS TO AVOID

The *one* type of diet most systems of medicine agree on is an anti-inflammatory diet. Part of activating super powers requires altering your eating to reduce and eliminate foods that cause inflammation. Inflammation is an immune response that happens when there is a perceived threat in the body. Often this shows up as joint pain and swelling, but many other symptoms including brain fog, depression, and anxiety can also be caused by inflammation. Some Power Types are more sensitive to gluten, while others need to be careful to avoid sugar and red meats. Every Rx you'll use in this book is designed to reduce inflammation so your unique super powers will be set free. The bulleted list below includes the main inflammation-causing culprits.

- **Gluten:** A protein found in wheat, gluten can trigger an immune reaction that damages the surface of the small intestine and can cause a variety of problems including interference with the absorption of nutrients, bloating, diarrhea, and sometimes constipation. People with sensitivity to gluten can experience anxiety, depression, mood swings, brain fog, fatigue, dizziness, migraine headaches, swelling or pain in joints.

- **Yeast:** Yeast is found in breads, rolls, croissants, pastries, doughnuts, beer, wine, cider, some stocks, and other fermented foods. People with sensitivities to yeast can experience abdominal bloating, constipation, diarrhea, anxiety, depression, hives, psoriasis, infertility, menstrual problems, respiratory issues, and weight gain.

- **Refined carbohydrates:** White flour, white rice, processed cereals, chips, crackers, French fries, and more are included on this list.

- **Lactose:** Lactose is the sugar found in milk and other dairy products. Lactose intolerance occurs in people who don't have enough of the enzyme lactase, which is needed to break down lactose. Lactose intolerance can cause stomach pain, gas and bloating, nausea, and diarrhea. Interesting fact: Plain Greek yogurt (which is my go-to yogurt) is 99 percent lactose free, so I find that many people who have this sensitivity are still okay with this product.

- **Milk:** Even if they don't have lactose intolerance, some people have a sensitivity to milk and dairy products that can cause an allergic reaction ranging from rashes, hives, itching, and swelling to more severe issues such as wheezing and trouble breathing.

- **Meat:** People with sensitive stomachs can have trouble digesting pork and red meats and, less often, poultry. This is especially true of factory-farmed, grain-fed, and antibiotic-infused animals. That's why my recommendation for all meats is for grass-fed, humanely raised, antibiotic-free products. It's the bacterial toxins in meat that most often trigger endotoxins in the blood.

- **Sugar:** Processed sugars are empty calories and just bad all around—they spike your blood sugar and are void of any valuable nutrients. Besides causing weight gain, they trigger the release of inflammatory messengers called cytokines and can cause suppression of white blood cells, which makes you more susceptible to getting sick. Inflammation caused by sugar has also been linked to certain cancers.

- **Alcohol:** All alcoholic beverages cause inflammation in your liver, your gut, your joints, tissues, and blood vessels. Alcohol is also associated with heart disease, stroke, cancer, and other digestive problems. Best to be avoided.

- **Saturated and trans fats:** These fats can trigger fat tissue inflammation in the body, which is an indicator of heart disease and is also linked to arthritis pain. Trans fats also trigger inflammation; they are most often found in fast foods, fried products, and processed snack foods.

- **Artificial sweeteners:** Aspartame, found in diet sodas, is a neurotoxin that causes inflammation in the brain, and Splenda has been shown to spike blood sugar and increase the release of insulin (not good for anyone at risk of diabetes).

- **Processed foods:** Most packaged foods have been altered for a long shelf life with preservatives, colorings, and artificial flavorings, all of which trigger inflammation in the body. If it comes in a box or bag and has a brand name, chances are good that it's bad.

"I used to crash in the afternoons and early evenings, but shortly after I added the B vitamins recommended by Dr. Taz, I noticed that I was feeling happier and more energetic—and those predictable energy slumps disappeared!"—Beth, 34, mom to two toddlers, project manager

- **Folic acid, 800 micrograms:** reduces the risk of birth defects, protects against anemia

- **Biotin, 2,500 micrograms:** works to strengthen and thicken hair and nails

◆ **Probiotics** are important in rebalancing the microbiome. They are naturally found in certain foods, which you'll see incorporated into the plans. Probiotic-rich foods include yogurt, kefir, bone broth, sourdough bread, and kombucha (a fermented drink thought to have originated in Russia), but probiotics can also be taken as supplements. You want a probiotic that is well labeled, with five or six strains of bacteria and at least 20 billion CFU (colony-forming units).

◆ **Digestive enzyme** supplements work to break down your food into smaller particles, making it easier for you to process and to absorb the nutrients from all the great foods you'll be eating. I recommend that women with digestive issues include one or two caplets of digestive enzymes with their heaviest meal. Take a digestive enzyme with amylase (an enzyme that breaks down starch), lipase (an enzyme that breaks down fat), and protease (breaks down protein). If you've had your liver or gallbladder removed, look for a product that includes ox bile, since it helps with fat absorption and processing. Each enzyme is dosed differently and in different units, so it is often best to start with just one capsule per meal—if the enzyme gives you a lot of gas and/or discomfort, back down to half a capsule. Pick capsules rather than tablets, and if you are taking half a capsule, just open it and take half the powder.

◆ **Magnesium,** or as I call it, the "miracle micronutrient," is a cofactor for hormones and neurotransmitters and helps with sleep and anxiety. The ideal amount of supplementation is 200 to 400 milligrams of chelated magnesium. You can also use Epsom salts baths for a great source of magnesium, or a topical magnesium oil.

Labs You Need to Know

You should definitely have these tests each year, in addition to cholesterol, blood pressure, and blood sugar evaluations and weight checks. There are also specific screenings you should have at certain ages. The following are my recommendations (conventional medical standards often recommend less frequent screenings). At 21, you should start annual cervical cancer screening; at age 40, it's time for your yearly mammograms; at 50, get ready for a colonoscopy and then repeat it every 10 years; and I recommend a baseline screening for osteoporosis at 50, and then a screening to follow every 10 years thereafter. In addition, request the following labs at your yearly physical.

LAB	IDEAL VALUES
Vitamin D	50–70 ng/ml
B_{12}	>500 pg/ml
Ferritin	50–70 ng/ml
Magnesium	>2.2 mg/do

Inflammation Markers

LAB	IDEAL VALUES
Homocysteine	<10 umol/l
C-reactive protein (CRP)	1–2 mg/hr
Erythrocyte sedimentation rate (ESR)	<10 mm/hr

Hormone Balance

LAB	IDEAL VALUES
Thyroid-stimulating hormone (TSH)	1–2 U/ml
Free triiodothyronine (free T3)	3–5 ng/do
Estradiol	50–150 pg/ml
Progesterone	0.5–2.0 ng/ml
Estrone	<150 ng/do
DHEA	100–200 ng/ml
C-peptide	1–3 ng/ml
Leptin	5–15 umol/l

THE FIVE GLANDS YOU NEED TO KNOW

Glands are organs throughout your body; some are responsible for secreting certain chemicals (think sweat, saliva, or breast milk), while others release hormones that tell your body what to do, how to work, or how to grow. Other glands release antibodies and substances to help you fight off illnesses. Let's take a look at the glands that we'll balance using the Super Woman Rx!

1. **Adrenal glands:** You have two adrenal glands, one on top of each of your kidneys. The hormones produced by your adrenals are the ones most often out of balance. These include adrenaline (also called epinephrine and norepinephrine) and cortisol. Weight imbalances, chronic stress, fatigue, anxiety, and infertility can all be signs of imbalanced adrenals.

2. **Pineal gland:** This is your sleep gland and responds to stimulation from light. Melatonin is the hormone secreted from the pineal gland and is thought in Ayurvedic and Chinese medicine to be connected to the "third eye," or the center of intuition and wisdom. Today, we know that your pineal gland secretes melatonin when the sun goes down, which makes you feel drowsy—if all is in balance. And the opposite applies in the morning: Light inhibits the pineal gland's melatonin production.

3. **Thyroid:** This critical gland for women sits in the base of the neck. Thyroid hormones triiodothyronine (T3) and thyroxine (T4) regulate metabolism, weight, energy, hair, mood, and many other hormones—in other words, they are important!

4. **Pancreas:** The insulin regulator, the pancreas produces insulin and the digestive enzymes that break down food, especially lipase, which keeps fat balanced in our bodies. If the pancreas takes a hit, our blood sugar levels become destabilized and we cannot digest or absorb our foods. The ultimate risk? Diabetes.

5. **Ovaries:** These glands help produce and regulate estrogen and progesterone, the essential female hormones. A decline or change in ovarian hormones is the culprit behind infertility, weight gain in perimenopausal women, and the androgen excess responsible for polycystic ovary syndrome (PCOS), cystic acne, and hair loss.

Other Tests

LAB	IDEAL VALUES
Liver function	
–Aspartate aminotransferase (AST)	<40 u/l
–Alanine aminotransferase (ALT)	<40 u/l
Sex hormone binding globulin (SHBG)	100–150 nmol/l
Total cholesterol	150–180 mmol/l

HOW YOU'LL TRACK YOUR PROGRESS

The best way for you to see your progress, catch mistakes or make necessary corrections, and stay motivated is by tracking some things on a daily basis and others weekly. With that in mind, the chapters in the next section include a variety of steps and tracking suggestions based on your specific Power Type. Different tracking measures are used depending on your particular super woman needs.

NOW you have all the super tools you need to begin your 3-Week Power Plan. There's just one last tip I want to offer you on your path to becoming the Super Woman you deserve to be: Stick with the results of your Power Type test! If you tested as a Nightingale, follow the Nightingale 3-Week Plan. A Gypsy Girl? Stick to the Gypsy Girl plan!

"I used to feel regularly bloated, and every day I'd feel drained around 2 p.m.—so I'd regularly reach for some chocolate—but once I started Super Woman Rx, not only did I cut out all dairy and gluten, I went 100 percent sugar free. I'm thrilled—I've gotten a ton of compliments from my coworkers saying I look thinner, that my skin looks great, and that my overall attitude is so positive. The bloating has melted away, and my clothes are fitting better! Before Super Woman Rx, I never exercised, and I'd be wiped by the time I got home from work. Now I have the energy to exercise after work, to cook healthy dinners, get the laundry done, and enjoy playtime with my son. I'm so revved up that I signed up for a triathlon event and am beginning training for it now!"
—Kelly, 34, super mom and an elementary schoolteacher

Even if you identified with more than one Power Type back in Chapter 4—and that's actually pretty normal—it's important that you follow only the 3-Week Power Plan that is in accordance with your test results. So, let's say that you tested as a Boss Lady, but you also feel like you have some significant issues with being a big-time caretaker like an Earth Mama or Nightingale. Or perhaps you are 99.9 percent Gypsy Girl and have been most of your life but recently have been struggling with weight gain. If you tested as a Gypsy Girl, follow the Gypsy Girl plan in Chapter 6, and so on. Once you've followed your current Power Type's plan for 3 weeks, you'll retake the test. If you've balanced out some of your issues, you may very well test as another type—this will be the time to go back and try another Power Plan. Otherwise, you'll get too overwhelmed.

It's still a good idea to familiarize yourself with all Five Power Types discussed in Chapters 6 through 10, but please only follow one plan at a time.

Ready? Read on!

Gypsy Girls: See Chapter 5.

Boss Ladies: See Chapter 6.

Savvy Chicks: See Chapter 7.

Earth Mamas: See Chapter 8.

Nightingales: See Chapter 9.

PART

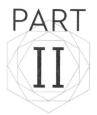

II

YOUR 3-WEEK
SUPER WOMAN RX

NOW IT'S TIME to go deep to learn all there is to know about what makes you uniquely you. In the next five chapters, you'll learn all the rich and intricate aspects of your unique Power Type and your personal Super Woman Rx: Your 3-Week Power Plan. Understanding your distinctive characteristics will address all you need to know to reach peak energy, balance, health, and happiness. Keep in mind: Your dominant Power Type is an important starting point, but just remember that you'll eventually want to familiarize yourself with all Five Power Types. You'll find clues, solutions, and characteristics about yourself in every super woman.

Each of the five 3-Week Power Plans is unique and customized, but all share certain things in common: All are separated into three 1-week phases, and each phase employs three strategies to keep you on track and moving toward better health, happiness, and energy—a weekly checklist of action steps, a shopping list, and a weekly menu for your Power Type.

By now, you should have completed the Power Type Test and should know which Power Type you fall into right now (if not, turn to page 18 and take the test before moving forward).

In regard to the shopping lists, please note that I haven't dictated exactly how many bananas, onions, etc., you should buy each week. I know that you are an experienced shopper with unique decisions to make about quantities you'll need, depending on the number of family members you are shopping for and whether you'll be choosing to prepare these meals for just yourself or for your entire clan.

Before you begin each week, it's a good idea to do some prep work.

WHAT'S KRYPTONITE?

In Superman's fictional world, kryptonite is a radioactive rock from the super hero's home planet that weakens him by draining him of his super powers.

Your kryptonite will be the "rock" you have a tendency to pick up that drains you of your energy and strengths. Your Power Type comes with specific forms of kryptonite that can zap your strength and vitality. Get too close to your kryptonite and you'll lose all your super powers. *Super Woman Rx* will show you how to conquer the unique kryptonite threats in your world.

With that in mind, on the Saturday or Sunday before you start your week, create a shopping list full of healthy foods for the week (you can also use the shopping lists provided in the following chapters). You'll adjust your list to fit your needs—maybe you'll double recipes for family members, or to make grab-and-go meals for later in the week. If you're using the recipes suggested in the 3-week menu, review the directions, and then set aside time to get some aspects of the recipes prepared for the week to come (for example, cook your chicken breasts and ground turkey ahead of time). Or wash, chop, and bag veggies and fruit for easy healthy eating.

Let's get started!

CHAPTER 5

THE GYPSY GIRLS' 3-WEEK RX

IMAGINATIVE, CREATIVE, AND expansive, Gypsy Girls spend a lot of time in the air or in a creative space—somewhere in their minds. This is why most Gypsy Girls are associated with the air element (a Gypsy Girl's main source of energy)—wide, spacious, and hard to catch with your hands. The goal is to keep this creative energy flowing in a healthy and balanced manner, but not to the extent that you become disconnected or find yourself overly anxious, sad, or irritable.

To fully understand your plan and effectively treat your issues, you first need to know about the most common Gypsy Girl medical risks and energy drains. Having seen more than 10,000 patients now, I've seen that these are the conditions that frequently afflict my Gypsy Girls.

Gypsy Girl at a Glance

ALTER EGO: THE ARTIST

Super powers: Creativity, artistic talent: When in balance, Gypsy Girls express their powers in the form of strong bursts of creative energy. When working at their optimum, these Power Types are fearless, passionate, and productive. They excel at translating their creativity into amazing works of art, music, or literature.

Kryptonite: Anxiety, fear, lack of structure, lack of sleep, overcommitting. Gypsy Girls have a tendency to get caught up in their creativity, so caught up that they forget basic care such as eating, exercising, etc. Gypsy Girl types are prone to pushing themselves too hard, and when they do they get overwhelmed and can experience dizziness, excessive fear, and the feeling of being disconnected from their bodies.

Elements: Air/Wind/Metal. These elements represent motion and flow and the season of autumn.

Personality: Creative, artistic, passionate, anxious, restless dreamer.

Body type: Thin, wiry, lean. Gypsy Girls tend to have a lighter frame and excellent agility. This Power Type also struggles with dry skin and hair and cold hands and feet. Gypsy Girls are prone to weight loss, joint pain, and weakness.

Celebrity example: Audrey Hepburn. How is Audrey Hepburn a Gypsy Girl? Well, she definitely had the body type—slim, waiflike, and graceful—and she was obviously highly creative. In addition to being a world-famous actress, she was also a trained ballerina and dancer. Hepburn described herself as an introvert, a definite characteristic of the Gypsy Girl, as was her grace and flair in her appearance and fashion sense. Physically, Hepburn also showed conditions of a Gypsy Girl. She suffered several miscarriages and was said to suffer bouts of anxiety and stress.

Colors: Yellow and sky blue. The blue sky carries the yellow sun. This follows through on the theme of the creativity, energy, and restlessness of Gypsy Girls.

COMMON GYPSY GIRL CONDITIONS

The fact that you are a Gypsy Girl does not mean that you will automatically suffer from any one of the conditions that follow. One thing I have learned from years of working with other systems of medicine, such as Traditional Chinese Medicine (TCM) and Ayurvedic medicine, is that we all have tendencies toward certain illnesses that manifest when we are out of balance. Let's look at the greatest hits for out-of-balance gypsy girls.

Anxiety

Global rates of anxiety and anxiety-related disorders have risen by nearly 50 percent over the last two decades, according to the World Health Organization. Anxiety disorders are consistently found to be the most prevalent class of mental disorders in the general population, and women are nearly twice as likely to suffer from anxiety as men. Many mental health practitioners believe that depression and anxiety are two faces of one disorder. In my experience, for Gypsy

Girls, this phenomenon shows itself most often as anxiety.

Anxiety presents with a range of symptoms, from overthinking (yes—the never-ending racing or circular thinking) to trouble sleeping, irritability, and even heart palpitations. Among the women I've worked with and met, Gypsy Girls are most prone to anxiety; it's a pattern I see over and over again in my work with this Power Type. By nature, a Gypsy Girl already has that mind-body disconnect that comes from living most often in a creative space. While there are many positive attributes to being highly creative, the risk is becoming ungrounded to the extent that the mind takes off and can't get back down to earth. This flightiness is associated with the air or wind element that Ayurveda and Chinese medicine often discuss. Your 3-Week Power Plan will soothe you and your nervous system by incorporating grounding moving meditations, establishing regular eating intervals and sleep times, using calming supplements, and incorporating mind-body strategies—all to bring you back to earth.

ADHD

Common complaints for Gypsy Girls are symptoms of ADHD, or attention deficit/hyperactivity disorder—the adult version. They often complain that they can't focus and may have had this struggle even in childhood. However, many Gypsy Girls report the onset of ADHD symptoms in adulthood, which leaves them feeling powerless when it comes to productivity, efficiency, and effectiveness. Some of my Gypsy Girls will seek medications, especially prescription stimulants such as Ritalin, Vyvanse, and Adderall, to help with focus and concentration. Others will use caffeine or energy drinks to try to power through a project or meet a deadline. Many of these ADHD symptoms are the presenting signs of a chemistry that is unbalanced—not just an imbalance of neurotransmitters, but an imbalance of the hormones and nutrients needed to make them! As you'll see when you begin your Super Woman Rx 3-Week Power Plan, you'll increase your ability to focus by incorporating healthy anchors and balancing strategies into your day through healthy eating, moving, supplements, and mind-body techniques that connect your mind to your physical body.

Eating Disorders

Women are twice as likely to have an eating disorder as men, and of all the Power Types I see, Gypsy Girls are at the greatest risk for anorexia, bulimia, and related eating disorders. Whether it is their anxiety or issues with focus that worsen self-esteem, anorexia nervosa and bulimia are not just issues for our teenagers—many women ranging in age from their twenties to their sixties suffer from these conditions.

In Ayurvedic and Chinese medicine, it's the sense of disconnection from the body that allows eating disorders to exist and persist. The mind is simply incapable of understanding or accepting the harm that is being done to the body. I am concerned that this is a silent epidemic for many women, with pressure on all of us to maintain the weight of our youth and fight the aging process with anything and everything we can find—even if it's destructive. Gypsy Girls can get so caught up in their creative endeavors that they forget all about healthy eating. I'll gradually show you, over the course of the next 3 weeks, how to establish regular, distraction-free times to eat nourishing meals.

Fatigue

Fatigue is common among women, with around a third complaining of a lack of energy, but it's a constant complaint I hear from Gypsy Girls. Most of my patients in this category complain of afternoon fatigue and often need a nap to make it through the evening. These women tell me that after work they are so exhausted that they can't follow through on exercise plans, get meals together, or do much other than press buttons on the remote and order pizza or takeout Chinese. In addition, when it comes to Gypsy Girl moms, I hear complaints that they don't have the energy it takes to soothe a grumpy or teething baby, supervise homework, or keep track of teen whereabouts. This fatigue will then sometimes turn into anxiety, depression or even destructive behaviors such as overeating or alcohol and/or substance abuse. Fatigue and insomnia (coming up next) are usually related, so it isn't surprising that they have shared solutions as well. Besides learning how to overcome energy slumps, you'll establish healthy and sustaining sleep patterns.

Insomnia

A Gypsy Girl may be tired in the evenings, but despite this she loves to stay up late, reading, writing, painting—whatever sort of creativity fits her mood. Insomnia is common in many Power Types, and more women than men suffer from insomnia (the National Sleep Foundation estimates that nearly 40 million Americans suffer from sleep disorders). Gypsy Girls find that late night is a time void of distractions and responsibilities. The night, with its quiet, is a Gypsy Girl's friend—until it's not. If you fall into this Power Type, you know: You might be able to get away with the 3 a.m. bedtime and the 7 a.m. wake-up temporarily but, I warn you, you'll eventually crash hard.

Irregular sleep, or lack of consistent sleep, wears on women's hormones, accelerates the aging process, and worsens many of the other conditions already discussed—including anxiety, ADHD, and risk for eating disorders. Trying to get my Gypsy Girls in bed at a reasonable hour is always a challenge. When they see a 10 p.m. bedtime on their treatment plans, my Gypsy Girl patients usually stare at me with an incredulous look that says I am taking their best friend away! I steady myself for what I know is invariably next: "I'm a night person Dr. Taz!" But when I succeed in convincing them to set, and stick to, a regular sleep schedule, the surplus of vitality they soon have proves the wisdom of the change quickly, and I am no longer the enemy. Phew!

Infertility

Infertility is yet another national epidemic, with countless numbers of women needing in vitro fertilization (IVF) or being told, even in their twenties, that they are in early menopause. This is so disheartening. I have watched many women struggle with infertility, feeling as if their hopes for a family are a disappearing dream.

"I cannot do this anymore," a patient will tell me, her eyes filling with tears. *"We have spent $40,000 with no success—I am exhausted. I just want a baby. I always wanted a family—I don't understand."*

I listen quietly when my sweet patients share these stories. I have to fight my own tears. I stare into the computer, pretending to take notes, so they cannot see my "unprofessional" response. My sadness? I know it does not have to be this way—but women come to me so beaten down, so fatigued and out of balance, that I feel like a fixer who never had a fair chance. The Gypsy Girl 3-Week Power Plan offers real hope, and will make real changes, so you have a fair starting point with your fertility.

Again, as with the ADHD symptoms discussed earlier, it is usually a chemistry imbalance at work here. Out-of-balance hormone signaling can put Gypsy Girls at increased risk for infertility, compared to other Power Types. Many systems of medicine can be helpful, but it takes work and dedication to reestablish fertility when the key elements—nutrition, hormone imbalances, and stress management—have been ignored for years. You may be walking around with high estrogen, low progesterone, and a sluggish thyroid and not even realize it. Incorporated into your 3-Week Power Plan are foods, supplements, and activities that will return your hormones to optimal levels—you just have to be willing to do the work.

Anovulatory (Missed) Cycles

Hormone imbalances that result in missed cycles are common in Gypsy Girls. They can be tied to nutritional deficiencies, can be the cause of infertility, and can cause fluctuations in weight and mood. Reestablishing menstrual cycles should be a goal for all women—but Gypsy Girls who are resistant to following the Super Woman Rx will often have the toughest time doing so. Taking actions that help you come back down to earth while still keeping your creativity revved is a challenge, but the payoffs from establishing a healthy routine are worth it.

Hair Loss

I know this one personally. The conventional medical term is *androgenetic alopecia*. Hair loss, secondary to nutritional and hormonal imbalances, is one of the most common complaints for Gypsy Girls. Hair loss can be diffuse, with hair thinning throughout the scalp or hair strands breaking easily when pulled. Often there is hair loss at the crown as well.

Again, the common imbalances in hormones and nutrition can affect the hair health of Gypsy Girls, leaving them feeling depressed and anxious about their health and their physical appearance. The supplements and nutrition recommendations, as well as the stress-relieving techniques, included in your 3-Week Power Plan will help to rejuvenate your hair, gradually restoring its luster, thickness, and shine.

Osteoporosis

Now considered an inflammatory disease, osteoporosis, a condition defined by low bone mass and increased bone fragility, is common among Gypsy Girls. Many of you may have a low body weight with a classic long, lean frame, and research shows that this increases your risk for osteoporosis. Building bone and preserving bone health are key health challenges for Gypsy Girls, making weight-bearing exercise Rx you will learn a critical part of your plan.

Chinese Meridian Diagnosis: Kidney Meridian Deficiency

If a Chinese medicine practitioner examined a Gypsy Girl, he would most likely conclude that she has a pattern that shows kidney meridian deficiency. Remember, in Chapter 4, you learned that, in Traditional Chinese Medicine (TCM), meridians are channels through which your qi (life energy) flows. The kidney meridian is seen as the center or seat of all energy and hormone function. The kidney meridian becomes depleted from chronic stress and anxiety, poor nutrition, excessive weight loss, and lack of sleep. When there is kidney deficiency, the hormone imbalances can result in the conditions already discussed, including infertility, missed periods, chronic fatigue, and hair loss. You'll address all of this in your 3-Week Power Plan by gradually incorporating potent nutritional strategies, healthy sleep patterns, grounding exercises, mind-body techniques, and more.

Ayurvedic Dosha Diagnosis: Vata

Remember, in Ayurvedic medicine, there are three main energies, or personality types, called doshas. Gypsy Girls are dominated by the vata dosha. The vata dosha in Ayurvedic medicine is known for movement and change (the wind or air element) and for having an energetic and a creative mind.

As is true of each of the doshas for each of the Power Types, there are positive qualities to the vata energy type, but these positive qualities can turn negative when overused. For instance, vata types, when in balance, are naturally creative, light, and active. However, if they become too active, they can go into overload, aggravate their dosha, and become anxious and exhausted—their creativity and light fly right out the window! Balance is always the key.

Adrenal Gland Imbalances

Out of all the glands that produce the hormones that work in synergy to keep us humming, the adrenals are the greatest risk for Gypsy Girls. The adrenal glands, with signaling from the pituitary, are responsible for cortisol and adrenaline regulation, hormones produced in response to stress (for more information, see "The Five Glands You Need to Know" on page 50). Cortisol, remember, is helpful in the right amounts, but levels that are too high or too low can cause a host of medical problems. Anxiety, weight imbalance, infertility, and even poor focus and concentration can all be related to this stress hormone. Too much cortisol from long-term chronic stress results in abdominal weight gain as well.

LAB FINDINGS

The most exciting part of the Super Woman Rx is that results from the lab work used in conventional medicine will match the predictions of older systems of medicine (TCM and Ayurvedic medicine). I find this fascinating—you can see the validity and relevance of Eastern healing practices in another light when they correspond with modern-day laboratory findings. How could TCM and Ayurveda be so on target that today we see the proof in lab results? I, to this day, am still amazed at the precision and accuracy of these old systems of medicine.

Here are the most common lab findings I see in my Gypsy Girls.

- Low B vitamins—including B_{12}, B_6, B_9 (folic acid)
- Low iron and low iron stores—serum iron, ferritin
- Low a.m. cortisol
- High p.m. cortisol
- Low cholesterol—total cholesterol less than 150
- Borderline thyroid function—TSH 3 to 4 uIU/mL
- Low amino acids
- Low fatty acids

I'll address these common deficiencies in the 3-Week Power Plan through healthy menus and supplements. See "Labs You Need to Know," page 49, for more information.

Nutritional Needs/Deficiencies

Based on the lab findings on the opposite page, Gypsy Girls need food and sometimes supplements that help to compensate for these deficiencies. Not only do nutritional deficiencies affect mood, energy, creativity, and the health conditions we discussed, but they also increase your long-term disease risk, as research continues to show how micronutrient deficiencies affect all aspects of health (see below).

As you begin your personal Power Plan, you will see how the plan focuses on your nutritional deficiencies. Foods high in B vitamins, iron, healthy fats, and protein can make or break a Gypsy Girl. Sometimes, even with the best food, supplements for specific deficiencies are still needed—since our food today is not as nutritionally replete as it was even one generation ago.

It's time to take action! Let's begin.

LONG-TERM DISEASE RISKS

Chronic micronutrient deficiencies can lead to disease, as we have mentioned before. So far I have focused mainly on how a Gypsy Girl may feel, not necessarily on the diseases she may develop. Nutritional deficiencies lead to functional medical imbalances like methylation and mitochondrial dysfunction—which often are the root of diseases like heart disease, cancer, and neurological conditions. Methylation is a metabolic process thought to be involved with repairing and regulating DNA genes and fighting infections; mitochondria are organelles that generate energy for your cells.

HOW THE GYPSY GIRL 3-WEEK RX WORKS

I recognize my Gypsy Girl patients quickly. It usually happens while I'm rattling off a bunch of medical information that I know will help alleviate my patient's issues. I'll look up and see eyes filled with tears, a flushed face, or a glazed look, and I'll know I'm talking to a Gypsy Girl. It took me a few years, but today I understand that a Gypsy Girl needs to first be given the space and freedom to breathe, and then a gentle nudge to get her more grounded in her body and less in her mind. For these reasons, I don't begin with an excessively detailed technical plan for Gypsy Girls. If you fit in this category, chances are that you are already feeling overwhelmed, fatigued, and disconnected, and if I start by giving you a bunch of numbers and grams to track and crunch, you might just fizzle out completely.

So how do I start? When I formulate a plan for a Gypsy Girl in my practice, my first aim is always to reconnect her to her physical body, her mind, and her energy. Many of my Gypsy Girls are so disconnected that they don't understand or are not even aware of the physical symptoms that are giving off warning signals until it is too late and they crash drastically, or get a disease or diagnosis that's tough to battle. My entire purpose for writing this book is to prevent this from happening to all Five Power Types. As a Gypsy Girl, your first goal begins with establishing a healthy relationship with your body and your mind so you can reconnect your fabulous spirit to the rest of you. So the first week is all about grounding, while the second week continues the steps you established and adds a focus on balancing. Week 3 brings it full circle by providing tools to keep you connected physically, mentally, and spiritually. Suggested menus and shopping lists are provided at the end of each week.

One last bit of housekeeping before we get started. While each week has its own focus, there are guidelines that I want you to follow starting on Day 1 and continuing for your entire 21-day Rx (details follow). Be dedicated to these foundational guidelines and you'll see the best and fastest results. Here they are.

The Gypsy Girl Rx Rules

1. **Wake up with a morning tonic and grounding exercise** (page 67).

2. **Meet your daily protein and fat goals.** Aim for 50 grams of protein, page 68, and 20 to 30 grams of fats each day. This means reading nutrient labels. If you don't want this extra homework, just follow the menus at the end of the chapter.

3. **Avoid bad foods.** Maintain an anti-inflammatory and gluten-free diet (see "Anti-Inflammatory Eating—Foods to Avoid," page 46), take the recommended supplements as listed in Action Step 4, and eat at regular intervals—ideally, every 3 to 4 hours.

4. **Limit daily calories.** Don't exceed 1,800 calories per day unless you are training for extreme sports.

5. **Sleep well.** Establish healthy sleeping habits (details on page 70). Gypsy Girls need to have a set wake-up time and a steady bedtime to be grounded.

6. Maintain a gluten-free diet. Gluten, the protein found in wheat and other grain, can worsen the vata or hormonal imbalance of a Gypsy Girl.

Note: If you follow the menus and recipes provided at the end of each week, you will meet all the Gypsy Girl nutritional guidelines and

THE 10 GYPSY GIRL ACTION STEPS AT A GLANCE

The following 10 steps outline the entire Gypsy Girl program. Please note that, during Week 1, you'll start with Action Steps 1 through 5, and you'll add further action steps in the second and third weeks. By the time you've completed the entire 3-Week Plan, you will have established all 10 of the following steps.

Step 1: Wake Up with a Morning Tonic

Step 2: Establish Grounding Exercises

Step 3: Power Up with Protein

Step 4: Supplement Your Mornings
- ☐ B-complex vitamins
- ☐ Omega-3 fats
- ☐ L-theanine

Step 5: Establish a Sleep Routine

Step 6: Boost Your Adrenals, 2 p.m. to 4 p.m.
- ☐ Snack
- ☐ Supplement (B_{12}, ashwagandha, and L-theanine)
- ☐ Catnap

Step 7: Fine-Tune Your Dinners

Step 8: Get Moving and Grooving

Step 9: Mind-Body Rx: Stay Connected

Step 10: Beauty: Replenish and Moisturize

action steps. In other words: You will automatically follow all Rx Rules.

To be sure to get the most out of super powered healthy eating, either implement the suggested menu and shopping lists I've created for each week, or you can create your own meals as long as you follow the Gypsy Girl Rx Rules. In addition, each week will focus on action steps that will teach you how to be the super woman you were meant to be. We'll build on these action steps over the next 21 days (see the summary on page 65). Stick with it and you'll activate your super powers each and every day!

Ready? Set? Go!

PHASE 1/WEEK 1: GROUND YOURSELF

Before taking on any full diet, supplement, exercise, or sleep routine, you're going to work on gaining a solid understanding and recognition of your physical body. This will help you grasp the connection between your mental and creative energy, and your physical and emotional health. Your goal will be to recognize and identify that line that often gets crossed from amazing energy to anxiety, creativity to paralysis, and/or joy to panic.

During your first week, you'll begin prioritizing reconnection. Phase 1 is all about reconnecting and grounding you back to your body. You'll move from that creative space in your mind to your physical body by incorporating a morning routine that includes gentle exercises, simple super powered meals throughout the day, helpful supplements, and a restful evening routine. You'll do this with five foundational action steps. I urge you to stay consistent with these first five strategies, because daily commitment and repetition will help cement these new behaviors into established and automatic habits that you'll learn to miss if you forget to do one.

Think back to Chapter 4, where we discussed the Ayurvedic vata principle of cold and elements of wind and air, and to this chapter's TCM concept that Gypsy Girls often have a deficiency in their kidney meridian deficiency (the master of all hormones). The first 7 days of the Gypsy Girl plan address this by focusing on warming up the body and providing the energy and comfort required to bring everything back together.

"The tonics are the best part of Super Woman Rx! Establishing the routine of having these warming drinks each morning gave me essential time for reflection and mental preparation for my day ahead. After just 3 weeks, it's become an automatic habit."—Nancy, 35, super mom and speech pathologist

Week 1 Action Steps

STEP 1: WAKE UP WITH A MORNING TONIC

6 a.m. wake-up: None of us likes waking to an alarm, but part of getting grounded and reconnected comes from establishing a regular wake-up time, so set your alarm for 6 a.m. the old-fashioned way, not on your phone. You can tweak this to be an hour earlier or later to fit your schedule, but no more, and be sure to add or subtract an hour to your bedtime relative to your wake-up time (we'll get to your evening routine soon). Once that alarm goes off, go ahead and get out of bed. Don't think! Just get up.

(Important: Do not check your phone, iPad, or any other electronic device prior to doing Step 1. I know it's tempting, but walk away!)

Warming tea tonic: Begin your day with a one-cup serving of a warming tea tonic to wake up your mind and your digestive system. Here are a few of my favorite morning options. You'll see these three tonics incorporated into your menu.

Ginger Tea

Honey Lemon Tea

Honey Turmeric Tea

STEP 2: ESTABLISH GROUNDING EXERCISES

Follow your warming tonic with 15 minutes of grounding work. For Gypsy Girls, it is best that this is something physical to force your energy out of your mind and through your body. I want you to get to know your own body—how do your hands, your feet, and your head feel? As part Gypsy Girl, I can leave my body easily and live in my head. Just recently, my mother-in-law pointed out that the heels of my feet were cracking and that I needed to do something about them—classic Gypsy Girl! The following exercises help by stressing the connection of your feet to the ground, using your breath to move energy, and increasing the flow of oxygen to all different parts of your body. My prescriptive picks for Gypsy Girl grounding exercises include:

◆ **Tai chi:** This ancient Chinese practice is characterized by a series of slow, fluid movements that flow one into the next to create a workout that's been shown to ease anxiety, improve concentration, and increase energy.
◆ **Qi gong:** Another Chinese tradition, qi gong is also characterized by flowing movements, but it is often more free flowing than tai chi and has a focus on wellness.
◆ **Yoga:** Developed in India nearly 5,000 years ago, yoga is a comprehensive system of physical, mental, emotional, and spiritual health. Focused on flowing and sometimes static poses, there are many different types of yoga, from ashtanga (more physically challenging) to hatha, kundalini, and more.

See pages 258, 265, and 266 in Chapter 11 for instructions and specific routines and further information on finding classes, apps, or videos for all three.

Okay, great job! You have already set the tone for your entire day—in under 20 minutes!

STEP 3: POWER UP WITH PROTEIN

Time to eat—not grab and go, not scarf down a protein bar, not chug down a diet shake—I'm talking about real eating here! The biggest challenge for a Gypsy Girl is remembering to eat, and even more importantly, remembering to eat high-protein meals (15 to 20 grams each) with a dash of healthy fats to help stabilize the production of the stress hormone cortisol and to limit wear and tear on the adrenals. We never know what the day ahead will entail, so plan ahead with your menu, page 72. Begin by taking advantage of your morning routine and eating the easy-to-make high-protein breakfast recipes, which will in turn help you manage your stress the rest of the day. The next step in keeping you balanced and energized is to include plenty of protein and also some healthy fats during the rest of your day. It is one thing to tell someone to eat high protein and another to actually translate that information into a meal. All of the daily breakfasts and lunches provided on your menu are packed with 15 to 20 grams of protein and at least 5 grams of healthy fat. You will notice that most of the meals repeat throughout the week and minimize refined carbs. The challenges for Gypsy Girls are making time to have regular meals and getting enough protein—and keeping those meals simple is key.

Being fueled and nourished properly will help you weather the ups and downs of any given day and keep you sharp and focused—moving that air energy to energy that can manifest itself in your life.

Note: Even though you will find lunch, snack, and dinner suggestions on the menu—they are optional. Just for this first week, you get a pass to continue eating any other meals and snacks later in the day the way you currently do.

STEP 4: SUPPLEMENT YOUR MORNINGS

Let's face it—we all have nutritional deficiencies despite our best attempts at eating well. Why? Well, that remains an ongoing debate involving everything from our genetics to the way our food is grown, manufactured, and processed to the quality of our soil, air, and water. The fact is that our food does not have the same nutritional quality that it may have had in the preceding generation, and our environment has changed dramatically as well.

I find that supplements can help, as long as they are targeted to your specific needs. I never want my patients buying so many supplements that they fill up a grocery bag or empty their bank account, and I certainly don't want you taking things you don't need. What you'll find below are the supplements I've found that help Gypsy Girls the most. Again, you are unique and individual and may have specific supplement needs in addition to those suggested here, but if you don't have access to full nutritional testing right now, this is a great starting point.

Take these each morning right after breakfast. As part Gypsy Girl myself, I notice that if I skip my supplements, even while sticking to other good habits, within a few days my energy drops, my mood shifts, and my skin and hair lose their shine and luster.

For more information on supplements, see Resources, page 316.

- ◆ **B-complex vitamins.** You will see B vitamins on all the different Power Type plans. I find that the potent role B vitamins play in women's health is undervalued. They are the key micronutrients involved in regulating hormone pathways and neurotransmitters, meaning that these miracle micronutrients can play a role in mood, sleep, energy, and beauty! See "Vitamins and Supplements You Need to Know," page 45.

- **Omega-3 fats (2 to 3 grams daily).** The omega-3 fats are as important for Gypsy Girls as they are for other Power Types because they nourish the brain and the hormones, keeping inflammation away. While there are many high-omega-3 foods, including salmon, nut butters, and chia seeds, getting these into your daily diet can be difficult. Choose a high-quality omega-3 supplement with at least 2 to 3 grams of EPA (eicosapentaenoic acid) and DHA (docosahexaenoic acid) each.

- **L-theanine (200 milligrams).** L-theanine is an amino acid that acts as a calming supplement, easing anxiety. It also improves cognition and focus by stimulating the production of the neurotransmitter GABA (gamma-aminobutyric acid). Get your L-theanine in the morning by adding a green, black, or oolong tea bag to your morning warming tonic. Often tea alone may not be enough to have a calming effect, so supplementing with an additional 200 milligrams of L-theanine daily can be helpful.

STEP 5: ESTABLISH A SLEEP ROUTINE

Correcting your sleep cycle is essential for a Gypsy Girl. That energy, those lists, the spark, the creativity—yes, we want to stay awake at all hours creating, transforming—uh—crashing. These first 7 grounding days are also an opportunity to correct your sleep cycle and get you to sleep much more consistently at night.

- **Evening supplements:** Take the following supplements an hour before bedtime: 200 milligrams of magnesium, which is calming, relaxing, and promotes sleep; and 500 to 1,000 milligrams of magnolia bark, an adrenal adaptogen that regulates and blunts the stress hormone cortisol to help you sleep restfully.

- **Bedtime:** Begin by establishing a regular bedtime. I think 11 p.m. is fair for a Gypsy Girl, but that means you need to be in your bed by 10 p.m. to give yourself time to unwind. If you are going to wake up earlier than 6 a.m., subtract an hour from your bedtime; if you are going to sleep in an extra hour, you can add an hour to your bedtime (i.e., go to bed by midnight)—but no matter what, always try to get to sleep by midnight and don't wake up prior to 5 a.m. In Chinese medicine, these are considered critical hours for women's health as practitioners believe all hormones are balanced during this time frame and the hormone regulator—the pituitary gland—needs these hours to rest, rejuvenate, and replenish.

These first five steps of the Gypsy Girl Rx will power up your energy, mood, and creativity. Listed below are suggested menus and shopping lists to help you put all your Week 1 steps together.

WEEK 1 SHOPPING LIST

PRODUCE

Fresh gingerroot, lemons, bananas, apples, pears, romaine lettuce, garlic cloves, radishes, carrots, baby carrots, celery, cucumber, cherry tomatoes, bell pepper, sweet potatoes, onions, cauliflower, eggplants, kale, limes, tomatoes

PROTEINS

Plain Greek yogurt, goat cheese, Cheddar cheese, tofu, 2 chicken breasts, ground turkey or beef, shrimp, stew beef, eggs, hummus

SWEETENERS

Honey, maple syrup

GRAINS

Quinoa, whole gluten-free bread (your choice)

SUPPLEMENTS

B vitamins (see page 45 for specifics), omega-3 fats, L-theanine, magnesium, magnolia bark

HERBS AND SPICES

Turmeric, cinnamon, garlic powder, salt, pepper, arrowroot powder, oregano, cumin, coriander, paprika, garam masala

OTHER/MISCELLANEOUS

Frozen mixed berries, walnuts, chocolate and vanilla protein powders (recommendations are on page 196), instant coffee, coconut or rice milk, black or green tea, olive oil, coconut oil, balsamic vinegar or favorite salad dressing, marinara sauce, tomato paste, almond flour, coconut flour, nutritional yeast, lentils, chickpeas (garbanzo beans), almonds, olives, a 16-ounce mason jar, skewers for kabobs

PHASE 1/WEEK 1 MENU

DAY	PRE-BREAKFAST WARMING TONIC (see page 67)	BREAKFAST	LUNCH	SNACK	DINNER
MONDAY	Ginger Tea (page 199)	Walnut-Berry-Yogurt Parfait (page 212)	Mason Jar Salads, Var. 1, with chicken (page 216)	Hummus and Veggies (page 255)	Sweet Potato Noodles with Cauliflower-Quinoa Meatballs (page 250)
TUESDAY	Honey Lemon Tea (page 199)	Cinnamon Banana Smoothie (page 196)	Lettuce Roll-Ups with turkey, shrimp, or chicken (page 222)	10 almonds and ½ cup baby carrots	Cauliflower-Quinoa Meatballs (page 243) and a small green salad
WEDNESDAY	Honey Turmeric Tea (page 200)	Mocha Banana Jump Start (page 197)	Snack Kebabs, 2 servings (page 254)	Hummus and Veggies	Paleo Shepherd's Pie (page 242)
THURSDAY	Ginger Tea	Walnut-Berry-Yogurt Parfait	Mason Jar Salads, Var. 1, with chicken	Nut butter toast (page 73)	Spiced Lentil Cakes with Chickpeas (page 246) and a small green salad
FRIDAY	Honey Lemon Tea	Cinnamon Banana Smoothie	Lettuce Roll-Ups with turkey, shrimp, or chicken	½ cup plain Greek yogurt, ½ sliced banana, 1 tsp maple syrup	Sweet Potato Noodles with Cauliflower-Quinoa Meatballs
SATURDAY	Honey Turmeric Tea	Mocha Banana Jump Start	Snack Kebabs, 2 servings	10 almonds and ½ cup baby carrots	Spiced Lentil Cakes with Chickpeas and a small green salad
SUNDAY	Ginger Tea	Walnut-Berry-Yogurt Parfait	Mason Jar Salads, Var. 1	Hummus and Veggies	Paleo Shepherd's Pie

Ready for Phase 2 of your Power Plan? Here we go!

PHASE 2/WEEK 2: BALANCE YOUR HORMONES

Now that you've had 7 solid days to work on getting grounded, it's time to take it to the next level by addressing your most common hormonal imbalances. For Gypsy Girls, they are centered in your glands (for a review, see page 50). As you embark on Phase 2, remember that you will maintain your five foundational steps from Phase 1, building onto them.

This week you'll get a plan for battling the kryptonite-like afternoon adrenal slump that strikes many a Gypsy Girl down.

That's right: As a Gypsy Girl, your adrenals are taxed more easily and cortisol is usually the first adrenal hormone to go haywire. This stress hormone triggers anxiety, irritable bowel syndrome, and fatigue—especially in the afternoon. We'll build on the work from last week by paying special attention to adrenal-balancing strategies at snack time and dinner that preserve and optimize cortisol regulation, which is essential to having a healthy, not hair-triggered, fight-or-flight response.

Week 2 Action Steps

STEP 6: BOOST YOUR ADRENALS, 2 P.M. TO 4 P.M.

Okay—so all the previous steps have been an attempt to prevent the afternoon adrenal crash and to keep cortisol regulation humming. Still most Gypsy Girls need help with the afternoon slump or adrenal crash. A key strategy to help prevent the crash or treat it if it is already there is your next step—the 2 p.m. to 4 p.m. boost. Set your phone alarm to go off between these hours and then follow the next three adrenal-boosting strategies.

1. **Eat an adrenal-amplifying snack.** Again, my preference is to use food to boost energy, so start with a high-protein snack with around 10 grams of protein. This should be something portable, easy to store in your car, purse, or desk. Here are a few of my favorite examples.

   ☐ 10 almonds

   ☐ Nut butter toast: 1 tablespoon almond butter or natural peanut butter on one piece of whole grain toast

   ☐ Hummus and Veggies (page 255)

2. **Supplement to sustain energy.** For an afternoon energy boost, add the following supplements.

   ☐ Vitamin B$_{12}$ (500 to 1,000 micrograms) to sustain afternoon energy

   ☐ Ashwagandha (1 to 2 grams daily) to keep the adrenals supported

   ☐ L-theanine (200 milligrams) to reduce anxiety and improve focus and concentration

3. **Catnap.** If you can, consider taking a short nap—even a 15-minute catnap can help boost the adrenals without interfering with nighttime sleep. Napping longer than 45 minutes can disrupt your nighttime routine.

STEP 7: FINE-TUNE YOUR LUNCH AND DINNER

Have a scheduled midday and evening meal so you don't forget to eat. Again, it's important to reiterate and reinforce a focus on high-protein foods—aim for at least 20 grams of protein each at lunch and dinner, not necessarily from meat, but from high-protein grains or alternatives like lentils, beans, or nut butters. Include healthy fats such as olive oil or ghee here as well to help support the adrenals.

Dinner should also include some complex carbohydrates—think quinoa, sweet potatoes, or brown rice, even oatmeal. I find many patients skip carbohydrates completely, which affects the sleep neurotransmitters (and not in a good way), leaving night-owl Gypsy Girls even more sleepless and restless. As with your other meals, I've done the legwork for you to keep dinner full of all the necessary, balanced components (see the menu).

Week 2 has incorporated steps that address your adrenals and pump up your lunches and dinners. With that in mind I've designed the following meal plan and shopping list to maintain your Week 1 goals and incorporate the two new action steps just discussed.

WEEK 2 SHOPPING LIST

PRODUCE

Fresh gingerroot, lemons, bananas, romaine lettuce, salad greens, apples, pears, grated carrots, avocado, garlic cloves, cucumbers, radishes, cherry tomatoes, bell peppers, cauliflower, onions, sweet potatoes, eggplant, limes, kale, tomatoes

PROTEINS

Plain Greek yogurt, goat cheese, boneless chicken or turkey breasts, ground turkey, grass-fed ground beef, shrimp, Cheddar cheese, hummus, firm tofu, stew beef, eggs

SWEETENERS

Honey, maple syrup

GRAINS

Gluten-free whole grain bread, quinoa, ground flaxseeds

SUPPLEMENTS

B vitamins (see page 45 for specifics), omega-3 fats, L-theanine, magnesium, magnolia bark, ashwagandha, L-theanine

HERBS AND SPICES

Turmeric, cinnamon, salt, pepper, onion powder, oregano leaves, ground cumin, ground coriander, garam masala

OTHER/MISCELLANEOUS

Frozen mixed berries, walnuts, almonds, chocolate or vanilla protein powder (choose one from page 196), instant coffee, coconut or rice milk, black or green tea, olive oil, balsamic vinegar, black or Greek olives, natural almond or peanut butter, almond flour, arrowroot powder, nutritional yeast, coconut oil, marinara sauce, tomato paste, chopped canned tomatoes, dried lentils or split peas, yellow split peas, coconut flour, flax meal, canned chickpeas, BBQ sauce, canned corn, wooden skewers

PHASE 2/WEEK 2 MENU

	PRE-BREAKFAST WARMING TONIC (see page 57)	BREAKFAST	LUNCH	SNACK	DINNER
MONDAY	Ginger Tea (page 199)	Walnut-Berry-Yogurt Parfait (page 212)	Mason Jar Salads, Var. 1, with chicken or shrimp (page 216)	10 almonds	Sweet Potato Noodles with Cauliflower-Quinoa Meatballs (page 250)
TUESDAY	Honey Lemon Tea (page 199)	Cinnamon Banana Smoothie (page 196)	Lettuce Roll-Ups (page 222)	Nut butter toast (page 73)	Cauliflower-Quinoa Meatballs (page 243) and a green salad or steamed veggies
WEDNESDAY	Honey Turmeric Tea (page 200)	Mocha Banana Jump Start (page 197)	Snack Kebabs, 2 servings (page 254)	Hummus and Veggies (page 255)	Paleo Shepherd's Pie (page 242)
THURSDAY	Ginger Tea	Walnut-Berry-Yogurt Parfait	Mason Jar Salads, Var. 1, with chicken or shrimp	10 almonds	BBQ Chicken Salad (page 217)
FRIDAY	Honey Lemon Tea	Cinnamon Banana Smoothie	Lettuce Roll-Ups	Nut butter toast	Spiced Lentil Cakes with Chickpeas (page 246) and a small green salad
SATURDAY	Honey Turmeric Tea	Mocha Banana Jump Start	Snack Kebabs, 2 servings	Hummus and Veggies	BBQ Chicken Salad
SUNDAY	Ginger Tea	Walnut-Berry-Yogurt Parfait	Mason Jar Salads, Var. 1 with chicken or shrimp	10 almonds	Persian Eggplant with Yellow Split Peas and Dried Lime (page 245)

PHASE 3/WEEK 3:
MANAGE YOUR MIND AND STAY CONNECTED

Okay! You have grounded your energy and balanced your adrenals. The next step? Mind control! That's right, if you can master your mind and stay not just grounded, but connected—training that amazing brain of yours to stay present, focused, and clear—your energy level will be transformed, and will transform those around you (I know—I do this everyday)! The last phase of the Gypsy Girl Power Plan is all about managing your mind and navigating your moods and thoughts, so you can catch all the sparks of creativity and see them manifested! You'll use some specific types of exercise and incorporate mindful tools during this third week to solidify your Power Plan. Let's continue building on the foundation of the last 2 weeks, meaning you will continue with Steps 1 through 7, and you'll add your final action steps, Steps 8 through 10. While Phase 1 was about grounding your energy and Phase 2 about balancing your adrenals, this last week will emphasize connection by training your mind to stay present and focused. We will use exercise and mindful strategies—so all of your powerful creative energy is grounded and super charged to energize you instead of spinning you off to a crash.

By now, you are already seeing a boost in your energy. You are feeling a bit more mentally sharp. It's time to amp this up even more.

Week 3 Action Steps
STEP 8: GET MOVING AND GROOVING

In this step, I want you to begin and/or modify your exercise routine to focus on activities that balance the adrenal glands and the production of cortisol—and force the brain to connect to the rest of the body. All this will help to invigorate without exhausting your energy stores. This step does not necessarily need to be done every day, but do it at least four times this week. The exercise I'm recommending here is an expansion of your morning grounding exercises, meaning that I want you to keep doing your 15 minutes of grounding exercise in the morning, and to add in 30 to 45 minutes of other healthy movement to your days, for a total of four to six times a week (see the following chart). My favorite adrenal-balancing exercises include walking, yoga, swimming, and biking. Many of my Gypsy Girls love to run, but I feel that this is a tough exercise for this Power Type because it wears down the immune system, taxes the adrenals, and ultimately becomes yet another stressor to the body. Walking is still a weight-bearing exercise and can help to reverse a Gypsy Girl's risk for having low bone density and increased bone fragility without causing an inflammatory response to flare up. Ditto for including some strength training, which may also help strengthen your bones. If you love running and don't want to give it up entirely, limit it to twice a week to keep your adrenals balanced and inflammation tamped down. Best times to exercise include early morning, after the morning routine, or after 4 p.m. If you choose to do a longer yoga or tai chi routine, do it in the morning as an extended session of your grounding exercise. For more detailed exercise guidelines, see Chapter 11.

THE GYPSY GIRL EXERCISE RX

The focus is on grounding and stabilizing exercises, three times a week (all exercise routines and suggestions are in Chapter 11).	MONDAY	TUESDAY	WEDNESDAY
	Walking, workouts on page 267	Strength-training routine, page 271, or rest	Yoga, routine on page 258
THURSDAY	FRIDAY	SATURDAY	SUNDAY
Rest	Strength-training routine	Water aerobics, page 270, or rest	Tai chi routine or walking, pages 265 and 267, or rest

STEP 9: MIND-BODY RX: STAY CONNECTED

We'll continue your Rx with one more attempt to calm that vata, or air, element and keep you grounded, sharp, and focused. The more emotions or thoughts Gypsy Girls keep bottled up, the more anxious and disconnected these thoughts become—this is your kryptonite. Use this step of your 3-Week Power Plan to continue the work of connecting your brain to your body and staying present. Here are a few ways to keep your connection and grounding strong.

- ◆ **Journal before bed:** Even writing just a few pages per day is helpful to move all that nervous energy out of the mind and somewhere else—it is almost a decluttering, so to speak, which then allows the creative energy to flow. Turn to page 290 for specific instructions.

- **Self-massage:** If you hate journaling, try one of my personal favorite Gypsy Girl balancing treatments, shirodhara: Drops of warmed oil are applied to your third eye (this is a spot slightly above the bridge of your nose, between the eyebrows), which melts away stress and anxiety. You can even make a homemade version of this spa favorite by warming up coconut or olive oil and massaging it into your scalp. Sleep with this application on overnight and you'll feel your brain relax and slowly declutter.

- **Adopt an aromatherapy Rx:** Using aromas from essential oils is a great tool for your Power Type. Calming oils like lavender, bergamot, and sandalwood can be diffused into the air or rubbed into the temples and inhaled to lower cortisol and induce the relaxation response. For more information on aromatherapy and essential oils, see "The Essential Essential Oils," on page 312.

STEP 10: BEAUTY: REPLENISH AND MOISTURIZE

Dry hair and skin and premature wrinkling are a Gypsy Girl's biggest beauty concerns. Fortunately, there are simple, natural, and healthy moisturizing fixes to foster your outer beauty that are simple and easy on your wallet. Many of the available over-the-counter cleansers and moisturizers contain harsh chemicals and drying agents—you don't need them. The beauty routine I recommend remains fairly consistent for all Power Types: cleansing, toning, and moisturizing for your face each morning and night, washing and moisturizing your body, and washing and conditioning your hair. The difference comes from the simple recipes I've created that are customized for your unique beauty needs. Follow the Gypsy Girl beauty Rx on page 299 in Chapter 13, where you'll find easy-to-make recipes for cleansing, nourishing, and moisturizing from head to toe.

Read on for this week's suggested shopping list and menu, and be sure to incorporate the last three steps to power up your fitness, mind, and body.

WEEK 3 SHOPPING LIST

PRODUCE

Fresh gingerroot, lemons, bananas, romaine lettuce, salad greens, apples, chicken breast, grated carrots, avocado, garlic cloves, cucumber, radishes, cherry tomatoes, bell peppers, cauliflower, onions, red onions, sweet potatoes, eggplant, limes, kale, tomatoes, spinach, green beans (fresh or frozen), parsley, shiitake mushrooms

PROTEINS

Plain Greek yogurt, goat cheese, Cheddar cheese, boneless chicken or turkey breast, ground turkey or ground grass-fed beef, stew beef, shrimp, sea bass, hummus, firm tofu, eggs

SWEETENERS

Honey, maple syrup

GRAINS

Gluten-free whole grain bread, quinoa, buckwheat noodles, flaxseed meal

SUPPLEMENTS

B vitamins (see page 45 for specifics), omega-3 fats, L-theanine, magnesium, magnolia bark, ashwagandha, L-theanine

HERBS AND SPICES

Turmeric, cinnamon, salt, pepper, onion powder, oregano leaves, ground cumin, ground coriander, garam masala, ground red pepper, ground sumac

OTHER/MISCELLANEOUS

Frozen mixed berries, walnuts, almonds, roasted pistachios, chocolate or vanilla protein powder (choose one from page 196), instant coffee, coconut or rice milk, black or green tea, olive oil, balsamic vinegar, red wine vinegar, black or Greek olives, natural almond or peanut butter, almond flour, arrowroot powder, nutritional yeast, coconut oil, marinara sauce, tomato paste, tomato sauce, chopped canned tomatoes, dried lentils or split peas, yellow split peas, coconut flour, canned chickpeas, BBQ sauce, canned corn, chicken broth or ingredients for bone broth (page 226), wooden skewers

PHASE 3/WEEK 3 MENU

	PRE-BREAKFAST WARMING TONIC (see page 67)	BREAKFAST	LUNCH	SNACK	DINNER
MONDAY	Ginger Tea (page 199)	Walnut-Berry-Yogurt Parfait (page 212)	Oven "Grilled" Sea Bass with Wilted Spinach (page 234)	10 almonds	Sweet Potato Noodles with Cauliflower-Quinoa Meatballs (page 250)
TUESDAY	Honey Lemon Tea (page 199)	Cinnamon Banana Smoothie (page 196)	Bissara (page 231)	Nut butter toast (page 73)	Cauliflower-Quinoa Meatballs (page 243) and a green salad or steamed veggies
WEDNESDAY	Honey Turmeric Tea (page 200)	Mocha Banana Jump Start (page 197)	Buckwheat Noodle and Kale Stir-Fry (page 244)	Hummus and Veggies (page 255)	Paleo Shepherd's Pie (page 242)
THURSDAY	Ginger Tea	Walnut-Berry-Yogurt Parfait	Warm Quinoa and Green Bean Salad (page 222)	10 almonds	BBQ Chicken Salad (page 217)
FRIDAY	Honey Lemon Tea	Cinnamon Banana Smoothie	Chickpea Salad (page 218)	Nut butter toast	Spiced Lentil Cakes (page 246)
SATURDAY	Honey Turmeric Tea	Mocha Banana Jump Start	Snack Kebabs, 2 servings (page 254)	Hummus and Veggies	BBQ Chicken Salad
SUNDAY	Ginger Tea	Walnut-Berry-Yogurt Parfait	Chicken Saag (page 237) and a small green salad	10 almonds	Persian Eggplant with Yellow Split Peas and Dried Lime (page 245)

CONGRATULATIONS! NOW YOU HAVE your foundation! These 3 weeks are your keys to helping you move forward to innovate, create, and harness your energy. Keep the steps together—all 10 of them—until they become second nature and daily, automatic habits. With practice, these 10 steps will unleash your hidden super powers and lead you to the life you were meant to live!

I suggest that you continue to follow the 3-week plan for two more rotations—for a total of 9 weeks, or about 2 months. Feel free to mix and match using any of the recipes in Chapter 10 that have comparable calories and protein. As you get more comfortable with the plan you may decide to substitute your own recipes instead, which is great—as long as they are Gypsy Girl Approved.

After you've followed the plan for a total of three months through, go back and retake both the Mojo Meter in Chapter 2 (page 9) and the Power Type Test in Chapter 3 (page 18). You may have moved to a different Power Type by shifting your chemistry. If so, head to that Power Type's chapter and give that 3-week plan, menu, and action steps a try. If you are still a tried-and-true Gypsy Girl, come back and continue this 3-week Rx. Once you feel you've mastered your plan and all 10 action steps have become a habit for you, you can ease up on the strict menus, but make sure that you continue to eat at set times and get plenty of protein. If you feel like you are falling out of balance, are going through a stressful time, and/or have shifted to another Power Type, retake the tests and follow the directions. Don't forget to familiarize yourself with all Power Types, and check out Part III for more super woman strategies for exercise, mindfulness, and beauty.

CHAPTER 6

THE BOSS LADIES' 3-WEEK RX

IF YOU'RE A Boss Lady, then you know by now—you're determined, invincible, and strategic. You set your sights on something and get it done. My Boss Lady patients are often known for their intellect and wit, but the demands they place on themselves are what ultimately affect their health and happiness.

I know a Boss Lady when I see one. Direct and to the point, they ask pertinent questions and speak linearly, meaning that they move quickly from point A to B to C and are often—quite frankly—impatient. I see the glance at the watch, the tapping of the fingers, and I often make a quick mental note—I need to deliver my information quickly and efficiently or I will lose my audience.

As a Boss Lady, you are usually in your element when you are commanding, directing, and leading. But all that responsibility can take a toll, and when not aware, the Boss Lady starts to fray at the edges, becoming irritable, angry, and restless. The greatest medical risk for a Boss Lady is an imbalanced digestive system that only contributes to more irritability and anger. Irritable bowel syndrome, reflux, constipation, and diarrhea are just a few of the health challenges common to the Boss Lady.

Boss Lady at a Glance

ALTER EGO: THE COMMANDER

Super powers: When at peak performance, Boss Ladies are powerhouses—they have a strong drive, are competitive and intense, and like challenges. They tend to be athletic and often excel at skiing, hiking, tennis, and mountain climbing. At work they are leaders, able to accomplish tasks efficiently while commanding respect.

Kryptonite: Stress and anger. Boss Ladies can burn out and flare up when they get out of sync. Their power-draining weaknesses surface when they misplace their off switch. While they tend to love socializing, Boss Ladies can overdo it, talk too much, become restless, and have insomnia. Coffee, too many engagements, and the highly competitive exercises they love can all drain Boss Ladies.

Element: Fire. This represents joy, passion, intensity, and the season of summer.

Personality: Leader, doer, good decision maker. Expansive, intense, sharp-witted, acidic, short-tempered, argumentative, angry, intellectual, precise, direct, outspoken.

Body type: Medium size and weight. Thinning hair and hair loss are common. A Boss Lady tends to run hot in body temperature. In balance, Boss Ladies can have great complexions. When off-kilter, Boss Ladies can suffer from skin rashes.

Celebrity example: Kim Kardashian. This Boss Lady is known for her punctuality—she is up early and gets right to work. Sure, it's the work of having her hair, makeup, and wardrobe done, but for Kardashian, this is what's made her one of the world's top pop icons. Regardless of your feelings about this Boss Lady, it's clear that she is a brilliant businesswoman who has created a sparkling brand based entirely on herself and her family.

Colors: Red, orange, and gold. As fiery, passionate women, Boss Ladies gravitate toward these flamelike colors. These hues represent passion, strength, and happiness. Red represents a short temper on one hand and courage on the other, and it's also a color linked to increased respiration and blood pressure. Orange represents a combination of yellow and red (happiness and energy)—vibrancy. Gold often symbolizes royalty and affluence.

COMMON BOSS LADY CONDITIONS

The following conditions are common amongst my Boss Lady patients. These are not certainties or absolute predictions; they are simply the patterns that I see over and over again when I work with Boss Ladies in my practice. Understanding these conditions helps you be better prepared to recognize them in yourself—and to reaffirm that you are the Boss Lady Power Type. Be aware of where and how these conditions are affecting you, and watch for the changes and improvements as you return to balance during your 3-Week Power Plan.

IBS

Irritable bowel syndrome, or IBS, is a common digestive condition that affects 25 million to 45 million Americans, and 10 to 15 percent of the global population. About twice as many women as men suffer from IBS. Symptoms alternate between bloating, gas, constipation, and diarrhea. The triggers for IBS are often debated. For some women, it is food or hormone fluctuations, while for others, stress plays a major role. Many women dismiss IBS, thinking it will go away or that it's just a temporary inconvenience, but the truth is that it can be a precursor to many different diseases and a player in inflammation. With all the recent research connecting your digestive health to inflammation and the gut microbiome, paying attention to IBS and trying to solve it have become critical. (See "The Gut Inflammation Cycle" on page 86.)

Reflux

Commanding, doing, and just, well, constantly moving, Boss Ladies are also at an increased risk for reflux or GERD (gastroesophageal reflux disease), which is a chronic condition in which your stomach's acidic contents come back up into your esophagus. Heartburn and a morning sore throat are some of the signs of GERD. Stress is a common trigger, but tough-to-digest foods like dairy, meat, or spicy and acidic foods can aggravate these symptoms as well. Hormone changes can also trigger GERD. Most women may reach for an acid blocker to help their symptoms, but like many medications these are only temporary solutions. Conversely, the 3-Week Power Plan will put you back into balance and keep your stomach acid where it belongs.

Constipation

Another digestive complaint common to Boss Ladies is constipation—and as with IBS, it's a complaint that women often dismiss. Older systems of medicine teach us that we should have a daily bowel movement, as it was seen as cleansing and detoxifying. Chronic constipation also affects your microbiome—the ultimate driver in inflammatory diseases.

Joint Pain

With the tendency toward digestive issues, it is no surprise that many Boss Ladies also suffer from joint pain, one of the hallmark symptoms of inflammation. Many will only notice that their joints are slightly tender, or maybe occasionally swollen, while others will have significant swelling, warmth, and tenderness. Again, most women will dismiss this, only taking note when symptoms start to interfere with daily function.

Insomnia

Boss Ladies don't sleep—they don't! And sure enough, they will struggle with falling asleep since they are often overstimulated or just working away on their endless to-do lists. The hormone melatonin (the sleep hormone) can be out of balance, which not only keeps them awake but also can eventually interfere with hormone cycles—even affecting ovulation. All the "doing" does eventually takes a toll.

Acne

Acne, in its varying forms, affects a third of adult women, according to a recent study published in the *Journal of Clinical and Aesthetic Dermatology,* and can be an extra challenge for Boss Ladies. This skin condition is more than likely related to the gut inflammation cycle, where chronic digestive issues can trigger an inflammatory cascade. Acne is a symptom of this cycle. Remember, there are different types of acne, with acne on the jaw considered more hormonal and acne on the forehead more digestive. Older systems of medicine saw acne as a "heat"

THE GUT INFLAMMATION CYCLE

The explosion of research on the gut during the last few years is changing medicine and the way we will practice medicine in the future. A key medical concept to master is the connection between the gut and inflammation. When the gut is damaged or digestion affected, it literally switches on the inflammatory cascade, putting your body on the defensive. When this becomes chronic and inflammation really takes hold, then the disease process begins, presenting in different ways, depending on your body.

sign—too much stress on the digestive system—a sign that the body needed to cool down.

Chinese Meridian Diagnosis: Liver Meridian Deficiency

The liver meridian in Chinese medicine or TCM is a powerful energy channel that dictates everything from detoxification to hormone balance and metabolism. Boss Ladies often show a liver meridian deficiency, which can be improved by stimulating related acupuncture points found on the feet, the legs, the forehead, and scalp. The body, remember, is considered an interconnected web.

Again, according to TCM explanations, all the driving, commanding, and directing create stress and even anger. That internal anger generates heat, the heat disturbs the digestive system of which the liver is a critical part, and then the entire balance of the gut and hormones is disrupted. Chinese medicine understood this imbalance well—anger equals liver meridian disruption, which equals heat, leading to hormone disruption—which I see in lab work all the time: high estrogen levels, low progesterone, or even a haphazard thyroid. The Chinese medicine prescription? To force a Boss Lady to calm down, relax, and balance her nervous system. Acupuncture and specific Chinese herbs are often the first steps to rebalancing the liver meridian, and your hormones, from a TCM perspective. One of the first things I learned in Chinese medicine is the importance of sleep when dealing with women's hormones.

Sleep is critical! The liver meridian needs rest—especially through

Back when I was in my late twenties, sleep was a luxury I didn't have. What with completing my residency and being scheduled for emergency room night shifts, altered hours and minimal sleep were the norm. I didn't even think that my hair loss and sleep could be connected, and the doctors I sought for help (who had far more experience than I had at the time) didn't make the connection either. I remember staring at one doctor in disbelief. "Young lady," he said, "you will be bald by 30. Take this drug—it's your only option." He never asked about sleep or my hormones or understood how they were connected to my hair. My only option? Maybe he just didn't know. Now way past 30, I, thankfully, am not bald and not on medication.

the hours of 1 a.m. to 3 a.m. Without sleep during this interval, the cycle of hormone imbalances begins. I know this personally from my years of shift work in medical residency and my early emergency room days, which eventually caused my own hormone disruptions. I've designed your 3-Week Power Plan to address these issues directly through improving your nutrition, establishing healthy sleep times, incorporating exercise, introducing mind-body techniques, and more.

Ayurvedic Dosha Diagnosis: Pitta

I can spot a Pitta (what a Boss Lady would be called in Ayurvedic terminology) in about 3 seconds. Maybe because I am partly one and one of my sisters also falls into this category, this energy type is familiar to me. In Ayurvedic medicine, pittas are known for being extremely ambitious, confident, and good decision makers. If out of balance, pittas are known for being short tempered, argumentative, and stubborn, often getting angry and irritable.

The pitta type's propensity for constant doing, moving, and commanding can leave her out of balance very quickly. It is Ayurvedic medicine that first drew the connection between pittas and the pattern of

Knowing Your Type

I have noticed a pattern in myself as part Boss Lady. At the beginning of the week, I am pretty even and kind, but something seems to happen by Thursday. Everything starts getting on my nerves! Mind you, I love my office and my amazing staff, and as their CEO I know the responsibility I have toward them. That said, I've noticed that on Thursdays when I arrive at the center, I immediately notice what is wrong—that the music is not on, the elevator carpet doesn't look vacuumed, and the lights outside are too bright or dim. By the time I step off the elevator, I am internally fuming before I even hit my desk. Sure, these are things that should be taken care of—but they seem so much bigger on a Thursday than they would on a Monday after I've had the weekend to rejuvenate. After three challenging workdays, I start to unravel. Understanding this pattern helps me to be aware and to take proactive steps to stay in balance.

gut disturbances, and this is what I see in my Boss Ladies. This connection between the gut and stress is something Ayurvedic medicine realized thousands of years ago but cutting-edge science is just beginning to understand.

The Ayurvedic plan for pittas focuses on cooling them by having them eat cooling foods, which include yogurt, cucumbers, whole grains, and more—some of which you'll see on your eating plan. Adequate rest and body treatments that force relaxation are essential for pittas. The combination of these steps helps transition pittas back to their balanced state of commanding, doing, and leading—without tipping over or crashing.

Hormone Imbalances: Thyroid and Melatonin

The most common hormone imbalances for my Boss Ladies center around the thyroid gland and involve two thyroid hormones, T3 and T4, and your sleep-regulating hormone, melatonin (for more specifics on your thyroid and hormones, see "The Five Glands You Need to Know," page 50).

Melatonin disruption can be the primary hormonal cause of insomnia for my Boss Ladies. Even a small flicker of light—from the computer, tablet, or smartphone screen—can be enough to disrupt the pineal gland, sending the signal to delay or inhibit melatonin production. Think about it. When you, a Boss Lady, are chronically stressed from being in a demanding leading or commanding role, you are more than likely not able to wind down or get to sleep. Hence many of you will tell me you are a "night person," or that you've always stayed up late, whereas the reality may be that you are in a melatonin-disrupted state—with sleep-wake cycles that have been altered to meet your go-getter lifestyle. That might be great for hitting deadlines, but not so great for your health.

Boss Ladies can also have poorly functioning thyroid glands. The beauty of understanding the older systems of medicine is that they predict and connect the essential nature of a Boss Lady to all elements of her health—including her thyroid. Here is how it works: Long-term stress on the gut triggers inflammation, which then disrupts many hormones, but the thyroid most of all. There is a subtle dance in the hormone world between the adrenal glands, which secrete cortisol in response to stress, and the thyroid hormones—the harder the demands on one gland, the more the other gland is taxed. This is the pattern we are seeing in scientific studies that investigate how to best balance hormones. Another way to think about this is to examine what happens when the gut takes a hit from stress, lack of sleep, poor diet, and so on. When this happens it weakens the liver meridian, which then directly disrupts the thyroid. Hypothyroidism, or a sluggish thyroid, is common in my Boss Ladies, while swings from high to low hormone levels (Hashimoto's thyroiditis) are also common. All Boss Ladies should be vigilant and proactive when it comes to thyroid health. While it's a good idea to have your thyroid checked during your yearly physical, the 3-Week Power Plan for Boss Ladies incorporates dietary strategies, supplements, and mind-body work that will get all your hormones back in balance.

LAB FINDINGS

Can we match your tendencies, from your emotional makeup to your Eastern diagnoses, to your hormone imbalances? The answer is *yes*! And that is the most exciting part. The following findings are those I see most often in my Boss Ladies. If you've noticed these findings in previous lab work you've had done, it's more confirmation that you are a Boss Lady. Also, use the following list to request future lab testing when you do go for your doctor visits.

- **Low B vitamins:** especially B_1, B_2, B_5, B_6, B_{12}, and folic acid
- **Elevated inflammation markers:** including C-reactive protein (CRP), erythrocyte sedimentation rate (ESR), and homocysteine, and altered antinuclear antibodies (ANA)
- **Elevated or altered cholesterol metabolism:** including high triglycerides and lipids (total cholesterol and LDL)
- **Elevated liver function tests:** aspartate transaminase (AST), alanine transaminase (ALT), and sex hormone– binding globulin (SHBG)
- **Low thyroid:** high TSH, low T4, low T3
- **Altered estrogen/progesterone ratios:** estrone, estradiol, and progesterone
- **Altered melatonin production**

Nutritional Needs/Deficiencies

Your gut, liver, and thyroid—the words are probably buzzing around in your head right now. Many of the nutritional needs of the Boss Lady are tied to the conditions we just discussed. For example, your gut needs

LONG-TERM DISEASE RISKS

Let's assume you feel great today. What I keep warning my patients about is that great today is not necessarily great tomorrow, and you have to be proactive and in prevention mode to guard against the following disease risks.

Gut risk: Chronic neglect and stress can trigger conditions like small intestinal bacterial overgrowth (SIBO) and candida or bacterial overgrowth, accelerating gut-based diseases like inflammatory bowel disease, diverticulitis, pancreatitis, gallbladder and liver dysfunction, and even colon or gut-based cancers.

Inflammation: Most of us understand this word now, but chronic inflammation, a Boss Lady risk factor, can be the precursor to any of the many autoimmune diseases that plague us today—lupus, rheumatoid arthritis, Sjogren's syndrome, psoriatic arthritis, to name just a few.

Hormone risk: Depleted thyroid hormones and malfunctioning melatonin will impact fertility, endometriosis, ovarian cysts, conditions like PCOS (polycystic ovary syndrome), and mental health, contributing to anxiety and depression.

foods high in healthy bacteria or probiotics, your liver needs greens for good detoxification, and your thyroid needs its main nutrients—selenium, iron and iodine—to stay healthy and humming. I will address these nutritional needs and more in your 3-Week Power Plan, coming up next!

HOW THE BOSS LADY 3-WEEK RX WORKS

So now to the Boss Lady plan—how to get you commanders and directors back in balance? When it comes to working with my Boss Lady patients, the challenge for me is getting these women to spend a fraction of their high-powered intellect on themselves and their own health. The world is yours and I want you to *own it!*

To get started, Boss Ladies need to focus on building and rebalancing their gut—better known as *command central* for many systems in the body and seen as a key driver of disease in Chinese and Ayurvedic medicine (something that conventional medicine is finally acknowledging, thanks to scientific research). During Week 1, you'll focus on resetting your system via a cleansing and detoxifying eating plan that will get your gut back in primed condition. In Week 2, you'll shift your focus to rebuilding your gut with a reintroduction of healthy meals and added supplements. Finally, during Week 3, you'll bring it all together by learning to cool your Boss Lady fire through further healthy eating strategies but also adding cooling exercise and relaxing mindful strategies and techniques. You'll find suggested Boss Lady menus and shopping lists at the end of each week.

To keep things simple, I'm going to start you off with guidelines that will cover what you need to do immediately to activate your Boss Lady super powers. While you'll build on these foundational guidelines in the later weeks of your program, begin with these rules and you'll see your health, energy, and happiness soar.

The Boss Lady Rx Rules

1. **Reset your pH in the morning.** Choose a drink from page 94 to ease inflammation and improve digestion.

2. **Detox with dairy- and yeast-free smoothies.** These smoothies detox your gut and minimize your digestive load. The result is an enhanced ability to absorb nutrients. Smoothie recipes are on page 194. (See "Anti-Inflammatory Eating—Foods to Avoid," on page 46 for more information on dairy and yeast.)

3. **Skip red meat but get 40 to 50 grams of protein per day.** The Boss Lady menus at the end of this chapter are designed to provide you with enough protein per day—40 to 50 grams—but ease the load that red meat can put on your digestive system (poultry and fish are okay).

4. **Eat a lot of fiber.** Boss Ladies need at least 40 grams of fiber per day, which is the equivalent of 6 to 8 servings of fruits and vegetables.

5. **Limit daily calories.** Limit your intake to 1,800 calories a day unless you exercise vigorously more than an hour a day.

6. **Maintain a dairy-free diet.** Dairy can be difficult to digest in an already vulnerable digestive system.

Note: If you follow the menus found in this chapter, you'll meet all the above guidelines.

At the beginning of each of your three weeklong phases, you'll see action steps for that week. There are just three to focus on in the first week, but each week you'll be adding empowering steps to perfect your health, happiness, and energy. Be sure to follow them to the letter to be *super powered* each and every day!

In addition, at the end of each week you'll find menus and shopping lists that you can use to make sure you are following all Boss Lady suggestions.

THE 10 BOSS LADY ACTION STEPS AT A GLANCE

The following 10 steps provide an overview of the complete Boss Lady 3-Week Rx. You won't be doing all 10 action steps until you complete all 3 weeks, but I want you to have a sneak peak at what living looks like for fully powered Boss Ladies.

Step 1: Reset Your PH, 6 a.m. to 7 a.m.

Step 2: Ease Digestion with Breakfast and Lunch Smoothies

Step 3: Skip Red Meat

Step 4: Build Your Microbiome by Eating Foods That Boost Good Bugs

Step 5: Seal a Leaky Gut, Fortify with Supplements
- ☐ Probiotics
- ☐ Digestive enzymes
- ☐ Glutamine

Step 6: Flush Toxins with a Liver Lover Smoothie

Step 7: Master Midday Meals

Step 8: Cool Your Fire with Food

Step 9: Cool Your Fire with Exercise

Step 10: Cool Your Fire with Mind, Body, and Beauty Regimens
- ☐ Mind—aromatherapy and meditation
- ☐ Body—choose one per day: massage, acupuncture, Epsom salt bath, or amla
- ☐ Beauty—follow directions on page 302

PHASE 1/WEEK 1: RESET YOUR GUT

The first step of the Boss Lady plan is to clear up and *CLEAN OUT* the belly. Older systems of medicine such as Traditional Chinese Medicine and Ayurvedic medicine not only believe that good gut health is paramount to optimal health but also address it methodically, beginning with a belly cleanup, and that begins with resting your gut—giving it a break. How? *By lowering the work of digestion.* This is exactly what you are going to do. Your first week will begin with a detox that works to heal, rest, and reset your stomach. The Boss Lady Phase 1—your first 7 days—focuses on balancing out the alkalinity and acidity of your digestive system, removing hard-to-digest foods and replacing them with foods that are easier on the digestive system. You will also take a short break from red meat, which can be hard to digest, especially when the digestive system may already be compromised. Your details and action steps for Phase 1 follow.

Week 1 Action Steps
STEP 1: RESET YOUR PH, 6 A.M. TO 7 A.M.

Your first action step on your 7-day detox is to start your day with a pH balancer, or "belly tonic." This tonic will help to shift you to a more alkaline pH, which improves digestion and minimizes inflammation. For more information on pH levels, turn to "What Is PH and Why Does It Matter?" on page 44. Enjoy one of the following pH tonics between 6 a.m. and 7 a.m. each morning.

- **Apple cider vinegar and water:** It's so easy—but I'm not promising tasty. Mix 1 tablespoon raw and organic apple cider vinegar with 3 tablespoons water and drink quickly. If you can tolerate larger amounts, try 1 ounce of the vinegar in 4 ounces of water.

- **Lemon water:** Squeeze half a lemon into 6 ounces of warm water and stir. If you cannot stand the taste, it's okay to add ½ teaspoon of honey. For even more fun, try frothing this concoction—yum! I crave this in the winter.

- **Pomegranate juice:** This is a bit of work to make on your own, but it's worth it. Cut a pomegranate and scoop out half of it. Blend with 8 ounces of water and enjoy (you can strain the juice, but it's not necessary). Not only is this drink tasty, it's absolutely beautiful. Make extra and you can store it in the fridge for up to 3 days.

◆ **Aloe vera juice:** Drink 1 to 2 ounces daily. This one is easiest to buy over the counter. (See Resources, page 316, for brand recommendations.)

STEP 2: EASE DIGESTION WITH BREAKFAST AND LUNCH SMOOTHIES

Next on your 7-day detox to-do list is the breakfast and lunch smoothie swap. For the next week, you'll replace your breakfast *and* lunch with one of the three smoothie recipes listed on page 97. You'll see suggestions for specific smoothies on your menu, but feel free to mix and match—if you prefer the Tropical Delight smoothie, for example over the chocolate, feel free to have it more often. You'll notice that the power drinks I recommend all have protein powder added—this is ideal for energy and nutrition, while being easy on the tummy. To choose a good protein powder, see "Dr. Taz's Favorite Protein Powders" on page 196.

The point of switching to smoothies during this 7-day detox is to minimize the work your body typically has to do to digest food, and to make it easier for your belly to absorb the nutrients you'll be consuming. I've also kept your menu dairy free, which makes digestion easier. As a Boss Lady, healing your gut should be your primary focus. While you may find the smoothies a little repetitive, you'll give your gut a much needed chance to rest and repair.

STEP 3: SKIP RED MEAT

Step 3 in your 7-day detox will be to pull all red meat out of your diet. This includes beef, lamb, and goat (poultry and fish are okay). Follow

"I usually depend on 32 ounces of soda in the morning and again in the afternoon. So I was scared of trading in that habit for two protein shakes a day, but I started to feel so much better after just a few days— so worth it! I started feeling really energized, which made me want to exercise, and in turn that made me feel better about myself, all of which added up to a better mood overall (even my boyfriend noticed). I lost 5 pounds in the first week, and I could tell that my pants were roomier around my belly and legs! All of that really motivated me to go on."—**Christine, 29, addiction prevention coordinator**

the suggestions in your menu. While many women, even Boss Ladies, need some animal protein, red meat is especially tough to digest, and tough to break down in the gut. When healing or trying to repair the gut, pulling out red meat for a short period of time helps to repair the lining and improve the motility or movement of the gut. *This is not necessarily something you need to do forever, since many Boss Ladies need some red meat for adequate iron intake.*

Follow these three basic steps to begin your path to balance. You can return to Phase 1 at any point if you feel like you need a simple and easy weeklong detox.

Note: You can use the warming tonics on page 199 to curb appetite and prevent mindless snacking throughout your day, another burden on the gut.

WEEK 1 SHOPPING LIST

PRODUCE

Lemons, pomegranates, bananas, frozen mangos, frozen pineapple, frozen blueberries, frozen strawberries, mint leaves, spinach, kale, romaine, tomatoes, onions, garlic, fresh or frozen green beans, limes, eggplants, cucumber

PROTEINS

Chocolate and vanilla protein powder (see page 196 for suggestions), dried lentils or split peas, dried yellow split peas, eggs, chickpeas, boneless chicken thighs or chickpeas and a package of firm tofu, boneless skinless chicken breasts, goat cheese

SWEETENERS

Honey, maple syrup

GRAINS

Quinoa, flax meal

SUPPLEMENTS

See Week 2

HERBS AND SPICES

Garam masala, paprika, cumin, coriander, herbal teas, mint

OTHER/MISCELLANEOUS

Aloe vera juice; coconut milk, rice milk, or almond milk; coconut oil; coconut flour; safflower oil or coconut oil; ghee; chicken broth or buy the ingredients for Dr. Taz's Spicy Bone Broth (page 226); red wine vinegar, balsamic vinegar, raw and organic apple cider vinegar; tomato paste; olive oil; canned corn; barbecue sauce; almond butter

PHASE 1/WEEK 1 MENU

	PRE-BREAKFAST pH Reset Drink (see page 94)	BREAKFAST	LUNCH	SNACK (Note: Drink water and herbal teas between meals for your first week)	DINNER
MONDAY	Apple cider vinegar and water (page 94)	Walnut-Berry-Yogurt Parfait (page 212)	Berry Bomb (page 195)	Water and herbal teas	Spiced Lentil Cakes with Chickpeas (page 246)
TUESDAY	Lemon water (page 94)	Tropical Delight (page 195)	Chocolate Protein Smoothie (page 194)	Water and herbal teas	Chicken Saag (page 237) and Warm Quinoa and Green Bean Salad (page 222)
WEDNESDAY	Pomegranate juice (page 94)	Berry Bomb (page 195)	Tropical Delight (page 195)	Water and herbal teas	Quick Cumin Chicken and Crunchy Kale Chips (page 241)
THURSDAY	Aloe vera juice (page 95)	Chocolate Protein Smoothie	Berry Bomb	Water and herbal teas	Persian Eggplant with Yellow Split Peas and Dried Lime (page 245)
FRIDAY	Apple cider vinegar and water	Tropical Delight	Chocolate Protein Smoothie	Water and herbal teas	Spiced Lentil Cakes with Chickpeas
SATURDAY	Lemon water	Berry Bomb	Tropical Delight	Water and herbal teas	BBQ Chicken Salad (page 217)
SUNDAY	Pomegranate juice	Chocolate Protein Smoothie	Berry Bomb	Water and herbal teas	Persian Eggplant with Yellow Split Peas and Dried Lime

PHASE 2/WEEK 2: REBUILD YOUR GUT

You'll continue most of the steps from the first week, but now we will focus more on strengthening and building your gut. Most of the problematic foods are out, so we can build on the success of the first 7 days. To that end, your next week will focus on gut-building foods and supplements.

Week 2 Action Steps

STEP 4: BUILD YOUR MICROBIOME BY EATING FOODS THAT BOOST GOOD BUGS

You want to keep your digestive system working with more regular (and *much improved*) eating habits. Part of keeping your belly healthy for the long run is including and learning to get comfortable with some probiotic-rich foods. Probiotics (the opposite of antibiotics) are good bacteria that can be taken in supplemental form and are used to essentially build your gut microbiome, or the population of good bacteria in your belly. Instead of relying only on supplements, I like to add probiotic foods—some of which you may never have heard of—to your lunch. I've included the following bug-boosters with your lunches on this and next week's menu.

- Nondairy yogurt (unsweetened), 1 cup*
- Nondairy kefir (unsweetened), 4 to 6 ounces*
- Kombucha, 1 cup (a fermented drink thought to have originated in Russia that contains lots of healthy bacteria that rebalance the gut)
- Dr. Taz's Spicy Bone Broth, 4 to 6 ounces (page 226)
- Organic sourdough bread (ideally made using organic grains), 1 slice

Ideally, you want to mix it up and try at least a few of the above choices during your week.

Note: While both yogurt and kefir do have dairy, try a nondairy version. Even people with dairy issues will tolerate these gut builders due to the population of helpful bacteria/probiotics.

*I love both yogurt and kefir as is, but if you like a touch of sweetness, add 1 teaspoon of honey or maple syrup.

STEP 5: SEAL A LEAKY GUT, FORTIFY WITH SUPPLEMENTS

Staying with the theme of rebuilding your gut, the next step of your plan is to add digestion-friendly supplements. Take all of the following for the remainder of your 21-day plan.

1. **Probiotics:** Choose a supplement with at least 50 billion CFU (colony-forming units). While there is much continued controversy over probiotics, I still find them helpful in regulating digestion and shifting to a healthier gut microbiome. Take a high-quality probiotic each morning with your breakfast smoothie, and consider rotating your probiotic every 6 weeks to maintain some bacterial diversity.

2. **Digestive enzymes:** These supplements work to break down your food into smaller particles, making it easier for you to process and to absorb the nutrients from all the great foods you're eating. I recommend taking one or two caplets of digestive enzymes with your heaviest meal, either lunch or dinner. Take a digestive enzyme with amylase (an enzyme that breaks down starch), lipase (an enzyme that breaks down fat), and protease (breaks down protein).

3. **Glutamine:** This is an amino acid and one of my favorite supplements since it helps with digestion and re-establishes the gut lining by literally sealing the gut. Plus, recent research suggests that glutamine is also good for muscle recovery after strenuous exercise—definitely a Boss Lady habit. Take 1 to 2 grams daily, in the morning or at whatever time you can take it most consistently.

STEP 6: FLUSH TOXINS WITH A LIVER LOVER SMOOTHIE

Boss Ladies need liver smarts. According to TCM, the liver is the powerhouse of all hormone production and metabolism, so we need to keep it healthy and humming. That means keeping your liver clean and unclogged. A simple step—add one green smoothie daily (see the Liver Lover Smoothie on page 198). Green drinks keep your liver flushed and cleansed by increasing your concentration of glutathione, an antioxidant that is critical in liver detoxification. I keep talking about hormones and the liver, and if you think about it for a second, it makes sense: If the liver does not have what it needs—the right antioxidants and the right nutrients—then it's like a dirty laundry bag where dirty clothes keep piling up. Enter your hormones, and they don't get broken down—instead, metabolites go down the wrong detoxification path, affecting your health and your super woman powers! Consider adding herbs like dandelion greens, parsley, or cilantro to your diet to further help flush and detoxify your liver.

STEP 7: MASTER MIDDAY MEALS

It's time to bring back the food, starting today. While you'll keep your morning breakfast smoothie and you'll continue to skip red meat during your second week, you will reintroduce a midday meal. You gave your gut a 7-day detox and now it's time to satisfy your joy of eating with a nourishing lunch! See lunch and dinner recipes suggested in your Week 2 menu on page 102, and then turn to the recipe pages in Chapter 10.

"I love the breakfast smoothies and the Liver Lover Smoothie! They make morning meals a no-brainer, and a great way to get more protein. I notice that I have more energy all day long. I'm sleeping better, and my family says I seem happier, and I know that I have far more patience with my kids than before the 3-Week Rx. Plus, my digestion has improved and my hair is shinier, my skin is clear, and my fingernails are thicker and stronger. I also have more mental focus and clarity during the day."—Jackie, 35, super mom to four young children, reading teacher

WEEK 2 SHOPPING LIST

PRODUCE

Lemons, pomegranates, bananas, frozen mangos, frozen pineapple, frozen blueberries, frozen strawberries, mint leaves, spinach, kale, romaine, tomatoes, onions, garlic, ginger, fresh or frozen green beans, limes, eggplants, cucumbers, celery, carrots, beets, dandelion greens, parsley, cilantro, zucchini, scallions, grape tomatoes, avocados, red onions, sweet potatoes, basil, bell pepper, cauliflower, dill, oregano, shiitake mushrooms, Brussels sprouts

PROTEINS

Chocolate and vanilla protein powder (see page 196 for suggestions), dried lentils or split peas, dried yellow split peas, dried mung beans, eggs, chickpeas, boneless chicken thighs, boneless skinless chicken breasts, chicken wings, salmon, plain nondairy yogurt, unsweetened nondairy kefir, chicken bones, goat bones, beef bones, salmon, tofu, turkey or veggie bacon, eggs, white beans

SWEETENERS

Honey, maple syrup

GRAINS

Quinoa, fermented bread (sourdough), lentil or soybean pasta, gluten-free lasagna noodles, buckwheat noodles

SUPPLEMENTS

Probiotics (page 99), digestive enzymes (page 99), glutamine (page 99)

HERBS AND SPICES

Salt and pepper, garam masala, paprika, cumin (ground and seeds), coriander, herbal teas, Thai red curry paste, arrowroot powder, onion powder, garlic salt, oregano, tandoori spice mix or ground chili pepper, garlic paste, ginger paste, turmeric, curry powder

OTHER/MISCELLANEOUS

Apple cider vinegar, aloe vera juice, cashew milk and coconut milk, rice milk and/or almond milk, coconut oil, coconut flour, almond flour, flax meal, safflower oil, ghee, chicken broth or Dr. Taz's Spicy Bone Broth (page 226), red wine vinegar, tomato paste, olive oil, canned corn, barbecue sauce, kombucha, butter (grass-fed), almond butter, fish sauce (tamari or coconut aminos work too), cashews, almonds, sesame oil, hot sauce, mustard, nutritional yeast flakes, capers or anchovies, garlic salt, pine nuts, kalamata/Greek olives, Dijon mustard, canned white beans, almond flour, shredded unsweetened coconut flour, marinara sauce, tomato sauce, pistachios, almond butter

PHASE 2/WEEK 2 MENU

	PRE-BREAKFAST pH Reset Drink (see page 94)	BREAKFAST	LUNCH	SNACK	DINNER
MONDAY	Apple cider vinegar and water (page 94)	Chocolate Protein Smoothie (page 194)	Paleo Pad Thai (page 240) and 1 cup kombucha	Liver Lover Smoothie (page 198) and sliced cucumbers	Sweet Potato Noodles with Cauliflower-Quinoa Meatballs (page 250)
TUESDAY	Lemon water (page 94)	Tropical Delight (page 195)	Chicken Wings and Crunchy Kale Chips (page 238, 252) and 1 cup Dr. Taz's Spicy Bone Broth (page 226)	Liver Lover Smoothie and Sprouted Mung Beans (page 255)	Greek Salad with Chickpeas (page 221)
WEDNESDAY	Pomegranate juice (page 94)	Berry Bomb (page 195)	Salmon-Kale Caesar Salad (page 220) and 1 slice sourdough toast	Liver Lover Smoothie and Dr. Taz's Spicy Bone Broth	Faux Fried Coconut Chicken (page 236) and Roasted Cauliflower and Brussels Sprouts Chips (page 253)
THURSDAY	Aloe vera juice (page 95)	Chocolate Protein Smoothie	Kale Pesto and Eggplant Lettuce Wrap (page 223) and 1 cup plain Greek yogurt	Liver Lover Smoothie and Crunchy Kale Chips (page 252)	Spinach and Kale Lasagna, made with tofu (page 249)
FRIDAY	Apple cider vinegar and water	Tropical Delight	Super Woman Cobb Salad (page 219) and 1 slice sourdough toast	Liver Lover Smoothie and cucumbers	Spiced Lentil Cakes (page 246)
SATURDAY	Lemon water	Berry Bomb	Snack Kebabs with chicken or shrimp, omit cheese, 2 servings (page 254), and 1 cup kombucha	Liver Lover Smoothie and Dr. Taz's Spicy Bone Broth	Buckwheat Noodle and Kale Stir-Fry (page 244)
SUNDAY	Pomegranate juice	Chocolate Protein Smoothie	Vegan Pasta with "Cheese" Sauce (page 248) and 1 cup kefir	Liver Lover Smoothie and Crunchy Kale Chips	Tandoori-Spiced Salmon with Yogurt Cucumber Sauce (page 233) and Sprouted Mung Beans

PHASE 2/WEEK 3: RELAX!

Yay! You've arrived at Day 14 of your 21-day Power Plan. You now have the foundation to build and maintain a better gut. But don't forget—there is a brain in your gut, and part of balancing a Boss Lady is to reestablish not just digestive health, but the entire gut-brain connection. This will help you to thrive and feel like you are sailing through life.

Fiery, aggressive, almost masculine? A boss lady often hears such labels in regard to her personality when stressed. Once you've done the work in the first two phases to settle and cool your digestive system, it will be time to turn your attention to the gut-brain axis (see "Understanding Your Gut Microbiome" on page 36) to reestablish the connection between your mental health and your digestive health. We have spent the last 2 weeks working on the chemistry of your digestion. Now it is time to turn to the other challenge for Boss Ladies—shutting down the stress hormone cortisol. There is no Boss Lady, with her roster of responsibilities, who does not battle her internal stress response (I know—remember, I am part Boss Lady myself. I have felt it when I get overtaxed, from the racing heart to the troubled mind.) None of us are good leaders when we lead from *that* place.

This week you'll shift gears and work on the stress management part, the emotional part of being a Boss Lady. You are going to zone in on the stress hormone cortisol and make it cooperate—shifting you from frazzled to fresh, angry and irritable to peaceful and serene. You'll also notice that I've included two meals with red meat (Wednesday's dinner and Saturday's lunch). If you have any digestive protest or discomfort with red meat, you can substitute one of the chicken or meatless meal recipes from other days of the week. Are you ready?

Week 3 Action Steps

STEP 8: COOL YOUR FIRE WITH FOOD

Remember the Ayurvedic description of the Boss Lady? Pitta—with a tendency toward too much internal heat (for a review, see page 42). Look closely at your face. For many Boss Ladies, the telltale crease between the eyebrows is the hallmark of a Boss Lady in overdrive. This corresponds with the liver region in Chinese and Ayurvedic medicine, and is also connected closely to the heart region, which sits on the bridge of the nose. If you notice changes here, your fire, passion, and work drive may be burning too hard, taxing your liver and creating the emotion of anger.

We want to "cool" this fire, and there are so many different foods that do this. I've incorporated one of the following cooling foods per day into the remainder of your menu. In Ayurveda, cooling foods are foods that are often steamed lightly and/or are easy to digest. Choose from any of the following:

- Cucumbers—10 slices
- Ghee—1 teaspoon
- Salads—pick your favorite from pages 216 to 217
- Greens—1 to 2 cups of kale, Swiss chard, or arugula (see recipes on page 220)
- ½ cup Sprouted Mung Beans (page 255)

STEP 9: COOL YOUR FIRE WITH EXERCISE

For all my Boss Ladies, exercise is an outlet, but it should not always be an aggressive, adrenaline-pumping one. Trust me, I get that we need some harder workouts to blow off steam, prevent weight gain, and build muscle tone—I love them—but in excess, strenuous exercise sessions worsen the whole stress/cortisol cycle. That's simply because vigorous exercise itself becomes a stressor on the body! With that in mind, I recommend that you limit adrenaline-pumping, competitive workouts to two to three times per week and incorporate adrenaline-calming exercises (think yoga, Pilates, or swimming) a few times per week. Boss Ladies need the mental relief that exercise provides, but they also need sports that cool their inner fire rather than aggravate it further. Use the following chart as a guide. For more details on exercise, read Chapter 11.

THE BOSS LADY EXERCISE RX

The goal is to alternate grounding exercises with cardio and strength training. Find workouts on pages 267 to 271.	MONDAY	TUESDAY	WEDNESDAY
	Strength, 30 minutes	Cardio, 45 minutes	Yoga, 45 minutes
THURSDAY	**FRIDAY**	**SATURDAY**	**SUNDAY**
Cardio, 45 minutes	Strength, 30 minutes, or Rest Day	Yoga, 45 minutes	Cardio, 45 minutes

ADRENALINE-PUMPING VERSUS RELAXING EXERCISES

Boss Ladies should limit adrenaline-pumping exercise to three times per week.

ADRENALINE-PUMPING	RELAXING
Running or sprinting	Walking
Spin class	Easy cycling
Kickboxing	Tai chi or qi gong
Ashtanga yoga	Gentle yoga
Competitive racquetball, tennis, or other team sport	Swimming
Rock climbing	Going for a nature walk
Shoveling snow	Gardening

STEP 10: COOL YOUR FIRE WITH MIND, BODY, AND BEAUTY REGIMENS

Getting out of your head, turning off list making, and just relaxing can be tough for a Boss Lady. With a little bit of this in my temperament, I can relate to how difficult it is to just calm down or cool down. Here are a few of my favorite tricks to cool my fire. You don't have to do all of these, but pick a few that resonate with you.

Mind

- **Aromatherapy:** Sandalwood and rose essential oils are perfect for cooling your Power Type. Aromas influence the limbic portion of the brain, which increases relaxation and lowers stress. Try applying a small amount to your wrists and temples throughout the day, or use a diffuser in your office or home. For more information, see "The Essential Essential Oils," page 312.
- **Meditation:** Set aside 10 minutes a day to calm and cool your mind. You can simply sit and focus on your breath, use a guided meditation from an app such as Insight Timer or The Mindfulness, or follow the simple meditation on page 288.

Bodywork

- **Massage:** Like acupuncture, massage has also been shown to reduce stress and protect the immune system. Boss Ladies often benefit from neuromuscular massage to help release tense trigger points exacerbated by stress. For more information, see page 295.

◆ **Acupuncture:** By targeting "blocked" acupuncture points and sluggish meridians, acupuncture is a wonderful way to lower cortisol, manage stress, and rebalance and heal a Boss Lady's digestive system. As a licensed acupuncturist, I have seen the benefits of this ancient modality firsthand. I recommend at least once-a-week visits for the high-stress Boss Lady. For more information, see "Build Your Body's Force Field with Bodywork," page 294.

◆ **Epsom salt soaks:** The magnesium in Epsom salts is a wonderful way to get the body to calm down and relax. Twice a week, fill up a warm bath and add 2 cups of Epsom salts, then soak for 20 minutes—doctor's orders!

◆ **Amla** (Indian gooseberry): Amla is an herb long used in Ayurvedic medicine that is thought to "cool" the body. It is high in vitamin C, antioxidants, and B vitamins—helping both the liver and the gut. It can be eaten whole (amla fruit), juiced, or taken as a supplement, 500 milligrams per day. (See Resources, page 316, for brand recommendations.)

Beauty: Calm and Cool

Boss Ladies need to pay close attention to their skin, including the skin on the scalp. Learn how to use simple household ingredients such as apple cider vinegar, lemons, yogurt, and more to cool and calm your skin and hair. See page 302 in Chapter 13 for your full Boss Lady Beauty Regimen.

WEEK 3 SHOPPING LIST

PRODUCE

Lemons, pomegranates, bananas, frozen mangos, frozen pineapple, frozen blueberries, frozen strawberries, mint leaves, spinach, kale, romaine, tomatoes, onions, garlic, ginger, fresh or frozen green beans, limes, eggplants, cucumber, celery, carrots, beets, dandelion greens, cilantro, parsley, zucchini, scallions, grape tomatoes, avocados, red onions, sweet potatoes, basil, bell pepper, cauliflower, dill, oregano, thyme, rosemary, mint, mushrooms, sumac, avocados, Brussels sprouts

PROTEINS

Chocolate and vanilla protein powder (see page 196 for suggestions), dried lentils or split peas, dried yellow split peas, dried mung beans, eggs, chickpeas, black beans, kidney beans, boneless chicken thighs, mung beans, boneless skinless chicken breasts, chicken wings, grass-fed ground beef or lamb, stew beef, plain nondairy yogurt, unsweetened nondairy kefir, chicken or goat or beef bones, salmon, shrimp, tofu

SWEETENERS

Honey, maple syrup

GRAINS

Quinoa, fermented bread (sourdough), lentil or soybean pasta, gluten-free lasagna noodles, buckwheat noodles, corn tortillas, flax meal

SUPPLEMENTS

Probiotics (page 99), digestive enzymes (page 99), glutamine (page 99)

HERBS AND SPICES

Salt and pepper, garam masala, paprika, cumin (ground and seeds), coriander, herbal teas, Thai red curry paste, arrowroot powder, onion powder, garlic salt, oregano, tandoori spice mix or ground chili pepper, garlic paste, ginger paste, turmeric, curry powder

OTHER/MISCELLANEOUS

Apple cider vinegar, aloe vera juice, coconut milk, rice milk, almond milk, coconut oil, coconut flour, almond flour, safflower oil, ghee, chicken broth or buy the ingredients for Dr. Taz's Spicy Bone Broth (page 226), red wine vinegar, tomato paste, olive oil, canned corn, barbecue sauce, kombucha, butter (grass-fed), almond butter, fish sauce (tamari or coconut aminos work too), cashews, almonds, sesame oil, hot sauce, mustard, nutritional yeast, capers or anchovies, garlic salt, pine nuts, kalamata olives, Dijon mustard, canned white beans, almond flour, shredded unsweetened coconut flour, marinara sauce, tomato sauce, pistachios, fire-roasted tomatoes, navy beans, salsa

PHASE 3/WEEK 3 MENU

	PRE-BREAKFAST pH Reset Drink (see page 94)	BREAKFAST	LUNCH	SNACK (Note: The Grocer's Green Drink is another liver-cleansing option that I've added here for variety.)	DINNER
MONDAY	Apple cider vinegar and water (page 94)	Chocolate Protein Smoothie (page 194)	Vegan Curry in a Hurry (page 239) and 1 cup plain Greek yogurt	Liver Lover Smoothie (page 198) and cucumbers	Black Bean Soup and Portable Tacos (page 227)
TUESDAY	Lemon water (page 94)	Tropical Delight (page 195)	Bissara (page 231) and 1 cup kombucha	Liver Lover Smoothie and Sprouted Mung Beans (page 255)	Greek Salad with chickpeas (page 221)
WEDNESDAY	Pomegranate juice (page 94)	Berry Bomb (page 195)	Snack Kebabs with chicken or shrimp, omit cheese, 2 servings (page 254), and 1 cup Dr. Taz's Spicy Bone Broth (page 226)	Liver Lover Smoothie and a small green salad with 1 tsp dressing or a squeeze of lemon juice, tsp of olive oil, and salt and pepper to taste	Paleo Shepherd's Pie (page 242)
THURSDAY	Aloe vera juice (page 95)	Chocolate Protein Smoothie	Spiced Lentil Cakes (page 246) and 1 cup fat-free plain kefir	Grocer's Choice Green Drink (page 197) and Dr. Taz's Spicy Bone Broth	Chicken Saag (page 237) and Roasted Cauliflower and Brussels Sprouts Chips (page 253)
FRIDAY	Apple cider vinegar and water	Tropical Delight	Chicken Wings of your choice (page 238), Crunchy Kale Chips (page 252), and 1 cup Dr. Taz's Spicy Bone Broth	Liver Lover Smoothie and cucumbers	Mason Jar Salads, your choice (page 216)

SATURDAY	Lemon water	Berry Bomb	Paleo Shepherd's Pie (page 242) and 1 cup kombucha	Liver Lover Smoothie and Sprouted Mung Beans	BBQ Chicken Salad (page 217)
SUNDAY	Pomegranate juice	Chocolate Protein Smoothie	Chicken Wings of your choice, Crunchy Kale Chips, and 1 cup plain Greek yogurt	Grocer's Choice Green Drink and Crunchy Kale Chips	Persian Eggplant with Yellow Split Peas and Dried Lime (page 245)

YOU ARE AMAZING! NOW that you've completed all 3 weeks of your Power Plan, I suggest that you repeat the Boss Lady 3-Week Rx for two more cycles, or about 2 months (9 weeks). As you get more comfortable with the plan, you may decide to create your own Boss Lady–approved meals.

If you are tiring of the recipes in the 3-week menus in this chapter, you can swap in other recipes from Chapter 10. (Just keep breakfast foods for breakfast, and so on.) You can use these 10 steps to keep your energy balanced for whatever demands are placed on you. After the 21 days, continue to follow the key elements of your plan, prioritizing specific sections as you need to (for example, emphasize cooling foods or exercise if you are feeling overly aggressive, or return and take a week to just do the detox to settle your gut). It does not matter—it only matters that you continue to use the plan and build on it to lead and command! After you've followed your plan for a couple months, go back and retake the tests in Chapter 2 and 3, and if you have shifted Power Types, switch to the appropriate plan and update your action steps accordingly. For now, turn to Part III to read on through to the end for tips and strategies to round out your plan with plenty of healthy exercise, home and mind-body tips, recipes, and beauty recommendations.

CHAPTER 7

THE SAVVY CHICKS' 3-WEEK RX

I LOVE ALL the Super Woman Power Types, but I have a special affinity for Savvy Chicks, maybe because I am one. I can relate firsthand to the needs and demands of this Power Type. This super woman is a blend of the previous two Power Types—equal parts ethereal artist and commander in chief. The combination is fascinating but challenging at the same time. A Savvy Chick often fluctuates between her two selves, with one being stronger than the other at different times. If you haven't done so yet, I recommend that you turn back to Chapters 5 and 6 and familiarize yourself with both sides of your Power Type—the Gypsy Girl and the Boss Lady.

The *gift* of being a combination of two types is what I call "translational creativity," or creativity that manifests in objective or tangible ways, such as the ability to create a new business or an innovative product. At her most powerful, the Savvy Chick is a true visionary—a woman who is an inspired, ingenious inventor. However, when out of balance, the medical *challenges* of this combo Power Type can be daunting, since the mix of the free-spirited gypsy and the structured commander comes with double the stressors and booby traps. Let's take a look first at the risk factors for you Savvy Chicks, and then we'll move into your 3-Week Power Plan, which will get you back to creating and innovating with energy and healthy passion.

Savvy Chick at a Glance

ALTER EGO: THE VISIONARY

Super powers: When in optimal balance and health, Savvy Chicks can have powers from both the spheres of Gypsy Girls and Boss Ladies. That can mean potent creativity and passion, plus a strong drive and work ethic. This combination can manifest itself in a true inventor and creator of bold businesses, products, or progressive families.

Kryptonite: With twice the blessings come twice the burdens, in some cases. A Savvy Chick's ultimate weakness is that her emotions pull her in two different directions. The artist in her wants to stay true to her visions and dreams and to follow the flow of creative energy, but the commander in her demands productivity, results, and structure. The Savvy Chick vacillates between creativity and inspiration and ordered schedules and tangible outcomes, all while insisting on adherence to her busy regimen—which can add up to burnout, blowups, and exhaustion.

Elements: Wind/Fire/Water. This combo type can experience both the motion and flow of the Gypsy Girl, as well as the passion and intensity of the Boss Lady—this can add up to amazing creativity and innovation, or complete meltdowns. Winter and summer, the seasons associated with Savvy Chicks, represent both cold and hot, hibernation and passion, the place where innovative thinking and ideas surface.

Personality: Savvy Chicks have a tendency to be both dreamers and doers. While they can be energetic and effective leaders, creators, and inventors, they have to watch for moodiness, restlessness, depression, anxiety, and irritability.

Body type: Medium to underweight. Savvy Chicks are prone to poor circulation and to cold hands and feet. Their skin is often rough, dry, and oily. Savvy Chicks often have large pores and hair that tends toward dryness.

Celebrity example: Jessica Alba. Successful actor Alba, a Golden Globe nominee, mom to two girls, and also the cofounder of The Honest Company, a multimillion-dollar consumer goods company that promotes healthier and safer baby and household products.

Colors: Indigo and purple (combinations of reds and blues). These colors represent stability, energy, dignity, royalty, power, and ambition. Think of the sea, of depth and stability. Darker blues also are colors of confidence, integrity, wisdom, and tranquility.

COMMON SAVVY CHICK CONDITIONS

As I've mentioned in the last two chapters, being a certain Power Type doesn't mean that you'll automatically have all of that type's issues, but these are the most common complaints I hear from my Savvy Chick patients. With these conditions in mind, I've designed the 3-Week Power Plan to bring my Savvy Chicks back into balance and soaring toward health and happiness.

Anxiety

Part Gypsy Girl, the Savvy Chick patients in my practice have a tendency toward anxiety, worry, and even a fearful mind-set as they dream, plot, and plan. When in balance, the wellspring of creativity flows, but out of balance, artistic endeavors can turn to obsessive worry, compulsive behaviors, or phobias. The common physical signs of anxiety often reported by a Savvy Chick are chest pain, palpitations, insomnia, and trouble focusing.

Because they are part Boss Lady, anxiety in a Savvy Chick can also express itself as anger rather than the depression that can overwhelm a Gypsy Girl. Helping Savvy Chicks with anxiety is a personal mission for me, since I know firsthand how it can block their awesomeness. Creativity and innovation are stifled when anxiety takes over—the sweaty palms, trouble focusing, racing heart, and sleepless nights all snowball, leaving Savvy Chicks paralyzed and ineffective.

Migraines

Migraine headaches are common amongst Savvy Chicks and while they can be the result of hormonal, nutritional, and digestive imbalances, they are also a sign of a Savvy Chick in overdrive. Many Savvy Chicks will come into my practice listing off a cocktail of multiple migraine medications that have been prescribed over the years in an attempt to manage the debilitating symptoms, often without success. The reason: The root of the migraines has never really been addressed.

IBS/Constipation

Like Boss Ladies, Savvy Chicks struggle with digestive issues, especially irritable bowel syndrome (IBS). Savvy Chicks are still commanders and leaders—and there is a great deal of stress that accompanies those responsibilities. Just as with Boss Ladies, the stress disrupts the gut-brain axis, as chronic stress halts digestion and bloodflow to the gut. Just picture your gut tightening into a tight, knotted ball every time you are stressed! Bloating, abdominal pain, constipation, and diarrhea are just a few of the digestive symptoms that a Savvy Chick may battle.

Amenorrhea/Infertility

Skipped menstrual cycles can be a common issue for Savvy Chicks, and this comes from the Gypsy Girl side of the equation. Like Gypsy Girls, Savvy Chicks are plagued with hormone imbalances and nutritional deficiencies as the result of *too much thinking and doing!* Because of these imbalances, fertility can be an issue. Balancing hormones, gut function, and nutrition can improve signaling for fertility hormones and regular menstrual cycles in my Savvy Chicks. Additionally, digestive issues can be at the root of polycystic ovary syndrome (PCOS), a condition characterized by imbalanced levels of estrogen and progesterone. PCOS affects 5 to 10 percent of women of childbearing age and is responsible for 70 percent of infertility issues in women who have trouble ovulating. It's something I see in increasing numbers in the young super women I treat, especially my Savvy Chicks.

TMJ/Increased Muscle Tension

Temporomandibular joint dysfunction, or TMJ, is common in Savvy Chicks and refers to the chronic tension and pain in the hinge that connects your upper and lower jaw. This is another one that, unfortunately, I am all too familiar with. I can recall at least three episodes when severe stress left my jaw tight and painful to the point that my ears rang. Symptoms like these are a definite wake-up call for a Savvy Chick! TMJ can be caused by chronic stress, lack of the muscle-relaxing mineral magnesium, or lower than optimal levels of progesterone. Progesterone is a female hormone that is also a natural anti-inflammatory and a muscle relaxer. In addition to TMJ, increased muscle tension is something that many Savvy Chicks face—especially in the neck and back.

Insomnia

Just like Boss Ladies and Gypsy Girls, Savvy Chicks tend to have trouble sleeping. You might experience the inability to both fall and stay asleep.

Savvy Chicks can have the low/altered melatonin of the Boss Lady Power Type, with the interrupted sleep of a Gypsy Girl, waking up between 1 a.m. and 3 a.m. Talk about an innovation stumper! The chronic lack of healthy sleep can dampen any creative vision and just leave a Savvy Chick plain old tired.

Eczema/Psoriasis

Alternating between the oiliness of a Boss Lady's complexion and the dryness of a Gypsy Girl's, Savvy Chicks have a tendency toward a combination skin type. A Savvy Chick may find that she is oily in the summer and dry in the winter. For this reason the skin barrier breaks down, and conditions like eczema or psoriasis can take root. According to conventional medicine, eczema is a chronic, noncontagious inflammatory skin condition that presents with dry, itchy skin that can weep clear fluid. Psoriasis, on the other hand, is an autoimmune disease characterized by raised, red, scaly patches on the skin. Other systems of medicine—such as Chinese medicine and Ayurvedic medicine—see both skin conditions as an indicator that your entire system is out of balance or that you—like the Boss Ladies—are simply generating *too much heat* (remember that word from the last chapter?). During the 3-Week Power Plan, we will nourish your skin using the wisdom of the best medical and healing practices from around the world. Part of your Savvy Chick Power Plan will be learning to maintain a healthy skin and hair barrier so that it stays moist and intact, using the right food, supplements, and products.

Chinese Meridian Diagnosis: Liver-Kidney Meridian Deficiency

The meridian imbalance of a Savvy Chick is typically a blockage in the flow of energy through the liver and kidney meridians. For example, the liver meridian in Traditional Chinese Medicine (TCM) balances and detoxifies hormones. The kidney meridian, on the other hand, is the seat of energy and the hormone factory in TCM. In Savvy Chicks, there is a tendency for both of these meridians to be out of balance, affecting hormone regulation. For a Chinese medicine practitioner, seeing the liver meridian out of balance is a signal that the body needs cleaning and detoxifying, while an imbalanced kidney meridian indicates the need to build the body, or to "strengthen" the blood, through diet, rest, and mind-body work. Remember, from a TCM perspective, you always aim for balance by using *all* of these avenues. We will tackle this in your Power Plan!

Ayurvedic Dosha Diagnosis: Vata-Pitta

The Savvy Chick blend of Gypsy Girl and Boss Lady is expressed beautifully in the Ayurvedic doshas (energy types) vata and pitta. Both doshas are predominant in your constitution, and the pull between these two types can increase your tendency to fall out of balance. For example, vatas are light, cool, and dry while pittas are hot, sharp, and oily. In a good sense, the heat of pitta can balance the coolness of vata, but under duress, the two elements clash. This can affect energy balance and concentration or focus. Getting back into balance then becomes a priority—with an increased commitment to promoting good habits for each Ayurvedic type. Ayurvedic literature even mentions focusing on balancing the vata element in fall and winter and the pitta element in spring and summer.

Hormone Imbalances: Adrenals and Thyroid

The most common hormone imbalance for Savvy Chicks is, not surprisingly, a blend. You have the tendency to burn out your adrenals like a Gypsy Girl, but you can also have thyroid abnormalities like a Boss Lady. Adrenal fatigue and hypo- and hyperthyroidism are conditions I see often in my Savvy Chick patients (see "The Five Glands You Need to Know," page 50, for more information about adrenal and thyroid glands).

The constant pull on the adrenals and the thyroid creates a demand on the other hormones as well. Adrenal fatigue, in its later stages, often leads to low progesterone levels, while the chronic thyroid imbalance, even at low levels, will disrupt estrogen metabolism. For more information, see the hormone imbalance information on Gypsy Girls (page 60) and Boss Ladies (page 89).

LAB FINDINGS

I love how all this data—the meridians, the doshas, the hormones—is quantifiable. It all adds up and can be proven in lab work! Low energy or low kidney qi often presents as low thyroid hormone or low B vitamin levels in lab testing, while a liver meridian imbalance may correlate to high cholesterol, high liver function enzymes, or high sex hormone–binding globulin. Here are the common lab findings in my Savvy Chicks.

- **Low B vitamins**—B_5, B_6, B_{12}, and folic acid, which often presents as lack of energy and poor concentration
- **Low magnesium level,** which often presents as fatigue and weakness, mood swings, insomnia, and trouble going to the bathroom
- **Low iron (ferritin, serum iron) levels**
- **Abnormal thyroid numbers** (TSH, T4, T3—free and total)
- **Low a.m. cortisol**
- **High nighttime cortisol,** causing irritability, anxiety, or depression; fatigue
- **Low progesterone,** causing everything from shorter menstrual cycles to irritability and insomnia
- **Low DHEA** (dehydroepiandrosterone), which affects libido
- **Altered FSH** (follicle-stimulating hormone), affecting ovulation
- **High estrogen**
- **Borderline high celiac antibodies**

(For more information on a specific lab, see "Labs You Need to Know" on page 49.)

Nutritional Needs

After evaluating so many Savvy Chicks, I know that one of the first steps to bringing them back to balance is using food as medicine. Just take a

LONG-TERM DISEASE RISKS

I think the greatest long-term disease risk for Savvy Chicks is the disruption of the digestive and hormonal systems. Big concepts like hormone failure, digestive dysfunction, inflammation, and poor methylation are all long-term disease risks contributing to autoimmune disease, osteoporosis, and breast and colon cancer. By starting to establish lifelong balance through the 3-Week Power Plan, you will be ahead of the game when it comes to preventing the common diseases that many women battle. Understanding how to eat and care for your Power Type is a prescription for long-term prevention as well.

look at the list of common lab values above. Many of these can be corrected with the right diet: foods high in B vitamins, iron, and protein—all critical in nourishing Savvy Chick hormones like cortisol and thyroid. Healthy fats are critical for a Savvy Chick, since a weak kidney meridian calls for more healthy fats to support optimal hormone production. Finally, many Savvy Chicks need to be gluten free. Gluten plays a role in altered thyroid function, either due to the processing of modern-day wheat with bromide—an industrial chemical that displaces thyroid-friendly iodine—or by affecting gut function. (For more about gluten, see "Anti-Inflammatory Eating—Foods to Avoid" on page 46 of Chapter 5.)

Savvy Chicks, like Boss Ladies, also need to guard their digestive systems by bringing in more probiotics and probiotic-rich foods to help digestion. The immunology of the gut and the microbiome is just as important for Savvy Chicks as for Boss Ladies.

HOW THE SAVVY CHICK 3-WEEK RX WORKS

While you are a blend of a dreamer and a doer, a Gypsy Girl and a Boss Lady, you, like all Savvy Chicks, need your own plan—in its own order—to balance the wellspring of talent that lies beneath the surface. Get ready—once Savvy Chicks get balanced, they really do change the world! You've got a lot of work ahead of you—remember, you are twice the woman in some respects. In some ways that means twice the effort, but it also means twice the payoff!

Read on to see the guidelines that I want you to begin adhering to from Day 1. You'll follow these rules throughout the entire plan. I include these for the women (especially those with high Boss Lady tendencies) who don't have patience for preparing the recipes I included. If you stick to these recommendations you'll see your health, happiness, and energy soar.

The Savvy Chick Rx Rules

1. **Don't use electronics until after breakfast.** It's important for Savvy Chicks to minimize their electronic usage. You'll incorporate steps to budget these resources wisely (details in Steps 1 and 2).

2. **Drink a daily warming tonic.** Wake up with a morning tonic. Recipes are in Chapter 10.

3. **Incorporate daily grounding exercise.** You'll alleviate mental stress and stimulate good digestive function.

4. **Meet your daily protein and fat goals.** Stick to 50 to 60 grams of protein and 20 to 30 grams of fat each day. You'll need to read nutrient labels, or you can simply follow the menus in this chapter.

THE 10 SAVVY CHICK ACTION STEPS AT A GLANCE

Here is your entire plan at a glance. These are all the action steps you'll be learning in the next 3 weeks. These differ from the overall rules in that they include *ALL* the steps for the entire program. You won't incorporate these all at once. In Week 1 you'll start with the first four steps, then build from there in Weeks 2 and 3. By the time you've completed all 21 days, you will have all these actions steps empowering you each and every day.

Step 1: Wake Up in an Electronics-Free Zone

Step 2: Drink a Warming Tonic

Step 3: Connect to the Ground

Step 4: Eat a High-Protein Breakfast

Step 5: Eat Power Lunches for Your Adrenals

Step 6: Eat to Boost Your Thyroid
- ☐ Eat an iron-rich dinner
- ☐ Go nuts
- ☐ Boost iodine stores
- ☐ Bulk up magnesium

Step 7: Supplement Your Adrenal and Thyroid Glands
- ☐ B-complex vitamins
- ☐ Iron
- ☐ Adrenal adaptogens
- ☐ Magnesium

Step 8: Eat Probiotic-Rich Foods for Good Gut Bacteria

Step 9: Supplement to Protect Your Gut Lining
- ☐ Take slippery elm, glutamine, or aloe vera juice every morning
- ☐ Optimize your digestion by adding a digestive enzyme

Step 10: Take a Mindful Gadget Break

"Every day or two, I slice and dice a bunch of fresh vegetables including broccoli, celery, carrots, and cauliflower to have on hand for a quick, easy, and crunchable snack—it really keeps me on track!"
—Sarah, 65, retired music teacher

5. **Focus on fiber.** Eat 30 to 40 grams of fiber every day. This is important for Savvy Chicks because it protects your digestive system, helps regulate blood sugar, and balances your gut and hormones.

6. **Avoid gluten and dairy.** Both are common irritants for Savvy Chicks' sensitive digestive systems. If you use the suggested recipes in the menus, make sure that you always use the gluten- and dairy-free options I've provided.

7. **Limit daily calories.** Don't exceed 1,800 calories unless you are exercising vigorously for more than an hour a day.

Note: The suggested menus in this chapter will help you follow the rules.

At the beginning of each phase/week, you will learn about that week's action steps, then see a suggested menu for effortless healthy eating and a shopping list that includes everything you'll need to have on hand for that week. You can swap out the recipes for your own favorites if you find it easier: Just make sure that your meals provide similar nutrients, protein, and fat. Incorporate all these tools to activate all your super powers every day!

PHASE 1/WEEK 1: GROUND YOURSELF

As part Gypsy Girl, it's often most beneficial to have Savvy Chicks start by addressing a common need of all creative types—to be grounded. Not so grounded that you crush your flair for innovation, just enough so you won't float away entirely. There's an inclination for Savvy Chicks to get lost somewhere in their heads, to be so busy creating and innovating in that mental space that they aren't present. More importantly, this detachment can disconnect you from your body and your physical health.

With that in mind, you'll start the first 7 days of your 21-day plan by working on grounding your energy using many of the same strategies employed by Gypsy Girls in Chapter 6.

Week 1 Action Steps

STEP 1: WAKE UP IN AN ELECTRONICS-FREE ZONE

Start by establishing and being consistent with a routine—set your alarm (on an old-fashioned clock—no phone alarms) for a 6 a.m. wake-up call. *Do not* touch your e-mail, cell phone, or any other electronic or battery-operated device. I know there are businesses to run and innovations to complete—but *stop*—don't drain your energy before you've even had a chance to wake up. Begin each morning of your 21-day plan by simply opening your eyes, stretching your arms up overhead and your legs down, pointing and flexing your toes, sitting up slowly, feeling the ground under your feet, looking around, and looking outdoors. Now, move on to your second step. That's right—still no electronics. Your e-mails, texts, and voice mails will still be there after breakfast, after you've had a chance to build a solid foundation from which to create.

STEP 2: DRINK A WARMING TONIC

Head to the kitchen to boil some water and to make a warming tonic that will send a signal to your sleepy body that you are awake and ready for your morning meal. These tonics not only help jump-start digestion for the day, they also help Savvy Chicks warm up mentally and emotionally. Choose one of three warming tonics—Ginger Tea, Honey Lemon Tea, or Honey Turmeric Tea. See your Week 1 menu for your daily tonic.

STEP 3: CONNECT TO THE GROUND

Once your warming tonic is inside you, you will probably be feeling more awake. Take the next 15 minutes to connect your energy from your head to the ground. Grounding is often discussed in older systems of medicine such as Chinese and Ayurvedic medicine and works to keep your energy stable and steady as you prepare for and move through the day. The following grounding choices are all often called moving meditations, or meditation in motion, because they work to connect your breath, mind, and body through gentle, flowing movements and positions.

- Tai chi
- Qi gong
- Yoga

See descriptions, routines, app suggestions, and information for finding a class in Chapter 11, starting on page 257.

STEP 4: EAT A HIGH-PROTEIN BREAKFAST

Eat the high-protein breakfast entrees in the Week 1 menu on page 122. You need protein to sustain the challenges of the day. Protein stabilizes your insulin and blood sugar levels, making sure you are focused and energetic.

OVER THE NEXT 7 DAYS, practice these steps over and over again—keeping yourself grounded and your energy balanced—and you will be shocked at the difference a mindful morning will make.

This week's suggested shopping list and menu follow. These two charts incorporate everything nutrition-wise discussed in your first four steps to help you to wake up, balance out, and maximize your energy all day long.

WEEK 1 SHOPPING LIST

PRODUCE

Ginger, lemons, bananas, frozen pineapple, frozen mango, onions, garlic, leeks, mushrooms, spinach, arugula, tomatoes, basil, cilantro, bell pepper, sweet potatoes, avocados, cucumbers, lime, Brussels sprouts, kale, carrots, celery, cauliflower, parsley, mint, portobello mushrooms

PROTEINS

Vanilla protein powder (see page 196), eggs, boneless skinless chicken breast, chicken or turkey sausage, chicken or turkey preservative-free lunch meat, salmon, sea bass, goat cheese, ground beef or lamb, chicken or beef or pork bones, black beans, plain nondairy yogurt, hummus, black beans, chickpeas, lentils

SWEETENERS

Honey

GRAINS

Pancake mix (paleo or gluten free), quinoa, corn tortillas, brown rice cakes, rice noodles, rice paper wrappers

HERBS AND SPICES

Turmeric, sea salt, pepper, nutmeg, arrowroot powder, vanilla extract, paprika, ground red pepper, Mexican or regular oregano, cumin, thyme, garlic salt, Italian seasoning

OTHER/MISCELLANEOUS

Chocolate chips, walnuts, unsweetened coconut flakes, carton of coconut milk (rice or almond milk okay too), coconut oil, ghee, olive oil, balsamic vinegar, salad dressing (your choice), chia seeds, canned coconut cream, canned coconut milk, green olives, canned crushed tomatoes, tomato paste, red enchilada sauce, mung beans, chicken broth, nutritional yeast flakes, almond flour, large mason jars

PHASE 1/WEEK 1 MENU

	PRE-BREAKFAST Warming Tonic	BREAKFAST	LUNCH	SNACKS (choose one)	DINNER
MONDAY	Ginger Tea (page 199)	Pancake Imposters (page 210)	Mason Jar Salads with chicken (page 216)	Hummus and Veggies (page 255) or Sprouted Mung Beans (page 255)	Paleo Shepherd's Pie with ground beef or ground lamb
TUESDAY	Honey Lemon Tea (page 199)	Tropical Delight (page 195)	Dairy-Free Tomato Soup (page 230) and Chicken Wings, your way (page 238)	Rice Cakes with Nut Butter (page 252) or 1 Pancake Imposter	Oven "Grilled" Sea Bass with Wilted Spinach (page 234) and Roasted Cauliflower and Brussels Sprouts Chips (page 253)
WEDNESDAY	Honey Turmeric Tea (page 200)	Paleo Quiche (page 203) with Sweet Potato Crust (page 204)	Paleo Shepherd's Pie (page 242)	1 Basil Roll (page 224) or Nut Butter Dream Bar (page 213)	Faux Fried Coconut Chicken with Honey Mustard Dipping Sauce (page 236) and Warm Quinoa Salad (page 222)
THURSDAY	Ginger Tea	Coconut Chia Seed Pudding (page 212)	Chicken Saag (page 237) and Kale Chips (page 252)	Sprouted Mung Beans or 3 Mini Protein Muffins (page 214)	Spiced Lentil Cakes with Chickpeas (page 246)
FRIDAY	Honey Lemon Tea	Festive Italian Frittata (page 206)	Bissara (page 231)	Dr. Taz's Spicy Bone Broth (page 226) or Hummus and Veggies	Middle Eastern Chicken Skewers with Quinoa Tabbouleh (page 235)
SATURDAY	Honey Turmeric Tea	Paleo Quiche with Sweet Potato Crust	Salmon-Kale Caesar Salad (page 220)	Grocer's Choice Green Drink (page 197) or 3 Mini Protein Muffins	Chicken Soup (page 228)
SUNDAY	Ginger Tea	Huevos Rancheros (page 208)	Portobello BLT with chicken (page 225)	1 Mini Roll-Up (page 254) or Dr. Taz's Spicy Bone Broth	Black Bean Soup and Portable Tacos (page 227)

PHASE 2/WEEK 2:
BALANCE AND OPTIMIZE KEY HORMONES

Being a Savvy Chick is big business—there is a lot to do and usually very little time to get it all done. What takes a hit? Your hormones, of course—like Gypsy Girls, Savvy Chicks are at great risk for adrenal fatigue, which usually shows itself by an irregular pattern of crashing adrenaline or altered levels of cortisol, the stress hormone that is released as we navigate the world. But it's not just the adrenal glands and adrenaline that crash—with Savvy Chicks, the thyroid also takes a major hit.

The combo of a Gypsy Girl and Boss Lady brings a one-two punch to your Power Type because the harder the adrenals work, the more stress and strain they create on the thyroid. Thanks to driven Boss Lady characteristics, over time, many Savvy Chicks battle thyroid irregularities—everything from hypothyroidism to the autoimmune conditions Hashimoto's thyroiditis and Graves' disease.

The aim of your Power Plan is to be proactive so you can continue to channel all your creative and intellectual energy, without taking the hormone hit. I know this is so important not just through my patients, but because I am a Savvy Chick, and I have had to deal with the consequences of not keeping my Power Type balanced. Yes, I have had the adrenaline crash and the thyroid hits, leaving me—well—not *me*. I don't want this for you! None of us wants to stop dead in our tracks and take a forced hiatus from our dreams. You don't have to—if you follow all the action steps from last week and combine them with new steps for this week.

In this phase of the Savvy Chick plan, your action steps are aimed at keeping your adrenals and your thyroid balanced using food, herbs, and even supplements.

Week 2 Action Steps

STEP 5: EAT POWER LUNCHES FOR YOUR ADRENALS

On your menu this week you'll continue to see lunch entrées with at least 15 to 20 grams of protein, and snacks with at least 7 to 10 grams of protein. You are also incorporating healthy fats—like coconut oil, olive oil, ghee, and grass-fed butter, which I call "hormone builders" because they provide the building blocks for all hormones in your body. Simply prepare and consume the lunches and snacks suggested on the Week 2 menu to heal and balance your adrenals and your thyroid.

STEP 6: EAT TO BOOST YOUR THYROID

You can protect and support your thyroid *before* you get a thyroid diagnosis. As we discussed previously, your thyroid numbers are specific to you—what is normal for one person is often not normal for another. You will see your thyroid numbers shift and change as *you* change—passing through each decade, pregnancy, and, finally, menopause—or as you experience life stresses, mixed with your particular genetics.

Start your thyroid protection plan *now*—begin choosing foods that support and help your thyroid. The key nutrients for optimal thyroid function include iron, selenium, magnesium, and iodine.

1. **Eat an iron-rich dinner.** At least two times a week, pick iron-rich foods including grass-fed beef or lamb. A 4-ounce serving of these proteins is plenty to get your quota of bioavailable iron.

2. **Go nuts.** Add Brazil nuts—packed with selenium—at least three times weekly.

3. **Boost iodine stores.** Use iodized salt or pink salt in your recipes or experiment with seaweed, adding fun sea vegetables like nori or kelp three times per week.

4. **Bulk up magnesium.** Have a daily dose of leafy greens, a small handful of almonds, or an occasional treat of dark chocolate to boost magnesium.

Hint: I've got you covered for all of these tips in your menu. You'll see beef and lamb incorporated into your dinners and the chia chocolates, kelp and kale chips, and trail mix on your snack menu do the rest of the work for your thyroid.

STEP 7: SUPPLEMENT YOUR ADRENAL AND THYROID GLANDS

Even the best intentions with food will sometimes still leave us nutritionally deficient. Why? I am often asked this, and there are a number of reasons—most of which I think go back to how our food is manufactured and processed today compared to 50 years ago. Our soil also does not have the micronutrient profile it once had, and that is part of the nutritional depletion as well.

In the Morning

- **B-complex vitamins:** Add a daily B-complex—look for one with a range of B vitamins, including B_1, B_2, B_5, B_6 (biotin), B_{12}, and folic acid. Remember, B vitamins support the adrenals and the thyroid, while influencing almost every other hormone and neurotransmitter axis (see "Vitamins and Supplements You Need to Know," page 45).

- **Iron:** Add 15 milligrams of elemental iron daily. Chelated or food-based forms of iron seem to work the best and are easier on the digestive system. A caveat: Iron supplements can cause constipation in some women. Start with a small dose, 15 milligrams, to make sure you tolerate this supplement with the iron-based foods included on this week's menu. If you still find that you experience constipation, skip this supplement and focus on the iron-rich foods I suggest in Step 6. For Savvy Chicks, iron really is essential, and I can share so many personal stories of how skipping iron resulted in hair loss, mood changes, or energy crashes.

In the Afternoon

- **Adrenal adaptogens:** Add any one of the following adrenal adaptogens (substances that help to manage stress and the stress response, improving your energy). You can also mix and match. These are my favorites.

  - Ashwagandha, 1 gram
  - Ginseng, 500 milligrams
  - Astragalus, 500 milligrams
  - Licorice root, 1 gram

Before Bed

- **Magnesium.** I cannot stress enough the importance of this super micronutrient. Magnesium is a key cofactor in hormone regulation and the neurotransmitters, just like the B vitamins. It also promotes sleep and eases anxiety. Add 200 to 400 milligrams of magnesium nightly as a part of a healthy Savvy Chick plan.

WEEK 2 SHOPPING LIST

PRODUCE

Ginger, lemons, bananas, peaches, berries, apples, pears, grapes, frozen mixed berries, frozen pineapple, frozen mango, onions, garlic, leeks, mushrooms, Brussels sprouts, spinach, arugula, romaine lettuce, tomatoes, basil, cilantro, mint, oregano, bell pepper, sweet potatoes, eggplant, avocados, limes, potatoes, zucchini or summer squash, celery, scallions, dill, cauliflower, kelp, kale

PROTEINS

Vanilla protein powder (see page 196), eggs, chicken or turkey sausage (beef and veggie okay too), ground beef or lamb, stew beef, goat cheese, plain nondairy yogurt, frozen boneless skinless chicken breasts and thighs, chicken breasts (bone in, skin on), lentils, dried split peas, black beans, chickpeas

SWEETENERS

Honey, brown sugar, maple syrup, coconut sugar

GRAINS

Pancake mix (paleo or gluten free), buckwheat flour (or other gluten-free flour mix), gluten-free bread, granola, gluten-free cornmeal flour, gluten-free lasagna noodles, lentil or soybean pasta, rolled oats or granola, corn tortillas

SUPPLEMENTS

B vitamins, iron, adrenal adaptogens, magnesium

HERBS AND SPICES

Turmeric, salt, pepper, nutmeg, arrowroot powder, vanilla extract, paprika, ground red pepper, Mexican oregano, cumin, baking soda, garlic powder, parsley, iodized salt or pink salt, garlic salt, Italian seasoning, cacao powder

OTHER/MISCELLANEOUS

Dark chocolate chips, chocolate chips, walnuts, unsweetened coconut flakes, coconut milk (rice or almond milk okay too), coconut oil, olive oil, ghee, grass-fed butter, chia seeds, coconut cream, green olives, diced tomatoes, canned crushed tomatoes, red enchilada sauce, sun-dried tomatoes, almond or cashew butter, sliced almonds, marinara sauce, nutritional yeast flakes, kalamata/Greek olives, Dijon mustard, white beans, chicken or veggie broth, Brazil nuts, almonds, cereal (your choice), coconut flour, skewers

PHASE 2/WEEK 2 MENU

	PRE-BREAKFAST Warming Tonic	BREAKFAST	LUNCH	SNACK	DINNER
MONDAY	Ginger Tea (page 199)	Greek Omelet (page 204)	Spinach and Kale Lasagna (page 249)	Thyroid Trail Mix (page 251)	Paleo Shepherd's Pie with ground beef or lamb (page 242)
TUESDAY	Honey Lemon Tea (page 199)	Protein Banana Bread with gluten-free flour (page 215)	Vegan Pasta with "Cheese" Sauce (page 248)	Kelp and Kale Chips (page 253)	Quick Cumin Chicken with Crunchy Kale Chips (page 241)
WEDNESDAY	Honey Turmeric Tea (page 200)	Nut Butter Sandwich with gluten-free bread (page 213)	Mason Jar Salads with chicken (page 216)	Chia Chocolates (page 251)	Black Bean Soup and Portable Tacos (page 227)
THURSDAY	Ginger Tea	Granola-Berry Parfait (page 211)	Bissara (page 231)	Snack Kebabs (page 254)	Oven "Grilled" Sea Bass with Wilted Spinach (page 234) and Roasted Cauliflower and Brussels Sprouts Chips (page 253)
FRIDAY	Honey Lemon Tea	2 or 3 Mini Protein Muffins with gluten-free flour (page 214)	Dairy-Free Tomato Soup (page 230) and Chicken Wings, your way (page 238)	Thyroid Trail Mix	Paleo Shepherd's Pie with ground beef or lamb
SATURDAY	Honey Turmeric Tea	Breakfast Skillet (page 205)	Chicken Salad with Avocado "Mayo" (page 218)	Kelp and Kale Chips	Sweet Potato Noodles with Cauliflower-Quinoa Meatballs in Tomato Sauce (page 250)
SUNDAY	Ginger Tea	It's Not Really French Toast with gluten-free bread (page 210)	Greek Salad with Chicken or Chickpeas (page 221)	Chia Chocolates	Chicken Soup (page 228)

PHASE 3/WEEK 3: RESET AND REBUILD YOUR GUT

Savvy Chicks have gut issues—many discussed previously, both in "Common Savvy Chick Conditions" at the beginning of this chapter and in Chapter 6, about Boss Ladies. Irritable bowel syndrome, reflux, constipation, and diarrhea are just a few of the many digestive ailments a Savvy Chick may battle. A gut check is important for Savvy Chicks, even if it is not their starting step, as it is with Boss Ladies. The gut issues of the Boss Lady are often expressed in Savvy Chicks as well—that's why it's important to prevent inflammation and help support the immune system in the gut. Savvy Chicks have the Boss Lady fire, so getting gut smart can prevent a lifetime of digestive issues.

Week 3 Action Steps

STEP 8: EAT PROBIOTIC-RICH FOODS FOR GOOD GUT BACTERIA

The same probiotic-rich foods that protect a Boss Lady's gut will make a good defense for Savvy Chicks as well. These are foods with a range of live bacteria that support the digestive system. You will rotate and alternate these power foods over the next 7 days and beyond to successfully build microbial diversity, which is a fancy way of saying that you will contribute to a range of helpful bacteria already living in your belly.

I make sure to eat one of the foods below each day—it's something I recommend to all my Savvy Chicks. To keep it simple, I've incorporated these foods into your Week 3 menu on page 132! Again, if you are not using the suggested menus, don't feel like you have to eat all of the probiotic foods listed below. You can pick and choose your favorites; just remember, the more variety, the better for your gut.

- 1 cup unsweetened nondairy yogurt in a breakfast berry parfait (see page 211 for recipe)
- 4 to 6 ounces fat-free unsweetened nondairy kefir in a breakfast smoothie (see page 194 for recipe ideas)
- 1 cup kombucha (see page 98 for more information)
- 1 slice fermented sourdough bread
- 1 cup Dr. Taz's Spicy Bone Broth (page 226)

STEP 9: SUPPLEMENT TO PROTECT YOUR GUT LINING

1. **Take slippery elm, glutamine, or aloe vera juice every morning.** Just like Boss Ladies, Savvy Chicks need to rebuild their gut lining to keep their digestive system humming at top-notch levels. Here are a few tricks to heal that leaky gut (for more information, see page 99). Choose ONE of the following supplements and take it for 2 or 3 days. If you tolerate it well, stick with it as a daily morning supplement. If you have any adverse reactions like diarrhea or abdominal pain, try one of the others. Once you find one that works well, stick with that.

   ☐ Slippery elm, 500 milligrams

   ☐ Glutamine, 2 to 3 grams

   ☐ Aloe vera juice, 1 to 2 ounces (not an aloe vera supplement)

   See Resources, page 316, for product information.

2. **Optimize your digestion by adding a digestive enzyme.** just like Boss Ladies, Savvy Chicks need to help their digestive systems digest. Business meetings, flights, lunches and dinners out and about at all different times—all of this can wreak havoc on your digestive system. Here is a Savvy Chick tip that I have found helpful: Carry digestive enzymes wherever you go. You can use these before or after a meal or during a week of stressful deadlines. I usually take one before my heaviest meal of the day, normally lunch. Digestive enzymes help to break your foods

"Before Super Woman Rx, I suffered chronically from bloating, constipation, and abdominal pain. After I started using glutamine, my symptoms all went away and I felt fantastic. My family has noticed that I have more energy and am spending more time with them, instead of napping on the couch. My daughter commented that my clothes were getting loose and fitting me better. The whole family has joined me in eating Dr. Taz's Super Woman Rx way—more veggies and less pizza—and everyone loves it."—**Julie, 56, super mom and window washer**

down a little more easily so your body can absorb the nutrients from all the great foods you are eating! For more information and recommendations, see "Vitamins and Supplements You Need to Know," page 45.

STEP 10: TAKE A MINDFUL GADGET BREAK

This last step gives my Savvy Chicks an extra boost to help them happily and healthfully navigate their world. I'm betting that this will be the most challenging step of all, since Savvy Chicks are usually inundated with e-mails and phone calls and deadlines, but *nothing* robs Savvy Chick energy faster than the multitasking electronic world. The demand to be both creative and a leader and strategist is draining, but creativity and expressive thought are robbed when the constant lure of e-mails, voice mails, and texts call to you. Trust me—I live this challenge daily. Stay off your electronics for at least 3 hours each day this last week of your plan. I am being generous because I don't want your businesses or projects to shut down—even one hour can be tough for some of us, but you can do it!

I know how you operate. There is probably no time when you are not thinking, plotting, or creating. Give these gadget breaks a try. I know it sounds counterintuitive, but I promise that you'll see your energy and brilliance soar. During this time I suggest that you try one of the following gadget-free mind-body practices.

- ◆ Add in an extra 15 minutes of grounding exercise from Step 3— yoga, tai chi, or qi gong. See page 258 for routines.
- ◆ Meditate for 10 minutes daily. Use meditation apps like Headspace or guided imagery and meditation tapes. More suggestions are on page 288.
- ◆ Journal. Putting pen to paper is powerful and can rewire the mind. Just write—get stuff out of your head and onto paper to declutter your mind. One of my all-time favorite books taught me to do this— *The Artist Way* by Julia Cameron, with her legendary morning pages. It has been instrumental in my own journey, and I have seen this book help so many of my patients. Also, be sure to see the writing exercises in Chapter 12, page 257, which are adapted from Cameron's book.

WEEK 3 SHOPPING LIST

PRODUCE

Ginger, lemons, bananas, peaches, berries, apples, pears, frozen mixed berries, frozen pineapple, frozen mango, onions, garlic, leeks, mushrooms, Brussels sprouts, spinach, arugula, romaine lettuce, tomatoes, basil, cilantro, mint, oregano, bell pepper, sweet potatoes, avocados, lime, potatoes, zucchini or summer squash, celery, scallions, dill, grapes, kelp, kale

PROTEINS

Vanilla protein powder (see page 196), eggs, chicken or turkey sausage (beef and veggie okay too), ground beef or lamb, goat cheese, plain nondairy yogurt, frozen boneless skinless chicken breasts and thighs, chicken breasts (bone in, skin on), chickpeas, lentils, dried split peas, 3 lbs bones (mix of chicken, goat, or beef), Cheddar cheese

SWEETENERS

Honey, brown sugar, maple syrup

GRAINS

Pancake mix (paleo or gluten free), gluten-free baking mix, buckwheat flour (or other gluten-free flour mix), gluten-free bread, granola, gluten-free cornmeal flour, gluten-free lasagna noodles, lentil or soybean pasta, rolled oats, quinoa, fermented sourdough bread (gluten-free preferred)

SUPPLEMENTS

B vitamins, iron, adrenal adaptogens, magnesium, digestive enzyme, glutamine, slippery elm, aloe vera juice (see Resources on page 316 for brand and buying suggestions)

HERBS AND SPICES

Turmeric, salt and pepper, nutmeg, arrowroot powder, vanilla extract, paprika, ground red pepper, Mexican oregano, cumin, baking soda, garlic powder, parsley, garlic salt, Italian seasoning, cinnamon, garam marsala

OTHER/MISCELLANEOUS

Chocolate chips, dark chocolate chips, walnuts, unsweetened coconut flakes, shredded unsweetened coconut, coconut milk (rice or almond milk okay too), coconut oil, olive oil, ghee, grass-fed butter, chia seeds, coconut cream, green olives, diced tomatoes, canned crushed tomatoes, tomato paste, red enchilada sauce, sun-dried tomatoes, almond butter, sliced almonds, marinara sauce, nutritional yeast flakes, Dijon mustard, white beans, chicken or veggie broth, chickpeas, Brazil nuts, almonds, cereal (your choice), coconut flour, skewers, fat-free unsweetened kefir, kombucha

PHASE 3/WEEK 3 MENU

	PRE-BREAKFAST Warming Tonic	BREAKFAST	LUNCH	SNACK (choose one)	DINNER
MONDAY	Ginger Tea (page 199)	Granola-Berry Parfait (page 211)	Spiced Lentil Cakes with Chickpeas (page 246)	Thyroid Trail Mix (page 251)	Curry in a Hurry with chicken or chickpeas (page 239)
TUESDAY	Honey Lemon Tea (page 199)	Coconut Chia Seed Pudding (page 212)	Middle Eastern Chicken Skewers (page 235) and 1 slice sourdough bread	Kelp and Kale Chips (page 253)	Paleo Shepherd's Pie, with grass-fed ground beef or lamb (page 242)
WEDNESDAY	Honey Turmeric Tea (page 200)	Breakfast Skillet (page 205)	Chicken Saag (page 237) and Crunchy Kale Chips (page 252)	Chia Chocolates (page 251)	Sweet Potato Noodles with Cauliflower-Quinoa Meatballs in Tomato Sauce (page 250) and 1 cup Dr. Taz's Spicy Bone Broth (page 226)
THURSDAY	Ginger Tea	Tropical Delight, made with kefir (page 195)	Bissara (page 231)	Snack Kebabs (page 254)	Faux Fried Coconut Chicken with Honey Mustard Dipping Sauce (page 236) and Warm Quinoa and Green Bean Salad (page 222)
FRIDAY	Honey Lemon Tea	Protein Banana Bread (page 215)	Mason Jar Salads with chicken (page 216)	Thyroid Trail Mix	Vegan Pasta with "Cheese" Sauce (page 248) and 1 cup Dr. Taz's Spicy Bone Broth
SATURDAY	Honey Turmeric Tea	Granola-Berry Parfait	Lettuce Roll-Ups with ground beef or lamb (page 222)	Kelp and Kale Chips	Paleo Shepherd's Pie, with grass-fed ground beef or lamb

	PRE-BREAKFAST Warming Tonic	BREAKFAST	LUNCH	SNACK (choose one)	DINNER
SUNDAY	Ginger Tea	Greek Omelet (page 204) and 1 slice fermented sourdough bread	Chicken Salad with Avocado "Mayo" (page 218)	Chia Chocolates	Persian Eggplant with Yellow Split Peas and Dried Lime (page 245)

IT'S JUST 10 STEPS over 21 days, but I know this plan will change you and your health—and most importantly—your life! Stick with this prescription for another 6 weeks (about 2 months total), and after that go back and revisit the Mojo Meter in Chapter 2 and the Power Type Test in Chapter 3. If you find that you test as a different Power Type, you can give that 3-Week Power Plan a try. If you remain a Savvy Chick, redo this 3-Week Power Rx by following the shopping lists, the 3-week menus, and all 10 action steps (see page 118). You can spice up the variety by substituting in new meals (an egg dish for an egg dish or a salad for a salad, for example) using the recipes in Chapter 10. Just be sure to choose options that have similar calories, protein, fat, and carbs.

CHAPTER 8

THE EARTH MAMAS' 3-WEEK RX

CARING, COMPASSIONATE, NURTURING—THESE are the words that come to my mind as I reflect on my Earth Mama patients. I know you natural caregivers thrive when thinking and doing for others, but too much giving—or playing the peacemaker and people pleaser—and you get drained and no longer feel *alive*. Keeping you Earth Mamas balanced and happy keeps you and your family humming, allowing you to be the epicenter for all—as you were meant to be.

There are so many Earth Mamas in my practice. As mothers and caretakers, many of us have an element of this nurturing energy in our psyche. But Earth Mamas are different. They live, breathe, and exist for others—they cannot help it, this is who they are. From being the sole caregiver of elderly parents to the busy mother of four children, my Earth Mamas give a lot. My own mother-in-law may be the ultimate Earth Mama—she is selfless and devoted. It took me a while to understand that she reveled in her ability to serve, and that what I saw as "chores" she saw always as an opportunity to help and serve others.

Out of balance, Earth Mamas lose the ability to give and are not able to be themselves. Not only can they no longer do the one thing that they are often the most passionate about—nurturing others—but they begin to retreat, withdraw, and become vulnerable to a host of medical conditions. Let's take a look.

||||||||||||||||||||||||||||||||||||||||||||||||||||||||||||||||||||||||||||||||||||||||||||||||||||||||

Earth Mama at a Glance

ALTER EGO: THE NURTURER AND THE PEACEMAKER

Super powers: When they're fully balanced, Earth Mamas are strong, steady, and stable—full of calm energy and great physical strength. Vibrantly healthy Earth Mamas are grounded, nurturing, and compassionate. These Power Types are known for bringing people together, make great mediators and peacemakers and reliable friends, and are the bedrock of the family.

Kryptonite: Overcommitting, people-pleasing, weight gain, isolation. Earth Mamas are prone to worry and meddling. When they get in an off-kilter state of mind, Earth Mamas are vulnerable to being taken advantage of, falling into the role of caretaker of the whole world, leaving no time to care for themselves.

Elements: Earth/Wood. The earth is a balance of both energies—yin and yang—and wood represents the nurturing quality of this element. The earth has a centering quality and is associated with hard work, nurturing, harmony, and practicality. When in the shadow of imbalance, this element can be over-protective (as in helicopter parenting) or have trouble setting boundaries.

Personality: Earth Mamas are caring and compassionate, the party organizers, full of warmth. Everyone gravitates toward them.

Body type: Large or heavy frame. Tendency to be overweight or obese when out of balance.

Celebrity example: Oprah Winfrey. Besides the entire world watching her weight struggles, Winfrey is known for being the quintessential down-to-earth best friend to women everywhere, and in some ways feels like the mother of us all. Winfrey has the luminescent skin and hair that I often experience in my Earth Mama patients. Personality-wise, this famous Earth Mama is known for her generosity (her Angel Network) and her compassion (her work in South Africa).

Colors: Brown, beige, and earth tones. These, of course, are all down-to-earth, comfortable tones that signify stability, structure, and support. They are grounding, nurturing, and warm.

||||||||||||||||||||||||||||||||||||||||||||||||||||||||||||||||||||||||||||||||||||||||||||||||||||||||

COMMON EARTH MAMA CONDITIONS

Below are the most common risks, illnesses, and conditions that I see in my Earth Mama patients. You may not be experiencing all the conditions listed, but they are the ones I see most often in the Earth Mamas I treat. If you identify with this Power Type, then chances are your days are filled with taking care of others, but not necessarily yourself. Read on to learn about a few of the red flags that can become roadblocks to your health and to your becoming your optimal self. I urge you to learn more about Earth Mama conditions and risk factors, then read on for the 3-Week Power Plan that will have you back to your happy, healthy, and grounded self.

Weight Gain/Obesity

While everyone has her own story, most of my Earth Mamas struggle in some form or fashion with maintaining a healthy weight. It may be weight they cannot lose or weight they've gained over many years; it could be that they've always carried extra weight—even as a child. The common denominator is that this weight is usually localized to the abdomen, arms, or back—classic places for insulin-based patterns of overweight and obesity. You can even see this in young children, where weight accumulates in their bellies.

The source of excess weight for Earth Mamas can be found in dysfunctional or imbalanced insulin regulation and its connection to the microbiome (aka: gut bacteria). It's important to note that this is also the reason that many of our kids are overweight (nearly 13 million in the United States), and why about 50 percent of women (not just Earth Mamas) today struggle with excess abdominal fat (which I discuss in my book *The 21-Day Belly Fix*). In many ways, insulin regulation, with its challenges and consequences, is a national epidemic. While doctors, researchers, and public health officials struggle to find the answers, most agree that insulin regulation is affected by the interaction of our food choices with our gut microbiome, hormones, stress, and sleep patterns—a complex web that can be tough to untangle and understand.

As we take a look at the medical conditions common to Earth Mamas, you'll see that the majority can be traced back to this insulin-microbiome connection and that this theme will continue to repeat itself. Altered insulin regulation triggers inflammation. Inflammation begins in response to a disrupted gut and causes obesity. In your Power Plan, we are going to tackle this insulin-gut connection head-on by taking time to work on your digestive health and to stabilize your insulin levels. Little things, like eating consistently, not eating late, and sleeping restfully, can make amazing differences in insulin and gut balance.

Depression

Earth Mamas out of balance get depressed—there really is no other way of saying it. They retreat, isolate themselves, almost disappear, and that is so contrary to the very thing that makes them tick—caring for people! Depression is a sign of disconnection from yourself, your spirit, and your purpose. It may start with feelings of frustration and disappointment but then transition to excessive sleep, dreading the day, and gaining weight due to disordered eating and lack of movement. It's a downward spiral because feeling bad, overeating, and being lazy feed into feelings of depression, which lead right back to more overeating and then not wanting to move.

Not on my watch! I am going to show you how to break the pattern and get back into the mix—back to being *you*. In your Power Plan, you will learn to care for yourself and guard against depression so that you will never find yourself battling this disease. Knowing this information allows you to be proactive—not reactive. By learning to listen to your body's clues, you will catch yourself before you fall into a cycle that leads to depression. I am going to help you learn your body, set boundaries, and stay balanced.

Cardiovascular Disease

With the dual tendencies toward insulin resistance and inflammation, it is no surprise that cardiovascular disease is a risk factor for Earth Mamas. It's almost like they are more prone to heartbreak—and heart disease. When we look to our ancestors in Chinese medicine and Ayurveda, they understood this connection: When the heart endures too much emotional stress, it results in disease. In fact, chronic stress to the heart meridian over time in Chinese medicine was a prescription—an Rx—for heart disease.

You can prevent cardiovascular disease—including clogged arteries, heart attacks, and plaque buildup—by following an Earth Mama diet and Power Plan.

Hypertension

Weight and chronic inflammation burden the heart and can lead to high blood pressure, since the heart has to work harder and harder to maintain good bloodflow. High blood pressure will affect energy, mood, and sleep. Many of the nutritional deficiencies of Earth Mamas can also trigger hypertension. Tracking your blood pressure and keeping it in a healthy range (100–120/60–80) should be a goal for all Earth Mamas. In your Power Plan, we will address the necessary diet and supplement changes to maintain good blood pressure.

Diabetes/Prediabetes

Insulin resistance, with belly fat and high blood pressure, completes the triad that makes up metabolic syndrome (also called syndrome X), a precursor to diabetes. Not surprisingly, Earth Mamas are at an increased risk for becoming diabetic. Irregular blood sugar levels trigger and alter insulin levels, first increasing blood glucose levels. These are then reflected in A1C levels—a lab marker that shows average blood sugar over a 3-month time frame. Early stages of prediabetes include weight gain, hypoglycemia (sudden drops in blood sugar), and changes in energy. Your 3-Week Power Plan will remove foods that trigger exaggerated insulin spikes and include foods to stabilize blood sugar. You'll also incorporate movement throughout your day, which helps increase insulin sensitivity and balance.

Joint Pain

Either due to the accumulation of weight or to the ongoing inflammation triggered by insulin irregularity, joint pain can be a common issue for Earth Mamas. Swollen, tender, or achy joints can be symptoms that affect the quality of life and energy for an Earth Mama. I have witnessed firsthand the frustration on an Earth Mama's face when she is desperate to exercise but completely limited by her pain and inability to move.

Constipation

Gastrointestinal issues, specifically constipation, affect Earth Mamas as well. Many Earth Mamas have altered microbiomes or an imbalance of good gut bacteria. This will affect the health of the GI tract and the ability to eliminate, again increasing inflammation. In fact, most Earth Mamas have an excess of candida, or overgrowth of yeast in the gut, further affecting insulin regulation.

Fatty Liver

Your liver is the largest organ inside your body, and it is involved with hormonal balance, immune system function, and the production of bile (involved in the breakdown of fat during digestion). It also regulates blood clotting; aids digestion; detoxifies alcohol, foods, supplements, and medications; and provides vitamins and minerals including B_{12}, iron, and copper. As you can see, the liver has a lot of demands to keep up with under the best circumstances. When the liver becomes overburdened by overweight and obesity and improper insulin function (in the case of diabetes or prediabetes), it accumulates fatty deposits that impair its ability to complete all its functions. An untreated fatty liver will continue to worsen insulin regulation, impair metabolism, and accelerate the cycles of inflammation.

Chinese Meridian Diagnosis: Spleen Meridian Deficiency

In Traditional Chinese Medicine (TCM), the spleen is known as the master digestive meridian—the regulator and the controller of the entire digestive system. The spleen is related to food and fluids and how they are transformed into usable nutrients. Spleen meridian deficiency is also associated with weight gain and digestive issues.

In Chinese medicine, when the spleen meridian is weak the body becomes damp (retains water), it holds on to fat, and there is a recognizable slowing of the entire digestive system. Worry, fear, and anxiety are the emotions that TCM believes lead to the spleen meridian dampening and weakening further.

Ayurvedic Dosha Diagnosis: Kapha

The Ayurvedic dosha kapha is known for protection, loyalty, and love and is the most dominant dosha in most Earth Mamas. When in balance, Earth Mamas are naturally calm and thoughtful. This Power Type, when in optimal health and balance, tends to be patient, steady, and supportive. Remember, Earth Mamas are the center of a community and a family. But when out of balance, kaphas can overstay and hold on to jobs and relationships, even when they become unhealthy and destructive. This can manifest as stubbornness and avoidance.

Kaphas, in Ayurvedic medicine (similar to Chinese medicine), hold on to water and fat and have slower metabolisms and a tendency to oversleep. Common recommendations for kaphas from an Ayurvedic practitioner would include eliminating or minimizing sugar, salt, and fat in the diet, not oversleeping, and incorporating some form of movement every day. You'll be doing all of the above in your 3-Week Power Plan.

Hormone Imbalances: Estrogen and Insulin

The most common hormone imbalances for kaphas center around estrogen and insulin. As promised, the theme of insulin regulation appears yet again! We know Earth Mamas struggle with insulin—the reason behind weight gain and fatigue—but they also battle higher-than-average estrogen levels, making the entire insulin issue worse. It's like a vicious cycle— high estrogen triggers or worsens insulin resistance, resulting in more weight gain and then—yes—more estrogen. Frustrating!

This cycle, known commonly as estrogen dominance, can trigger many high-estrogen symptoms, including tender breasts, weight gain in the hips, migraines, heavy periods, or even midcycle spotting.

LAB FINDINGS

The results of merging the Chinese medicine concept of spleen meridian deficiency with the Ayurvedic diagnosis of kapha actually match up with specific modern-day labs. Take a look at the common lab findings in my Earth Mamas (see page 49 for more).

- ◆ High cholesterol
- ◆ High inflammation markers—C-reactive protein (CRP), erythrocyte sedimentation rate (ESR), and homocysteine

- High insulin and C-peptides
- High estrone (an estrogen metabolite indicative of estrogen dominance)
- High estradiol (estradiol is a circulating hormone; high levels or poor metabolism result in estrogen dominance)
- Altered antinuclear antibodies, or ANA (another marker of inflammation)
- Positive *Candida* antibodies in blood or stool (a reflection of yeast in the gut)

Nutritional Needs/Deficiencies

The nutritional needs of Earth Mamas focus on foods and micronutrients that improve the digestive system, ease and prevent inflammation, and generate energy. For this reason, you'll see more protein and healthy fats in your 3-Week Plan and fewer carbohydrates. Earth Mamas tend to have a very poor carbohydrate tolerance. Further, micronutrient deficiencies, including not enough B vitamins, amino acids, magnesium, and omega-3 fats, are common to Earth Mamas, so these nutrients will be included in your plan.

Finally, probiotic-rich foods are a powerful help in balancing the gut microbiome. Dr. Taz's Spicy Bone Broth (page 226) can help the gut further and is also incorporated in your Power Plan.

LONG-TERM DISEASE RISKS

Problems with insulin regulation and estrogen metabolism are two well-defined hormone patterns for Earth Mamas. These patterns contribute to a greater risk of cardiovascular disease and diseases of inflammation. Inflammation is the driver of the majority of diseases we see today, but a key factor in the rise of cancer and autoimmune disease. Diabetes is a common Earth Mama risk as well.

Preventing these conditions makes following the plan so much more critical for an Earth Mama, as she is more vulnerable to these conditions over the long term, especially if insulin and estrogen issues go unchecked.

HOW THE EARTH MAMA 3-WEEK RX WORKS

Get ready, Earth Mamas—at the end of your plan, I know you will feel on fire and ready to reembrace your world. I will have you back to nurturing your friends, communities, or families—but this time, with better boundaries for yourself.

My biggest challenge with Earth Mamas is getting them to take care of themselves. Because of their unique mix of genetics, hormonal chemistry, and nutritional needs, I find that Earth Mamas often struggle with managing their weight and often fight depression. It's almost as if their bodies, as the Ayurvedic term kapha describes, hold on to water and fat, risking Earth Mama energy. Over time, weight challenges can lead to mood issues or vice versa, and the giving Earth Mama can become a shadow of her true self.

The Earth Mama Rx Rules

1. **Eat every 3 hours.** Pace your snacks and meals to come every 3 hours. If breakfast is at 7 a.m., a snack should come at 10 a.m., lunch by 1 p.m., and so on. Earth Mamas do best if they eat their breakfast by 9 a.m. at the latest.

2. **Track your daily food and calories.** I see my Earth Mamas succeed the best when they track their food and calories, especially while following their 3-Week Rx. That means writing down everything you eat and drink every day all day *and* counting your calories. Limit yourself to 1,800 calories per day.

3. **Get your protein from plant-based sources.** It's important for Earth Mamas to get the majority of their protein from plant-based sources, meaning mostly vegetables. Aim to get about 60 grams of protein each day. See "Best Nonmeat Sources of Protein" on page 147.

4. **Modify your carb and fat intake.** My Earth Mamas do best when they eat a diet that encourages their bodies to burn fat instead of carbs. You do this by limiting your carbohydrates to a daily maximum of 100 grams of whole grains, vegetables, and fruits and keeping fats to 20 to 30 grams per day from *healthy* sources. Examples are the omega-3 fats found in fatty fish like salmon and tuna, nuts, and seeds like chia and flax and

THE 10 EARTH MAMA ACTION STEPS
AT A GLANCE

The following 10 steps capture the Earth Mama's entire 3-week plan. Combine this checklist with the above Earth Mama Rules and you've got everything you need for super powered living in one place. Read on, and you'll see that I've chopped this down into weekly, bite-size segments that start with the first four steps in the first week and build from there. Remember, a complete suggested menu and shopping list follow each week's action steps.

Step 1: Eat Every 3 Hours

Step 2: Create a Better Plate
- ☐ Eat proper portions
- ☐ Eat the correct ratio of protein to carbs

Step 3: Go Sugar Free

Step 4: Remove Meat, Dairy, and Poultry

Step 5: Begin the Liver Lover Cleanse
- ☐ Apple cider vinegar (ACV) tonic
- ☐ Dandelion tea
- ☐ Liver Lover Smoothie

Step 6: Take Clean-Liver Supplements
- ☐ Probiotics
- ☐ Choline
- ☐ Digestive enzymes
- ☐ B-complex vitamins
- ☐ Magnesium

Step 7: Add Gut-Builders
- ☐ Bone broth
- ☐ Kitchari

Step 8: Evaluate Your Relationships

Step 9: Add Self-Nurture Time
- ☐ Part 1: Physical Nurturing
- ☐ Part 2: Emotional Nurturing

Step 10: Reconnect
- ☐ Cultivate healthy relationships
- ☐ Balance for beauty

medium-chain fats like coconut oil or ghee. Newer research is showing that fat actually stabilizes insulin, sometimes better than protein.

5. **Maximize fiber and go sugar free.** Aim for 40 to 50 grams of fiber per day, and eliminate all sugars from your diet. You can include two servings of whole fresh fruit per day, but avoid higher-sugar varieties like mangoes and bananas.

6. **Balance your protein-to-carb ratio.** This is important for Earth Mamas. When making your meals, limit your carbs to a quarter of your plate. Protein gets another quarter, and your vegetables should cover half your plate.

7. **Go dairy free.** Dairy can worsen yeast or candida in the gut affecting insulin.

Note: If you follow the suggested menus at the end of each week's plan, you'll succeed at reaching all these goals.

Each of the following 3 weeks will include and detail a set number of action steps, with Week 2 building upon Week 1, and Week 3 building upon the first 2 weeks. For each phase/week, you'll find that week's action steps, followed by a suggested menu and a shopping list of everything you'll need to have on hand for that week. Incorporate the above rules and the action steps that follow and you'll activate your super powers every day!

PHASE 1/WEEK 1: BALANCE YOUR INSULIN LEVELS

Insulin is a hormone produced in response to our food. If you eat too many high-sugar and/or refined carbohydrate foods, your insulin will respond by spiking up and then crashing down, which leaves you drained. Too many high-fat foods? Your insulin levels and your digestion will struggle to get cranking, almost like a car sputtering around as it runs out of gas.

We'll begin this first week by addressing insulin balance and regulation with a focus on getting your blood sugar balanced—no highs and lows—and that means no hitting the sweets or greasy food for comfort or energy. Instead you'll improve your insulin sensitivity by adopting specific food choices and eating patterns.

Are you ready to get back in balance, back to your nurturing, caring, energized self? With the spleen as the weakest meridian and kapha as the most dominant Ayurvedic element, for Earth Mamas, I have found that balancing insulin and blood sugar are the biggest medical challenges and the best places to start. Ready to feel amazing?

Week 1 Action Steps

STEP 1: EAT EVERY 3 HOURS

Eating at regular intervals is important for all of us, but unlike the other types, it's critical for Earth Mamas. This is a key step to preventing the highs and lows of fluctuating insulin levels and important to keeping your energy optimized. Many Earth Mamas will tell me that they don't eat breakfast or forget to eat all day—and then don't understand why they might be gaining weight or feeling "low." Often this is because an Earth Mama will skip breakfast and maybe even lunch, and then be so starving by dinner and on into the evening that she eats more than she thinks. Plus, insulin levels spike and plummet without consistent eating, which signals the body to store fat. The solution is to eat every 3 to 4 hours. That way you will keep your energy flowing and keep your meals more manageable.

STEP 2: CREATE A BETTER PLATE

Earth Mamas are more vulnerable than other Power Types to high carbohydrate loads and big portions. Think back to the overall slowing of the digestive system that both Ayurvedic and Chinese medicine describe for Earth Mamas. Our goal is to beat this natural inclination by helping you perfect your plate. This step is all about learning to monitor your protein-to-carbohydrate ratios. Earth Mamas, due to issues with insulin, have a very low carbohydrate tolerance. They thrive on a lower-carbohydrate, higher-protein, and healthy fat diet, which keeps insulin stable longer.

- **Eat proper portions.** This means smaller servings of food, and this is the second half of Step 1. Large meals are tough on an Earth Mama stomach, and they tend to happen when you restrict or skip eating for long periods of time, so yes, you'll do better when you eat smaller meals more often. An easy way to accomplish this is to simply switch your plates—trade out a large dinner plate for a smaller one, and downsize your bowls. Limit yourself to the food allowed in these smaller dishes rather than going back for more. Another trick is to simply eat half of your normal serving size.

◆ **Eat the correct ratio of protein to carbs.** Make protein and vegetables your dominant foods at every meal. Limit any carb to a quarter of your plate, or a quarter of what you are eating. For example, let's say you are out and decide on eating a sandwich—usually, two slices of bread with a side of something. Either remove a piece of bread and have a side of vegetables, or cut the sandwich in half. If you want to do the numbers, aim for 15 to 20 grams of protein and keep carbohydrates under 30 grams at each meal, while loading up on fresh, healthy veggies.

Of course, you have no worries if you eat directly from the menu on your 3-Week Power Plan, but these strategies come in handy if you have to attend a business lunch or are traveling.

STEP 3: GO SUGAR FREE

Sugar is an energy zapper. There is no room for sugar in an Earth Mama's chemistry, and that means all sugars, including honey, stevia, Splenda, brown sugar, coconut sugar, and alcohol—you name it and I'd probably tell you to nix it from your menu. Some of these sugars may be less insulin provoking than others, but to get the best results over the course of the next 21 days, sugar in all its hidden forms—including alcohol—is out. So sorry to be the party pooper. The news isn't all a downer: Enjoy up to two pieces of fruit per day for natural sweetness.

Sugar creates a reaction in the body that results in a quick insulin spike and then a hard crash, giving you a momentary sensation of energy, comfort, and pleasure but quickly leaving you fatigued, dejected, and craving more—almost like chasing that crush you had back in school. Remember the guy who'd give you a few kernels of encouragement to hang on to but never enough to commit? You know the inner dialogue: from the high of "He likes me!" to the low of

"Wait, he's ignoring me." Anyhow, I digress. The bottom line is that highs and lows are *out* for the next 21 days. The payoff is worth it. You will change your taste buds and your entire energy equation by simply removing sugar—which I think is a prescription-free, unlabeled drug for all of us.

STEP 4: REMOVE MEAT, DAIRY, AND POULTRY

The sluggish digestion of the Earth Mama makes digesting meat, dairy, and poultry tough, adding to the burden of the digestive system and slowing down metabolism overall. This may seem reminiscent of what I've said about my Boss Ladies, but there is a critical difference—the Earth Mama does not necessarily have a lot of "fire" that needs cooling, or a digestive system that is necessarily out of balance due to stress. This is just the way your digestive system works—it's slower and more methodical. Chances are that you have more of a sleepy digestive system that needs to be stimulated. Meat is tough on Earth Mama stomachs; it takes longer to digest and can *deplete* rather than *reenergize*. I have included some easy-to-digest fish in a couple of your dinner entrées. We'll reintroduce meat later in the program, but for now you and animal protein (except eggs) are on a break. (See "Best Nonmeat Sources of Protein" below.)

Follow these first four foundational steps consistently over the next 7 days, and you'll lay the groundwork for your best self.

BEST NONMEAT SOURCES OF PROTEIN

FOOD	SERVING/PROTEIN	FIBER/SERVING
Mung beans	1 cup/14 g	15 g
Lentils	1 cup/18 g	16 g
Edamame	1 cup/16 g	8 g
Quinoa	1 cup/8 g	5 g
Chia seeds	1 ounce/6 g	10 g
Chickpeas	1 cup/12 g	12 g
Eggs	2 eggs/15 g	0 g

WEEK 1 SHOPPING LIST

PRODUCE

Ginger, lemons, bananas, peaches, fresh berries, apples, pears, frozen mixed berries, frozen pineapple, frozen mango, onions, red onions, garlic, leeks, mushrooms, Brussels sprouts, spinach, arugula, romaine lettuce, tomatoes, basil, cilantro, mint, oregano, bell pepper, sweet potatoes, avocados, lime, potatoes, zucchini or summer squash, celery, scallions, dill, grapes, kelp, kale

PROTEINS

Vanilla and chocolate protein powder (see page 196), eggs, vegetarian sausage, lentils, dried split peas, mung beans

GRAINS

Pancake mix (gluten free or whole grain), gluten-free baking mix, buckwheat flour (or other gluten-free flour mix), gluten-free bread, gluten-free granola, gluten-free cornmeal flour, brown or white rice, lentil or soybean pasta, rolled oats, quinoa

HERBS AND SPICES

Turmeric, nutmeg, arrowroot powder, vanilla extract, paprika, ground red pepper, Mexican oregano, cumin, baking soda, garlic powder, parsley, garlic salt, Italian seasoning, cinnamon

OTHER/MISCELLANEOUS

Walnuts, unsweetened coconut flakes, unsweetened shredded coconut, coconut milk (rice or almond milk okay, too), coconut oil, olive oil, ghee, grass-fed butter, chia seeds, coconut cream, green olives, diced tomatoes, canned crushed tomatoes, red enchilada sauce, sun-dried tomatoes, almond butter, sliced almonds, marinara sauce, nutritional yeast flakes, Dijon mustard, white beans, chicken or veggie broth, chickpeas, Brazil nuts, almonds, cereal (your choice), coconut flour, skewers

"I started out feeling unsure about all the new recipes. Would I like them? How would they taste? But everything was delicious—totally worth it. It's funny because my favorite part of the Earth Mama plan ended up being all the new recipes. I am in LOVE with the Bissara lentil soup—the flavor is amazing! I even froze up some extra so I could come back to it another day, and it was seriously just as good reheated! I also loved the Kale Pesto and Eggplant Lettuce Wrap. And the Avocado "Mayo"—I could have eaten it by the spoonful (so good)! Whenever I had any of the wraps for lunch I felt super light afterward—it made me feel like I could go for a run immediately after I ate. I never had that "heavy" feeling you get after some meals."—**Melissa, 21, student**

PHASE 1/WEEK 1 MENU

	BREAKFAST	MIDMORNING SNACK	LUNCH	MIDAFTERNOON SNACK	DINNER
MONDAY	Egg-Veggie Roll-Up (use gluten-free baking mix) (page 207)	Kitchari (page 247)	Mason Jar Salads with chickpeas (page 216)	Kale and Kelp Chips (page 253)	Black Bean Soup and Portable Tacos (page 227)
TUESDAY	Chocolate Protein Smoothie (page 194)	Hummus and Veggies (page 255)	Kale Pesto and Eggplant Lettuce Wrap (page 223)	1 piece Avocado Toast (page 209)	Oven "Grilled" Sea Bass with Wilted Spinach (page 234)
WEDNESDAY	Paleo Quiche with Vegetarian Sausage and Sweet Potato Crust (page 204)	Kitchari	Portobello BLT (page 225)	Kale and Kelp Chips	Bissara (page 231)
THURSDAY	Chocolate Protein Smoothie	Lettuce Roll-Up (vegan) (page 222)	Festive Italian Frittata (page 206)	Dairy-Free Tomato Soup (page 230)	Vegan Pasta with "Cheese" Sauce (page 248)
FRIDAY	Egg-Veggie Roll-Up (use gluten-free baking mix)	Kitchari	Buckwheat Noodle and Kale Stir-Fry (page 244)	Kale and Kelp Chips	Salmon-Kale Caesar Salad (page 220)
SATURDAY	Paleo Quiche with Vegetarian Sausage and Sweet Potato Crust	Hummus and Veggies	Kale Pesto and Eggplant Lettuce Wrap	Rice Cake with Nut Butter (page 252)	Lettuce Roll-Up (page 222)
SUNDAY	Huevos Rancheros (omit cheese) (page 208)	Berry-Spinach Power Punch (page 202)	Spinach and Kale Lasagna (page 249)	Crunchy Kale Chips (page 252)	Oven "Grilled" Sea Bass with Wilted Spinach

PHASE 2/WEEK 2: WAKE UP YOUR LIVER AND GUT

I have mentioned the sleepy digestive system of the Earth Mama a few times already—hopefully you are not rolling your eyes—but now it's time to get more specific. The chemistry of the Earth Mama is one where the body wants to hold on to everything—food, emotions, sleep, and people.

This week, continue all the steps for Phase 1, but now it's cleanup time, and any effective cleanup plan has to start with the liver and the gut: They are your body's construction workers and cheerleaders and you cannot succeed without them. You'll also add three supplements that improve your insulin function and that of your liver and your gut. The final step for this week will be to add two recipes to your repertoire that are rich in healthy fats and easy on an Earth Mama's digestive system.

Here we go!

Week 2 Action Steps

STEP 5: BEGIN THE LIVER LOVER CLEANSE

Next step? A liver cleanse—a way to jump-start your liver, which can be affected by the highs and lows of insulin regulation. Fatty liver can be a common Earth Mama condition—a condition where, due to poor digestion, excess weight, and sluggish insulin, fat accumulates on the liver itself, impacting many other systems in the body. I am going to make this the simplest liver cleanse you have seen.

- **Apple cider vinegar (ACV) tonic.** Start every day with an apple cider vinegar and water tonic. (In a small glass, mix together 1 tablespoon vinegar and 3 tablespoons water). Apple cider vinegar helps with fatty liver and gut health by improving the gut microbiome and helping in the metabolism of fat. The best brands of vinegar are raw and organic.

- **Dandelion tea.** Drink a cup of dandelion tea daily. Dandelion is a liver purifier and can help support the liver. You can use tea bags or take a few teaspoons of dried chopped dandelion root (available in health food stores) and boil them in water for 10 minutes. Strain the mixture before drinking.

- **Liver Lover Smoothie.** Include the Liver Lover Smoothie (page 198) as your afternoon snack for further liver-cleansing benefits.

Easy, simple, and doable—time to move on to the next step.

STEP 6: TAKE CLEAN-LIVER SUPPLEMENTS

Staying focused on liver and gut cleanup, I have found the following supplements to be the most helpful to my Earth Mamas in my practice. Plan on taking all the following after breakfast or dinner (whichever works better for you).

- **Probiotics, 50 billion CFU:** We have talked a bunch about the microbiome because digestion is a key theme for my Earth Mamas. Probiotics are a must-have for stubborn digestive systems, as research mounts daily linking the disturbed microbiome to insulin regulation, depression, and more. Add a high-quality probiotic to your daily regimen. Look for probiotics with at least 50 billion CFU (colony forming units) and multiple strains. Take one per day with breakfast. Note: I am not encouraging a lot of probiotic-rich foods for the Earth Mama, since they often contain yeast. Yeast overgrowth is another medical challenge for many of my Earth Mamas and the root of their inability to tolerate sugar, alcohol, or refined carbohydrates.*

- **Choline, 1 gram per day:** Choline is a phospholipid that helps to metabolize fat and regulate insulin. It is found naturally in eggs and organ meats like liver, but I often have Earth Mama patients add 1 gram of choline as a daily supplement to facilitate liver support.

- **Digestive enzymes:** I discussed these in the previous two chapters, and here they are again—digestive enzymes! Earth Mamas need them too. Your sleepy digestive system needs a push to break down foods and keep your metabolism humming. Look for a product containing amylase, lipase, and protease, which help you break down starch, protein, and fat. I have seen a few digestive enzymes that contain ox bile, which also helps further with fat metabolism, but they may be harder to find. Take this supplement just before, during, or after your heaviest meal of the day.*

- **B-complex vitamins:** Adequate amounts of B vitamins are needed for a healthy liver and increased energy overall.*

- **Magnesium:** This supplement is vital for a healthy body and liver! Western science shows that magnesium deficiency is common in people with liver disease, while Traditional Chinese Medicine practitioners associate magnesium with liver function.*

*See "Vitamins and Supplements You Need to Know" on page 45 and reputable supplement brand recommendations in Resources, page 316.

STEP 7: ADD GUT-BUILDERS

One more step in your Phase 2 liver-gut plan—time to add the gut-builders. Gut-builders continue the work of building and balancing the microbiome, improving the working of your digestion and metabolism (your body's calorie-burning engine). Gut-builders are foods rich in healthy fats and easy on the digestive system. Check out the list below and in your menu plan.

Introduce one serving of either of the following gut-builders into your daily diet over the next 7 days.

- **Bone broth.** Long known as a healing food in Chinese and Ayurvedic medicine, bone broth is still prescribed as medicine to the sick, nursing moms, and anyone who has had a traumatic life event. The thought then—as is scientifically proven now—is that as the broth simmers, the bones release nutrients, collagen, and good bacteria that help you to reestablish a healthy gut. Even though this recipe uses beef and chicken bones, it doesn't contain the actual meat that Earth Mamas find difficult to digest. See page 226 for a bone broth recipe that I like, or you can order bone broth and have it delivered to your home (see Resources, page 316). When I was a child my family regularly made bone broth that I ate grudgingly—only to now force it on my own children.
- **Kitchari.** This is a traditional Indian dish made of an easily digestible and highly nutritious mix of rice and mung beans. Soaking the mung beans overnight and then cooking them under pressure makes them an easily digestible source of protein. The rice is purposely cooked to an almost mushy consistency, so that it is easy on the digestive system. See page 247 in Chapter 11 for a recipe.

Okay—2 weeks down. Your liver and gut are in better shape, you have bid sugar adieu, and your forced break from meat hopefully has you experimenting with other sources of protein. One more week to go!

WEEK 2 SHOPPING LIST

PRODUCE

Ginger, lemons, bananas, peaches, berries, apples, pears, frozen mixed berries, frozen pineapple, frozen mango, onions, garlic, leeks, mushrooms, Brussels sprouts, spinach, arugula, romaine lettuce, tomatoes, basil, cilantro, mint, oregano, bell pepper, sweet potatoes, avocados, lime, potatoes, zucchini or summer squash, celery, scallions, dill, grapes, kelp, kale

PROTEINS

Vanilla and chocolate protein powder (see page 196), eggs, chicken or turkey sausage (beef and veggie okay too), goat cheese, plain dairy-free yogurt, use dairy-free alternative cheese, frozen boneless skinless chicken breasts and thighs, chicken breasts (bone in, skin on), lentils, dried split peas

GRAINS

Pancake mix (paleo or gluten free), gluten-free baking mix, buckwheat flour (or other gluten-free flour mix), whole grain or gluten-free bread, gluten-free granola, gluten-free cornmeal flour, gluten-free lasagna noodles, lentil or soybean pasta, rolled oats, quinoa, brown or white rice

SUPPLEMENTS

Probiotics, choline, digestive enzymes

HERBS AND SPICES

Turmeric, salt and pepper, nutmeg, arrowroot powder, vanilla extract, paprika, ground red pepper, Mexican oregano, cumin, baking soda, garlic powder, parsley, garlic salt, Italian seasoning, cinnamon

OTHER/MISCELLANEOUS

Walnuts, unsweetened coconut flakes, unsweetened shredded coconut, coconut milk (rice or almond milk okay, too), coconut oil, olive oil, ghee, grass-fed butter, chia seeds, coconut cream, green olives, diced tomatoes, canned crushed tomatoes, red enchilada sauce, sun-dried tomatoes, almond butter, sliced almonds, marinara sauce, nutritional yeast flakes, Dijon mustard, white beans, chicken or veggie broth, chickpeas, Brazil nuts, almonds, cereal (your choice), coconut flour, skewers

PHASE 2/WEEK 2 MENU

	PRE-BREAKFAST	BREAKFAST	MIDMORNING SNACK	LUNCH	MIDAFTERNOON SNACK	DINNER
MONDAY	Apple cider vinegar (ACV) tonic (page 150)	Festive Italian Frittata, omit cheese, and enjoy ¼ of pie (page 206) and dandelion tea (page 150)	Hummus and Veggies (page 255)	Spiced Lentil Cakes (page 246) and 1 cup Dr. Taz's Spicy Bone Broth (page 226)	Liver Lover Smoothie (page 198) and 1 Egg-Veggie Roll-Up	Kabocha Squash Soup with Cauliflower-Quinoa Meatballs (page 232)
TUESDAY	ACV tonic	Avocado Toast (page 209) and dandelion tea	Berry-Spinach Power Punch (page 202)	Bissara (page 231)	Liver Lover Smoothie and Crunchy Kale Chips (page 252)	Kale Pesto and Eggplant Lettuce Wrap and Kitchari (page 247)
WEDNESDAY	ACV tonic	Tofu Scramble (page 209) and dandelion tea	½ cup Kabocha Squash Soup (page 232)	Mason Jar Salads with chickpeas (page 216) and 1 cup Dr. Taz's Spicy Bone Broth	Liver Lover Smoothie and Rice Cake with Nut Butter (page 252)	Greek Salad with Chickpeas (page 221)
THURSDAY	ACV tonic	Egg-Veggie Roll-Up (page 207) and dandelion tea	Hummus and Veggies	Bissara	Liver Lover Smoothie and Kale and Kelp Chips (page 253)	Sweet Potato Noodles with Cauliflower-Quinoa Meatballs (page 250) and Kitchari
FRIDAY	ACV tonic	Avocado Toast and dandelion tea	Lettuce Roll-Ups, vegan (page 222)	Kale Pesto and Eggplant Lettuce Wrap (page 223) and 1 cup Dr. Taz's Spicy Bone Broth	Liver Lover Smoothie and Rice Cake with Nut Butter	Oven "Grilled" Sea Bass with Wilted Spinach (page 234)
SATURDAY	ACV tonic	Breakfast Skillet (page 205) and dandelion tea	Lettuce Roll-Ups, vegan	Buckwheat Noodle and Kale Stir-Fry (page 244)	Liver Lover Smoothie and Avocado Toast	Salmon-Kale Caesar Salad (page 220) and Kitchari

	PRE-BREAKFAST	BREAKFAST	MIDMORNING SNACK	LUNCH	MIDAFTERNOON SNACK	DINNER
SUNDAY	ACV tonic	Tofu Scramble and dandelion tea	Sprouted Mung Beans (page 255)	Portobello BLT and 1 cup Dr. Taz's Spicy Bone Broth	Liver Lover Smoothie and Dairy-Free Tomato Soup (page 230)	Tandoori-Spiced Salmon with Yogurt Cucumber Sauce (page 233)

PHASE 3/WEEK 3: SET BOUNDARIES

I have mentioned a few times that the need for connection and the inability to let go of some emotional baggage are common challenges for Earth Mamas. I know this from my patients and from the many Earth Mamas that support me in my life—including the male version that I see in my hubby (that is probably a different book).

This last week of your 3-Week Rx will round out your Power Plan by taking you into the world of boundary setting. Here you'll practice what can be the biggest challenge for you nurturing Earth Mamas—taking care of yourself!

Phase 3 may be the most important part of your plan since in many ways you might find these steps to be your biggest challenge. There is such a flux between our mind, our hearts, and our bodies—and all have to be connected and balanced to fully access your super powers.

Week 3 Action Steps

STEP 8: EVALUATE YOUR RELATIONSHIPS

Relationships are the crux for an Earth Mama, and relationships that are too demanding or one-sided drain her energy, affecting her chemistry and biology more so than any other Power Type's. Many times, we are surrounded by relationships that require us to be the epicenter but also drain us and are not replenishing. Use these next 7 days to look closely at your relationships and answer the following relationship balance questions. Hopefully these will help you to identify the energy drains in your life and show you where you need to take time to care for yourself. You can do all the diet, supplement, and medical steps, but if there is a constant, nagging drain on your energy, the results will be minimal.

1. You are the giver in almost every single one of the relationships in your life. (Y/N)

2. You always put the needs of others before your own. (Y/N)

3. You feel overwhelmed with guilt when someone helps you. (Y/N)

4. You apologize more than three times a day. (Y/N)

5. You rarely stand up for yourself or your needs. (Y/N)

6. You don't believe that your friends and/or family will love you if you say no. (Y/N)

7. When you are completely honest with yourself, a big part of your giving and doing is because of a desire to feel loved, liked, or admired. (Y/N)

Pay attention to these statements this week. If you notice a pattern of yes answers, you may not be giving yourself the self-care you need. Make sure that you prioritize the next two steps.

STEP 9: ADD SELF-NURTURE TIME

This is a two-part step that will address two critical needs for every Earth Mama—physical exercise and emotional nurturing. Earth Mamas tend to neglect their own needs in favor of their other life demands, family, work, and friends. You might not feel like you have time for both of these strategies, but making sure to take time for them will actually give you *more* energy all day long. When it comes to discussions about exercise, many of my Earth Mama patients cringe, but once they begin to cultivate exercise that is made to order for this Power Type, most come to love it.

Part 1: Physical Nurturing

In Chapter 11, on page 279, you'll find a specific chart dedicated to the Earth Mama Exercise Rx. Here you'll learn how to incorporate 10-minute mini bouts of activity all throughout your day to achieve 35 to 60 minutes of structured exercise most days of the week.

Part 2: Emotional Nurturing

For the remainder of your 21-day Power Plan and after, I want you to take 30 minutes every day to do something you love. I want you to think of yourself as your own child. What is it that your child needs? What do *you* need? What is it that nurtures you?

If you have no idea where to begin, start by using this time as a writing exercise—or if you are more of a visual person, try painting or drawing. Sometimes, doing a task that is not on the to-do list will create that lightbulb moment. For example, use your hands to make pottery, knit, or draw. I want you to get out of your body and your head so, rather than simply meditating, try any of the following:

- Walking in nature: a park counts, and so does a lake or even a pleasing neighborhood
- Playing a musical instrument
- Dancing to music
- Gardening
- Riding your bike

It does not matter which activity you do, just that your calendar allows 30 minutes for this every day—*just for you*. Some women have trouble with this step. Another option is to block out 3 hours weekly for appointments to do something that nurtures you, such as:

- Getting a massage
- Getting a facial
- Counseling
- Attending a support group
- Having a manicure/pedicure
- Taking a class—painting, drawing, dancing, cooking, pottery, origami, yoga, tai chi, music lessons

Don't even think about skipping this step! Both physical *and* emotional nurturing are vital to rev up your body's calorie-burning engine, to increase your energy, and to wake up your mind and mood. Your entire Power Plan will collapse without it.

STEP 10: RECONNECT

Connection is the fuel for an Earth Mama, so let's make sure you really are connected, both to others in a healthy and balanced manner and to yourself by setting aside "me" time.

Cultivate Healthy Relationships

Foster relationships with people who sustain and support you, not just need something from you. During the next 7 days, schedule connection time *at least twice* on nonconsecutive days (say, Tuesday and Thursday or Monday and Friday). Some ideas:

- A date night with your husband/partner—make sure you are having amazing sex with the right person
- Playtime with your children
- A girls' night out
- If you are lacking community and family connections, work to build these relationships and create your own family—maybe it's your neighbors, a few great girlfriends, or your work family.

Balance for Beauty

This Power Type—when in balance—has the most beautiful skin and hair. Not surprisingly, however, Earth Mamas tend to shun their self-care, including morning and evening cleansing and nourishing, and when out of balance this Power Type can battle oiliness. Here I want you to take 5 minutes each morning and evening to follow the simple beauty steps that you'll find in Chapter 13, on page 308. I've included several simple recipes for cleansers, toners, moisturizers, and conditioners.

These 21 days are your ticket, your passport, back to *yourself.* As you move past the plan, stick with the parts you love and maybe let up a little on the no meat and no sugar. Return here when your energy and your psyche start to fray as a reminder to always work on the foundation, the roots of you, before you give yourself away.

WEEK 3 SHOPPING LIST

PRODUCE

Ginger, lemons, bananas, peaches, berries, apples, pears, frozen mixed berries, frozen pineapple, frozen mango, onions, garlic, leeks, mushrooms, Brussels sprouts, spinach, arugula, romaine lettuce, tomatoes, basil, cilantro, mint, oregano, bell pepper, sweet potatoes, avocados, lime, potatoes, zucchini or summer squash, celery, scallions, dill, grapes, kelp, kale

PROTEINS

Vanilla and chocolate protein powder (see page 196), eggs, chicken or turkey sausage, (beef and veggie okay too), goat cheese, dairy-free yogurt, dairy-free alternative, frozen boneless skinless chicken breasts and thighs, chicken breasts (bone in, skin on), feta cheese, lentils, dried split peas, chickpeas, bones (a mix of chicken, beef, and goat)

GRAINS

Pancake mix (paleo or gluten free), gluten-free baking mix, buckwheat flour (or other gluten-free flour mix), whole grain or gluten-free bread, gluten-free granola, gluten-free cornmeal flour, gluten-free lasagna noodles, lentil or soybean pasta, rolled oats, quinoa, brown or white rice, flaxseed meal

SUPPLEMENTS

B vitamins, probiotics, choline, digestive enzymes

HERBS AND SPICES

Turmeric, salt and pepper, nutmeg, arrowroot powder, vanilla extract, paprika, ground red pepper, Mexican oregano, cumin (ground and seeds), baking soda, garlic powder, parsley, garlic salt, Italian seasoning, cinnamon, garam masala

OTHER/MISCELLANEOUS

Walnuts, unsweetened coconut flakes, unsweetened shredded coconut, coconut milk (rice or almond milk okay too), coconut oil, olive oil, ghee, grass-fed butter, chia seeds, coconut cream, green olives, diced tomatoes, canned crushed tomatoes, red enchilada sauce, sun-dried tomatoes, almond butter, sliced almonds, marinara sauce, nutritional yeast flakes, Dijon mustard, white beans, chicken or veggie broth, chickpeas, Brazil nuts, almonds, cereal (your choice), coconut flour, skewers

PHASE 3/WEEK 3 MENU

	PRE-BREAKFAST	BREAKFAST	MIDMORNING SNACK	LUNCH	MIDAFTERNOON SNACK	DINNER
MONDAY	Apple cider vinegar (ACV) tonic (page 150)	Tofu Scramble (page 160) and dandelion tea (page 150)	½ serving Chocolate Protein Smoothie	Spinach and Kale Lasagna (page 249)	Liver Lover Smoothie (page 198) and ¼ cup Thyroid Trail Mix (page 251)	Oven "Grilled" Sea Bass with Wilted Spinach (page 234) and 1 cup Dr. Taz's Spicy Bone Broth (page 226)
TUESDAY	ACV tonic	Egg-Veggie Roll-Up (page 207) and dandelion tea	Sprouted Mung Beans (page 255)	Buckwheat Noodle and Kale Stir-Fry (page 244)	Liver Lover Smoothie and Rice Cakes with Nut Butter (page 252)	Spiced Lentil Cakes (page 246) and 1 cup Dr. Taz's Spicy Bone Broth
WEDNESDAY	ACV tonic	Chocolate Protein Smoothie (page 194) and dandelion tea	Berry-Spinach Power Punch (page 202)	Festive Italian Frittata (page 206)	Liver Lover Smoothie and Crunchy Kale Chips (page 252)	Vegan Pasta with "Cheese" Sauce and 1 cup Dr. Taz's Spicy Bone Broth
THURSDAY	ACV tonic	Avocado Toast (page 209) and dandelion tea	Lettuce Roll-Up (vegan) (page 222)	Kale Pesto and Eggplant Lettuce Wrap (page 223)	Liver Lover Smoothie and Dairy-Free Tomato Soup (page 230)	Salmon-Kale Caesar Salad (page 220) and Kitchari (page 247)
FRIDAY	ACV tonic	Chocolate Protein Smoothie and dandelion tea	Berry-Spinach Power Punch	Mason Jar Salad with chickpeas (page 216)	Liver Lover Smoothie and Crunchy Kale Chips	Kale Pesto and Eggplant Lettuce Wrap (page 223) and 1 cup Dr. Taz's Spicy Bone Broth
SATURDAY	ACV tonic	Huevos Rancheros (page 208) and dandelion tea	Sprouted Mung Beans	Vegan Pasta with "Cheese" Sauce (page 248)	Liver Lover Smoothie and Thyroid Trail Mix	Tandoori-Spiced Salmon with Yogurt Cucumber Sauce (page 233) and Kitchari

	PRE-BREAKFAST	BREAKFAST	MIDMORNING SNACK	LUNCH	MIDAFTERNOON SNACK	DINNER
SUNDAY	ACV tonic	Paleo Quiche with Sweet Potato Crust (page 203) and dandelion tea	Hummus and Veggies (page 255)	Buckwheat Noodle and Kale Stir-Fry	Liver Lover Smoothie and Rice Cakes with Nut Butter	Spiced Lentil Cakes and 1 cup Dr. Taz's Spicy Bone Broth

CONGRATULATIONS! YOU'VE ACCOMPLISHED SO much. Now that you've completed this chapter and your 3-Week Power Plan, I suggest that you repeat your Rx two more times for a total of 9 weeks (about 2 months). You can spice up the variety by swapping in other meals (breakfasts for breakfasts, for example) using the recipes in Chapter 10. After that, go back and retake both the Mojo Meter in Chapter 2 (page 9) and the Power Type Test in Chapter 3 (page 18). You may find that you've moved to a different Power Type by shifting your chemistry in these last 3 weeks. If so, follow the 3-week Rx for your new Power Type. If you are still an Earth Mama, come back and continue this 3-week plan from the beginning. Continue to practice Earth Mama steps and menus until they are truly a daily habit.

CHAPTER 9

THE NIGHTINGALES'
3-WEEK RX

THE NIGHTINGALE IS a blend of all types, with kapha-vata the most dominant, and some pitta. It is one of my favorite types and one that I am most in *awe of*. Nightingales are motivated by a constant selflessness and sense of service. In some ways, they represent all women and our longing to change and improve our world in some way, big or small. But the Nightingale goes beyond, always being in service to others and always selfless.

The problem: All that giving takes a toll. I clearly remember my pro-

It happened again. This was the third visit in a month for this patient. Strong, admirable—you might mistake her for a Boss Lady at first. But after years of giving and commanding as a missionary and public health worker, she was now a Nightingale. Her motivation had changed—it was no longer about building a successful business; it really was about changing the world, and she worked at it tirelessly. She sat looking at me, drawn and pale, with dark circles under her eyes. "I cannot clear this sinus infection," she told me. "I have taken antibiotics, decongestants, and used a nebulizer, but it's not going away." She had just returned from her third trip to Africa and was now headed to Asia for more mission fieldwork in public health. The first trips had been to help fight Ebola; now she was headed off on another to help conquer a mosquito-borne illness that was taking root.

My answer: "I have a great idea—how about some rest?"

fessor in my integrative fellowship emphatically telling us to guard our energy. "Imagine that you have an invisible shield around you, preventing you from getting too energetically drained," he instructed. I have learned that Nightingales need to take that lesson and magnify it a hundred times.

So goes my conversation with many a Nightingale. Their gift, their beauty, is the almost angelic quality with which they carry themselves through the world. Their kryptonite? Overcommitment and selflessness, which leads to depletion. They may sound like Earth Mamas, but Earth Mamas tend to be more methodical. Nightingales have the aspirations of a Boss Lady, the visions of a Savvy Chick, the creativity of a Gypsy Girl, and the heart of an Earth Mama.

The drain comes from an overworked and overwhelmed immune system, which puts Nightingales in a state of systemwide chronic inflammation that results in chronic illness. It is subtle at first—the occasional cold or cough—and then it crescendos into being sick "all the time" or developing one of our many conventional diagnoses: autoimmune disease, cancer, or a mental health disorder. I know where to start with Nightingales—reclaim your immune system!

First, it's helpful to have a good understanding of the conditions that frequently affect my Nightingale patients. Chances are, if you fit this Power Type, you'll relate to much of this. In addition to getting familiar with the following conditions, it's a good idea for you to get acquainted with Chapter 6, on Gypsy Girls, and Chapter 9, on Earth Mamas, since these ladies are close cousins to you. Once you have a clear understanding of your risk factors, you'll be ready to take action with your 3-Week Power Plan, which you'll begin in the second half of this chapter.

The Nightingale at a Glance
ALTER EGO: THE SAINT

Super powers: When a Nightingale has balanced energy, she will always save the day. Her super powers include those of an Earth Mama's steadfastness, nurturing, and compassion and also the Gypsy Girl's passion, determination, and artistic and creative expression. When balanced, Nightingales can access and express all these qualities.

Kryptonite: Immune deficiency, depression, isolation, anxiety. This combination Power Type can be thrown off by anxiety and fear, and to make matters worse, she can become overwhelmed by her Earth Mama characteristic of having flimsy boundaries. A pure Gypsy Girl tends to know that she needs downtime, and while the Nightingale's combination of types gives her some unique strengths, it also leads to some equally unique weaknesses. Earth Mamas enjoy caring for everyone else and can be energized by it, but their fragile, flighty Gypsy side can cause Nightingales to suffer terribly from low self-esteem and burnout.

Elements: Earth/Air/Wood/Water/Fire/Metal. This type is hard to pin down because she can be a blend of all types. Fluid, fiery, nurturing, visionary, and life giving are the many energies of the Nightingale.

Personality: Passionate, steady, compassionate, determined.

Body type: Nightingales can vary in body type, but usually have a small to medium build and are prone to either losing or gaining weight.

Celebrity example: Angelina Jolie. Academy Award–winning actress Jolie, mom to six children (three adopted and three biological), is known as an exceptionally talented and successful actress, an extremely nurturing mom, and repeatedly celebrated for her humanitarian work in conservation, education, women's rights, and advocacy for refugees.

Colors: Black and white. These two opposites of light and dark represent the fusion of Nightingales. White is associated with self-reliance, goodness, perfection, purity, and innocence. Black is associated with power, elegance, formality, mystery, fear, and emotional insecurities.

COMMON NIGHTINGALE CONDITIONS

The following conditions are the illnesses, challenges, and obstacles that can be roadblocks for Nightingales. That said, this list is not entirely definitive. You are an individual, and while I'd bet good money that you'll relate to many of the following issues, you probably won't have all of them—yet. Get familiar with these, and then take action with the 3-Week Power Plan for Nightingales to build up your own super powered force field and become bulletproof to illness and other immune-busters.

Frequent Coughs, Colds, and Respiratory Infections

Years of too much service and caretaking will deplete anyone's immune system. Not surprisingly, I find that my Nightingale patients, who have a tendency to be too willing to do for others, are especially susceptible. The warning signs are sometimes hard to see at first. What starts as the occasional cold or a cough soon progresses to being sick every month, and then every week. Sniffles turn into a sinus infection, pneumonia, bronchitis, or some other more severe illness that should have been fairly easy to fight off. Preventing colds and other viruses from taking hold and enhancing the immune system are essential for a Nightingale.

Allergies/Asthma

The depleted immune system also leaves a Nightingale more vulnerable to allergies. There is science here that connects these dots—in practice, we find that when there are low levels of immunoglobulins (antibodies that help to fight off illnesses), the histamine level increases. Histamine is the chemical produced by your cells in response to an allergen and causes coughing, a runny nose, hives, and trouble breathing. In fact, anyone with multiple food allergies, environmental allergies, or chemical sensitivities is more than likely immunodepleted, with higher than average histamine levels. Fighting allergies and asthma, both diseases of atopy (a more reactive, more sensitive than average immune system), is all about strengthening the immune system and healing the gut—both of which we will do in your Power Plan.

Insomnia

Just like Gypsy Girls, but unlike Earth Mamas, Nightingales usually have trouble both falling asleep and staying asleep. Overwork has led to alterations in their sleep-wake cycle, affecting both melatonin and cortisol, two hormones that determine the quality of our sleep. The air element of the Nightingale needs help—grounding her, lulling her, and coaxing her back to sleep.

Reflux

Digestive issues haunt the Nightingale as well. Abdominal symptoms including reflux and bloating are Nightingale issues. Reflux, I have found, is a condition where the digestive system has been disrupted and slowed due to a lack of digestive enzymes, good gut bacteria, and/or simply the wrong food. Chronic reflux, or gastroesophageal reflux disease, can lead to a condition known as Barrett's esophagus, where the lining of the esophagus becomes badly damaged, setting up a cycle of discomfort, inflammation, and digestive disorders.

Fatigue

Fatigue should come as no surprise to Nightingales, who have trouble setting limits and work themselves into the ground. Fatigue can present in so many different ways—the morning drag out of bed, the afternoon crash, or just the fight to get through the day. Usually accompanying symptoms, including allergies, frequent illnesses, or digestive discomfort, exacerbate this fatigue.

Anxiety/Depression

The Gypsy Girl is prone to anxiety and the Earth Mama, to depression. As a hybrid of these two types, the Nightingale can experience either or both, depending on life circumstances. It is the lack of personal—not societal—connection that is the Achilles' heel for the Nightingale. Nightingales often spend more time connecting to the demands of the world or to some larger purpose than they do on their own personal relationships or on themselves, which leaves them unwittingly without the support they need. Just like the Gypsy Girl, the Nightingale has to focus on being connected to her own body and aware of her physical needs, while her Earth Mama tendencies reinforce the need for emotional connection to her own family, partner, or children. She needs these connections to help her breathe—they refuel her, so to speak. Without these essential elements, the Nightingale can find her constant service and selflessness unrewarding, demanding, and personally unfulfilling.

Infertility

Because she yo-yos between the characteristics of a Gypsy Girl and Earth Mama, the Nightingale can have missing menstrual cycles and trouble both getting pregnant and maintaining a pregnancy. Managing key hormonal imbalances is critical in helping Nightingales get and stay pregnant—along with giving them license to rest!

Chinese Meridian Diagnosis: Spleen/Kidney Meridian Deficiency

Nightingales have spleen and kidney meridian deficiency in Traditional Chinese Medicine (TCM). They retain the Earth Mama issues of spleen meridian deficiency—dampness, poor digestion, and a sluggish metabolism. At the same time, they have the Gypsy Girl pattern of kidney meridian deficiency. The kidney meridian is the seat of all hormones, the source of energy that you are gifted with at birth, according to Chinese medicine. When the kidney meridian declines, the TCM understanding is that the raw materials to make hormones and to sustain energy are simply not present—and a life of too much work or service has depleted this energy faster than was originally intended.

Warming the kidney, removing dampness, and returning the flow of energy are the Chinese medicine goals for you Nightingales—and an Rx for keeping you balanced.

Ayurvedic Dosha Diagnosis: Kapha-Vata

Nightingales can be a blend of two Ayurvedic types: kapha, the Earth Mama nurturer, quiet and steady; and vata, the Gypsy Girl artist, who's not as grounded and can sometimes be disconnected from herself. As Nightingales, you may often dance between both of these types. Therefore, your Power Plan requires elements that work to provide balance. It is a challenge—finding balance between these two seemingly conflicting doshas—but definitely doable. Your 3-Week Power Plan will keep you steady, without going to either extreme.

Hormone Imbalances

The greatest hormone imbalances I see in my Nightingales are in plummeting cortisol levels, known as adrenal fatigue, along with insulin irregularity and low progesterone levels (see "The Five Glands You Need to Know," page 50, for more information). Conditions like chronic fatigue, adrenal fatigue, and prediabetes can all affect Nightingales, ultimately affecting their estrogen-to-progesterone ratios—and hence, their fertility. Melatonin and cortisol are affected as well, causing the sleep disturbances common to Nightingales. These hormones also affect fertility, blocking ovulation. In the next 3 weeks you'll learn to balance and optimize all levels of important hormones through food choices, supplements, bodywork, and more.

LONG-TERM DISEASE RISKS

The long-term disease risks of a Nightingale center around the immune system. Protecting your immune system prevents inflammation and mitochondrial dysfunction—where chronic depletion of antioxidants can lead to conditions like Alzheimer's, multiple sclerosis, and myopathies. It also protects against diseases that affect muscular and neurological health.

LAB FINDINGS

Here are the lab findings common to Nightingales.

- **Low B vitamins:** especially folate, B_1, B_2, B_6, and B_{12}
- **Low vitamin D:** specifically, D_3
- **Low iron or ferritin levels**
- **Low IGG levels** (these are immunoglobulins important for building the immune system)
- **Low IGA levels** (another key immunoglobulin that manages the immune system)
- **High histamine levels**
- **High nighttime cortisol**
- **High TSH** (thyroid-stimulating hormone)
- **Low progesterone**
- **High estrogen:** estradiol, estrone

See "Labs You Need to Know" on page 49.

Nutritional Needs/Deficiencies

Given the background and potential imbalances of Nightingales, their nutritional needs focus on antioxidant-rich foods and foods that strengthen the microbiome, often considered command central of the immune system. Adding probiotic-rich foods and foods high in antioxidants, including most brightly colored fruits and vegetables, improves a Nightingale's energy. At the same time, pulling back on insulin disruptors like alcohol, caffeine, and sugar is a key nutritional strategy for Nightingales.

HOW THE NIGHTINGALE 3-WEEK RX WORKS

Now that you've got a good handle on your risk factors, common lab findings, and the different ways TCM and Ayurvedic medicine view your Power Type, it's time to take action. During the following weeks, we will build your immune system, reduce inflammation, and balance your hormones, getting *you* back to *you* and all the great work that you long to do.

Immune support is the focus of your first week. We will focus on food, supplements, and lifestyle tips to help you rebuild your immune system. Leveling out your hormones is the goal for the next week. And finally, Week 3 brings us to strategies for improving emotional balance and boundaries, physical activity, mindfulness, relaxation, self-nurturing, and self reflection—all necessary to keep your Nightingale spirit soaring.

The Nightingale Rx Rules

1. **Drink a daily immune booster.** Choose one of three drinks found on page 171, or follow the suggested menus.

2. **Take immunity-protecting supplements.** Nightingales need to take B vitamins, astragalus, and probiotics. See page 171 for details.

3. **Stick to your protein and fat parameters and avoid refined sugars.** Aim to eat 50 to 60 grams of protein and 20 to 30 grams of fat daily, and avoid refined sugars (whole natural fruits are okay).

4. **Eat an anti-inflammatory diet.** Avoiding foods that cause inflammation will power up your body's natural defenses. See "Anti-Inflammatory Eating—Foods to Avoid" on page 46. Also, limit yourself to a total of 1,800 calories a day unless you are training for an extreme sport or sporting event.

5. **Treat yourself to weekly bodywork.** Massage and acupuncture are natural ways to nurture yourself and to improve your immunity. Schedule a session once a week. That's an order!

6. **Prioritize sleep.** Make sure that you are getting 7 to 9 hours of sleep a night, especially between the hours of 11 p.m. and 6 a.m.

Note: If you follow the suggested menus at the end of each week, you will automatically be meeting all of your nutritional goals.

Let's get to it.

THE 10 NIGHTINGALE ACTION STEPS AT A GLANCE

While the Nightingale Rx Rules work as your quick-start guide, the steps below give you an overview of your entire 21-day plan. You'll build on these steps week by week until you are fully super powered!

Step 1: Drink a Daily Immune Booster

Step 2: Incorporate Immune-Building Supplements
- ☐ B-complex
- ☐ Astragalus root
- ☐ Probiotics

Step 3: Add Acupuncture and/or Massage

Step 4: Prioritize Sleep

Step 5: Eat to Heal Adrenal Fatigue

Step 6: Go Sugar Free to Stabilize Insulin

Step 7: Build Your Hormones Back Up
- ☐ Ghee
- ☐ Chicken soup

Step 8: Exercise to Lower Stress Hormones

Step 9: Set Boundaries

Step 10: Create Service Ambassadors

PHASE 1/WEEK 1: BUILD YOUR IMMUNE SYSTEM

The immune system is often ignored until it's too late—especially by Nightingales. You frequently find yourself sick or get an illness that can be tough to beat. Not on my watch—I am going to teach you to protect and monitor your immune system so that you can spend more time giving rather than recovering.

Week 1 Action Steps

STEP 1: DRINK A DAILY IMMUNE BOOSTER

When I think of building an immune system, I am thinking about increasing your cellular oxygen levels to fight off viruses and bacteria, beating inflammation, and building up your nutrients. Your first step is to add one of the following three immune boosters to your daily regimen.

- Grocer's Choice Green Drink (page 197)
- Turmeric Pepper Honey Tea (page 200)
- Chicken Soup (page 228)

Each of these recipes contains either antioxidants or good gut bacteria to help you boost your immune system, and I've incorporated them all into your menu on page 174.

STEP 2: INCORPORATE IMMUNE-BUILDING SUPPLEMENTS

There are a lot of supplements that help to repair and restore a depleted immune system. I am including my favorite tried-and-true immune-boosting supplements for Nightingales as your second step. After seeing more than 10,000 patients in practice, I know these work! Add the following to your daily plan.

- **B-complex:** If you've looked at the other Power Type plans prior to this chapter, you'll see that I've included B vitamins in every one. Nightingales are no exception. I cannot stress enough the critical role these vitamins play in your health. B vitamins are powerhouses that work to keep your immune system primed and your energy replenished. If you can't find a multi–B vitamin supplement that has my recommended amounts, buy them separately. (For those amounts, see "Vitamins and Supplements You Need to Know," on page 45.)

- **Astragalus root:** One of my absolute favorites, astragalus root originally derives from the Chinese medicine pharmacopeia. It works to strengthen the immune system and also helps cells stay younger for longer. Much research is being done on astragalus root and its effects on telomeres, the marker on our DNA that can predict aging. For example, short telomeres indicate rapid aging, while longer telomeres are seen as more optimal. Take one dropper daily, and up to three droppers per day when feeling ill. One dropper typically contains 500 milligrams of astragalus root.

- **Probiotics:** Almost 75 percent of your immune system is in your belly! So add a high-quality probiotic to your daily routine. (See "Vitamins and Supplements You Need to Know," on page 45.)

BOOST YOUR IMMUNITY WITH IV VITAMINS

In our practice at CentreSpring MD, we do many IV infusions that support the immune system, especially during times of high stress and sickness. Many holistic and integrative doctors offer IV vitamin C and Myers' cocktails (an IV infusion of amino acids, magnesium, calcium, B vitamins, and vitamin C). These can help build up your body's disease- and inflammation-fighting defense system to help with asthma, migraines, fatigue, fibromyalgia, muscle spasms, respiratory infections, sinusitis, allergies, heart disease, and more. See Resources on page 316 for more information.

STEP 3: ADD ACUPUNCTURE AND/OR MASSAGE

For the next 3 weeks, pick between a weekly acupuncture or massage session. Both types of bodywork reduce stress, open up blocked channels of energy, and increase circulation to boost your body's natural disease-fighting abilities. A growing body of research shows how these modalities boost immune function and turn off inflammation—your key challenges. See pages 294 and 295 for tips on finding a certified acupuncturist and massage therapist.

STEP 4: PRIORITIZE SLEEP

We cannot repair any immune system without sound and consistent sleep. I know this all too well—my years in emergency medicine left me battling colds and getting sick all the time, simply because my sleep schedule was so altered.

Create a sleep environment for the duration of this plan and longer, and commit to establishing a consistent sleep schedule—no flip-flopping, no going to bed at random times. Pick your bedtime and stick with it. Sleep heals the immune system. Aim for 7 to 9 hours of sleep a night—definitely no less than 7. You need the restorative healing that only this sleep quota can provide. I know that everyone has different jobs and schedules, but try to stay close to the original Chinese recommendation for women: Sleep is critical from 11 p.m. to 6 a.m. For more ideas on improving your sleep and sleep environment, see page 284.

WEEK 1 SHOPPING LIST

PRODUCE

Kale, spinach, garlic, yellow onion, red onion, dill, parsley, cilantro, basil, bananas, frozen strawberries, frozen mixed veggies, kelp, arugula, mushrooms, leeks, tomatoes, bell pepper, avocados, limes, lemons, salad greens, romaine lettuce, sprouts, cucumbers, carrots, eggplants, chile pepper, shiitake mushrooms, grape tomatoes, baby carrots, celery, jicama, radishes, potatoes, zucchini or summer squash

PROTEINS

Mixed bones (chicken, beef, and goat), eggs, mung beans, chocolate protein powder (see page 196), turkey or chicken sausage, chicken leg quarters, boneless chicken breasts, salmon fillets, sea bass, Cotija cheese, chickpeas, tofu, vegan sausage, plain Greek yogurt, hummus, black beans, split peas or lentils, white beans

SWEETENERS

Honey—while sugar should be kept to a minimum, it is okay to have 1 teaspoon of honey when a craving strikes or to use a teaspoon or less per serving in a recipe

GRAINS

Brown or white rice, gluten-free pancake mix, rice noodles, buckwheat noodles, brown rice cakes, corn tortillas, lentil or soybean macaroni or rotini noodles, gluten-free bread, and rice, egg, or spaghetti noodles

SUPPLEMENTS

B-complex vitamins (see page 171), astragalus root (page 171), probiotics (page 171)

HERBS AND SPICES

Kosher salt, pepper, turmeric, ground red pepper, cumin seeds, garam masala, nutmeg, paprika, Mexican or regular oregano, ground cumin, Italian seasoning, garlic salt, sumac

OTHER/MISCELLANEOUS

Black and/or green tea, ghee, coconut oil, chicken broth, walnuts, unsweetened coconut flakes, red enchilada sauce, olives, pine nuts, almonds, cashews, green olives, 2 cans coconut milk, canned tomato sauce, canned diced tomatoes, roasted pistachios, mustard, anchovies or capers, turkey or veggie bacon crumbles, nutritional yeast flakes, chicken and vegetable broth, 1 carton coconut milk, tamari sauce, almond flour

PHASE 1/WEEK 1 MENU

	BREAKFAST	LUNCH	SNACKS (choose one)	DINNER
MONDAY	Pancake Imposters (gluten free and omit chocolate chips) (page 210)	Mason Jar Salads with chickpeas (page 216) and Chicken Soup (page 228)	Kitchari (page 247) or Kale and Kelp Chips (page 253)	Black Bean Soup and Portable Tacos, with chicken (page 227)
TUESDAY	Chocolate Protein Smoothie (page 194) and Turmeric Pepper Honey Tea (page 200)	Kale Pesto and Eggplant Lettuce Wrap (page 223)	Hummus and Veggies (page 255) or Avocado Toast (page 209)	Oven "Grilled" Sea Bass with Wilted Spinach (page 234)
WEDNESDAY	Paleo Quiche with Sweet Potato Crust (page 203) and Grocer's Choice Green Drink (page 197)	Portobello BLT (page 225)	Kitchari or Kale and Kelp Chips	Bissara (page 231)
THURSDAY	Chocolate Protein Smoothie and Turmeric Pepper Honey Tea	Mason Jar Salads with chickpeas and Chicken Soup	Lettuce Roll-Ups with hummus or tofu (page 222) or Dairy-Free Tomato Soup (page 230)	Vegan Pasta with "Cheese" Sauce (page 248)
FRIDAY	Egg-Veggie Roll-Up with gluten-free baking mix (page 207) and Grocer's Choice Green Drink	Salmon-Kale Caesar Salad (page 220)	Kitchari or Kale and Kelp Chips	Buckwheat Noodle and Kale Stir-Fry (page 244)
SATURDAY	Paleo Quiche with Sweet Potato Crust	Kale Pesto and Eggplant Lettuce Wrap	Hummus and Veggies or Rice Cake with Nut Butter (page 252)	Lettuce Roll-Up (vegan) and Chicken Soup
SUNDAY	Huevos Rancheros (page 208) and Grocer's Choice Green Drink	Portobello BLT	Berry-Spinach Power Punch (page 202) or Crunchy Kale Chips (page 252)	Oven "Grilled" Sea Bass with Wilted Spinach

"Before starting this plan, my energy levels would wane in the afternoon, and since I am not a daytime nap person, I would reach for cookies, candy, or a handful of chips to pick up my energy and tide me over until supper. The super power drinks and smoothies fixed all that. It was easy to double the batch when making them. I'd just seal up the extra portion, and then I'd have it around 3 or 4 p.m. for a healthy afternoon pick-me-up. After the first week, I found that my cravings for sweets had dwindled and that I wasn't dragging in the afternoons."—**Sarah, 65, retired music teacher**

Congratulations—you've completed the first week of your Power Plan! Now let's continue on to Phase 2.

PHASE 2/WEEK 2:
BALANCE YOUR ADRENALS AND INSULIN

Having worked a bit on the immune system over the last 7 days, let's shift focus to repair your levels of the two hormones that take the biggest hit when you're running low—the adrenal hormones and insulin. The stress hormones of the adrenals go haywire when much is demanded of the body physically, while erratic insulin can affect energy, mood, and focus.

Week 2 Action Steps
STEP 5: EAT TO HEAL ADRENAL FATIGUE

Follow the principle of eating for your adrenals: Eating at regular intervals, as well as choosing higher-protein breakfasts, lunches, and dinners, keeps your adrenal hormones balanced and steady. So don't forget to eat every 3 to 4 hours and to get plenty of protein. *Protein* is the key word here. Keep your total protein at around 60 grams per day, or 15 to 20 grams per meal and 7 to 10 grams per snack. You'll get plenty of protein by following your weekly menu.

STEP 6: GO SUGAR FREE TO STABILIZE INSULIN

Get sugar out of your daily diet. While the risk for the Earth Mama is erratic insulin levels, resulting in weight gain and depression, the risk for

Nightingales is further weakening of your immune system and worsening of inflammation. And, yes—all sugars are out, including alcohol. Sugar interferes with the disease-fighting properties of white blood cells, and refined sugars trigger the release of cytokines (inflammatory messengers) in your body. You can eat fruit, but limit it to two servings per day.

STEP 7: BUILD UP YOUR HORMONES

The concept of hormone "building" is unique to Traditional Chinese Medicine (TCM), but doctors of Eastern and Western medicine know that when the body becomes depleted, the hormones are the first to go—especially estrogen and progesterone, which make us feel alive and vital. The body goes into triage mode when chronically stressed or depleted, trying to determine what to keep and what can be sacrificed. Hormones hit the chopping block pretty quickly, so it's important to add one of the following hormone builders into your daily regimen over the next 7 days.

- **Ghee:** Ghee is a healthy fat that supports cholesterol, the foundation of all hormones. Consider adding ¼ teaspoon to ½ teaspoon of clarified organic ghee to your diet daily. (It's available in most health food stores.)
- **Chicken soup:** In TCM, soup is thought to "build blood and qi," which are seen as the key elements of hormone balance for women. Eating 1 cup per day was a common TCM "prescription," for hormone balance. Try the chicken soup recipe on page 229, and add some sliced ginger to the broth.

You've done a lot of work in the last 2 weeks—from changing your eating habits and incorporating supplements to using hormone-balancing recipes and strategies. Hopefully you are noticing a shift in your health—it may be an overall better sense of well-being or improved sleep and energy. Let's keep moving forward!

WEEK 2 SHOPPING LIST

PRODUCE

Kale, spinach, garlic, yellow onion, red onion, dill, parsley, cilantro, basil, oregano, bananas, frozen strawberries, frozen cherries, frozen blueberries, frozen mixed veggies, kelp, arugula, mushrooms, leeks, tomatoes, bell pepper, avocados, limes, lemons, salad greens, romaine lettuce, sprouts, cucumbers, carrots, eggplants, chile pepper, shiitake mushrooms, portobello mushrooms, grape tomatoes, baby carrots, celery, jicama, radishes, potatoes, zucchini or summer squash, Brussels sprouts, kabocha squash, shallots, ginger, cauliflower

PROTEINS

Mixed bones (chicken, beef, and goat), eggs, mung beans, chocolate protein powder (see page 196), grass-fed ground beef or lamb, turkey or chicken sausage, chicken leg quarters, boneless chicken breasts, salmon fillets, sea bass, Cotija cheese, feta cheese, chickpeas, tofu, vegan sausage, plain Greek yogurt, hummus, black beans, split peas or lentils, white beans

SWEETENERS

Honey—while sugar should be kept to a minimum, it is okay to have 1 teaspoon of honey when a craving strikes or to use a teaspoon or less per serving in a recipe

GRAINS

Brown or white rice, gluten-free pancake mix, rice noodles, buckwheat noodles, brown rice cakes, corn tortillas, lentil or soybean macaroni or rotini noodles, gluten-free bread, gluten-free cornmeal flour, flaxseed meal, quinoa, and rice, egg, or spaghetti noodles

SUPPLEMENTS

B-complex vitamins (see page 171), astragalus root (page 171), and probiotics (page 171)

HERBS AND SPICES

Kosher salt, pepper, Himalayan salt, turmeric, ground red pepper, cumin seeds, garam masala, nutmeg, paprika, Mexican and regular oregano, ground cumin, Italian seasoning, garlic salt, sumac, baking soda, arrowroot powder, tandoori spice mix or ground chili pepper, garlic paste, ginger paste

OTHER/MISCELLANEOUS

Black and/or green tea, ghee, coconut oil, chicken broth, walnuts, unsweetened coconut flakes, red enchilada sauce, olives, pine nuts, almonds, cashews, green olives, 2 cans coconut milk, canned tomato sauce, canned diced tomatoes, roasted pistachios, mustard, anchovies or capers, turkey or veggie bacon crumbles, nutritional yeast flakes, chicken and vegetable broth, 1 carton coconut milk, tamari sauce, almond flour, bone broth (page 226), kalamata/Greek olives, sun-dried tomatoes

PHASE 2/WEEK 2 MENU

	BREAKFAST	LUNCH	SNACKS (choose one)	DINNER
MONDAY	Greek Omelet (page 204)	Spiced Lentil Cakes with Chickpeas (page 246) and Chicken Soup (page 228)	Liver Lover Smoothie (page 198) or ½ serving Egg-Veggie Roll-Up	Kabocha Squash Soup with Cauliflower-Quinoa Meatballs (page 243)
TUESDAY	Avocado Toast (page 209) and Turmeric Pepper Honey Tea (page 200)	Bissara (page 231)	Berry-Spinach Power Punch (page 202) or Crunchy Kale Chips (page 252)	Portobello BLT
WEDNESDAY	Tofu Scramble (page 209) and Kale-Cherry-Berry Super Juice (page 202)	Mason Jar Salads with chickpeas (page 216)	½ cup Kabocha Squash Soup (page 232) or 1 Egg-Veggie Roll-Up	Greek Salad with Chickpeas (page 221)
THURSDAY	Egg-Veggie Roll-Up (page 207)	Bissara	Hummus and Veggies (page 255) or Rice Cake with Nut Butter (page 252)	Sweet Potato Noodles with Cauliflower-Quinoa Meat-balls (page 250) and Chicken Soup
FRIDAY	Avocado Toast and Kale-Cherry-Berry Super Juice	Kale Pesto and Eggplant Lettuce Wrap (page 223)	Lettuce Roll-Up (vegan) (page 222) or Kale and Kelp Chips (page 253)	Oven "Grilled" Sea Bass with Wilted Spinach (page 234)
SATURDAY	Breakfast Skillet (page 205) and Turmeric Pepper Honey Tea	Salmon-Kale Caesar Salad (page 220)	Lettuce Roll-Up (vegan) or Dairy-Free Tomato Soup (page 230)	Buckwheat Noodle and Kale Stir-Fry (page 244)
SUNDAY	Tofu Scramble and Grocer's Choice Green Drink (page 197)	Portobello BLT (page 225)	Sprouted Mung Beans (page 255) or ½ serving Berry Bomb (page 195)	Tandoori-Spiced Salmon with Yogurt Cucumber Sauce (page 233)

PHASE 3/WEEK 3:
FOLLOW THE NIGHTINGALE MIND-BODY RX

After rebuilding your immune system, fighting off inflammation, and building up your hormonal reserve, it's essential for you Nightingales to create a mind-body self-care routine that matches your passionate intensity about the work you do. These last 7 days will focus on strategies that protect boundaries, exercises that will energize you and eliminate toxic stress, and methods for delegating to keep you from sacrificing your personal energy or well-being.

Week 3 Action Steps
STEP 8: EXERCISE TO LOWER STRESS HORMONES

Those stress hormones—adrenaline and cortisol, and those affected by stress such as insulin—need time to rest. Excessive or aggressive exercise isn't the best for your needs and may actually deplete your immune system, while lighter exercise that celebrates movement in nature will replenish you! Choose from adrenaline-balancing workouts like a mixture of walking, yoga, tai chi, and/or qi gong daily for the next 7 days (see Chapter 11, page 257, for workouts).

Before a Nightingale chooses her daily exercise, it's important for her to check in, to see how she is feeling energy-wise. Remember, as part Gypsy Girl, you can have a tendency to become disconnected from how you feel, and as part Earth Mama you can lean toward skipping out on physical activity. Find your balance in the middle. See the Exercise Rx for Nightingales on page 281.

STEP 9: SET BOUNDARIES

Changing the world and being service oriented is endless work, made up of countless hours—but you have to set some boundaries! I know it's hard. Cut it off at a particular time, give yourself that 3-day weekend to recover, or simply take a vacation. Build this in, put it on the calendar—make it nonnegotiable. While I don't consider myself a Nightingale, someone once told me that every time you return from a fun activity or vacation you should schedule the next one because *life is short and you have to build in the breaks*. With that in mind, I want you to keep a written record of at least three things you do each and every week to set boundaries and make time for yourself (use a checklist like the following).

Day___ What I did to set a boundary: _____

Day___ What I did to set a boundary: _____

Day___ What I did to set a boundary: _____

STEP 10: CREATE SERVICE AMBASSADORS

Passionate about a project or mission? You don't have to do it alone. Create mini versions of yourself, and share your projects with others—this will move your vision forward without draining your energy and making you sick. Use this week to determine the best plan for creating your ambassadors and seeing your own vision expand.

- **Include all family members.** Everyone who lives under your roof should participate in household responsibilities. Even a 5-year-old can help fold clothes or do some simple dusting, and it helps build confidence and competence. Plus participating helps everyone understand the importance of contributing to the greater good. Ask your spouse or partner to take over at least one job—taking out the trash, making the bed each morning, getting the mail—and ideally more than one. And then (here's the hard part), hands off! Let him do it his way, and just say thank you.
- **Hire part-time mini me's.** Having even an hour or two of help several times a week can make a big difference! I use a part-time nanny to help with preparing dinner, supervising the kids, and some light cleaning.
- **Outsource a job.** Have your house cleaned every other week, your groceries delivered weekly, or your dog walked several times a week.

WEEK 3 SHOPPING LIST

PRODUCE

Kale, spinach, garlic, yellow onion, red onion, dill, parsley, cilantro, basil, bananas, frozen strawberries, frozen cherries, frozen blueberries, frozen mixed veggies, kelp, arugula, mushrooms, leeks, tomatoes, bell pepper, avocados, limes, lemons, salad greens, romaine lettuce, sprouts, cucumbers, carrots, eggplants, chile pepper, shiitake mushrooms, portobello mushrooms, grape tomatoes, baby carrots, celery, jicama, radishes, potatoes, zucchini or summer squash, Brussels sprouts, kabocha squash, shallots, ginger, cauliflower

PROTEINS

Mixed bones (chicken, beef, and goat), eggs, mung beans, chocolate protein powder (see page 196), grass-fed ground beef or lamb, turkey or chicken sausage, chicken leg quarters, boneless chicken breasts, steak, shrimp, salmon fillets, sea bass, Cotija cheese, feta cheese, chickpeas, tofu, vegan sausage, plain Greek yogurt, hummus, black beans, split peas or lentils, white beans, mung beans

SWEETENERS

Honey—while sugar should be kept to a minimum, it is okay to have 1 teaspoon of honey when a craving strikes or to use a teaspoon or less per serving in a recipe

GRAINS

Brown or white rice, gluten-free pancake mix, rice noodles, buckwheat noodles, brown rice cakes, corn tortillas, lentil or soybean macaroni or rotini noodles, gluten-free bread, gluten-free cornmeal flour, flaxseed meal, quinoa, and rice, egg, or spaghetti noodles

SUPPLEMENTS

B-complex vitamins (see page 171), astragalus root (page 171), probiotics (page 171)

HERBS AND SPICES

Kosher salt, pepper, Himalayan salt, turmeric, ground red pepper, cumin seeds, garam masala, nutmeg, paprika, Mexican and regular oregano, ground cumin, Italian seasoning, garlic salt, sumac, baking soda, arrowroot powder, tandoori spice mix or ground chili pepper, garlic paste, ginger paste, vanilla extract

OTHER/MISCELLANEOUS

Black and/or green tea, coconut oil and ghee, chicken broth, walnuts, unsweetened coconut flakes, red enchilada sauce, olives, pine nuts, almonds, chia seeds, cashews, green olives, 2 cans coconut milk, canned coconut cream, canned tomato sauce, canned diced tomatoes, roasted pistachios, mustard, anchovies or capers, turkey or veggie bacon crumbles, nutritional yeast flakes, chicken and vegetable broth, 1 carton coconut milk, tamari sauce, almond flour, bone broth (page 226), kalamata/Greek olives

PHASE 3/WEEK 3 MENU

	BREAKFAST	LUNCH	SNACKS (choose one)	DINNER
MONDAY	Tofu Scramble (page 209) and Kale-Cherry-Berry Super Juice (page 202)	Kale Pesto and Eggplant Lettuce Wrap (page 223)	½ Chocolate Protein Smoothie or Immunity-Boosting Chicken Soup, with ghee (page 229)	Oven "Grilled" Sea Bass with Wilted Spinach (page 234)
TUESDAY	Coconut Chia Seed Pudding (page 212) and Turmeric Pepper Honey Tea (page 200)	Buckwheat Noodle and Kale Stir-Fry (page 244)	Sprouted Mung Beans (page 255) or Immunity-Boosting Chicken Soup, with ghee	Black Bean Soup and Portable Tacos, with chicken (page 227)
WEDNESDAY	Chocolate Protein Smoothie (page 194) and Turmeric Pepper Honey Tea	Mason Jar Salads with chickpeas (page 216)	Berry-Spinach Power Punch (page 202) or Immunity-Boosting Chicken Soup, with ghee	Vegan Pasta with "Cheese" Sauce (page 248)
THURSDAY	Avocado Toast (page 209) and Kale-Cherry-Berry Super Juice	Kale Pesto and Eggplant Lettuce Wrap	1 Lettuce Roll-Up (vegan) (page 222) or Immunity-Boosting Chicken Soup, with ghee	Salmon-Kale Caesar Salad (page 220)
FRIDAY	Protein Banana Bread (gluten-free flour) (page 215) and Turmeric Pepper Honey Tea	Mason Jar Salads with chickpeas	Berry-Spinach Power Punch or Immunity-Boosting Chicken Soup, with ghee	Portobello BLT (page 225)
SATURDAY	Huevos Rancheros (page 208) and Kale-Cherry-Berry Super Juice	Vegan Pasta with "Cheese" Sauce (page 248)	Sprouted Mung Beans or Immunity-Boosting Chicken Soup, with ghee	Tandoori-Spiced Salmon with Yogurt Cucumber Sauce (page 233)
SUNDAY	Paleo Quiche and Sweet Potato Crust (page 203) and Turmeric Pepper Honey Tea	Buckwheat Noodle and Kale Stir-Fry	Hummus and Veggies (page 255) or Immunity-Boosting Chicken Soup, with ghee	Black Bean Soup and Portable Tacos, with chicken

WAY TO GO! NOW that you've completed all 3 weeks of your Power Plan, you are well on your way to establishing your super powers. I suggest that you continue to follow the 3-Week Rx by going back to the beginning and repeating it for two more cycles (a total of 9 weeks, or a little over 2 months). You can spice up the variety by swapping in meals (breakfasts for breakfasts, for example) using the recipes in Chapter 10. After 2 months, go back and retake the Mojo Meter in Chapter 2 (page 9) and the Power Type Test in Chapter 3 (page 18). Continue to retest yourself every few months and update your plan accordingly. If you find that you've shifted to a different Power Type, go to that chapter and follow *that* 3-Week Rx. Read on through to the end to round out your plan with plenty of healthy exercise, mind-body, and beauty tips.

Remember, Nightingales are a blend of all women, with all Power Types kind of mashed up together, but they still need their own unique plan. As you learned, you can fluctuate between all Power Types at different times or phases of your life. A Nightingale today may be an Earth Mama in a month. If you retake the Power Type Test (page 18) every few months or so you will stay connected with your inner super woman.

Calling all Nightingales—rest, build, go forth, and conquer!

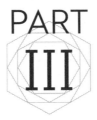

PART III

FORTIFY YOUR SUPER POWER ARSENAL

YOU MADE IT! You know your Power Type, you have your plan in hand, and you may already be feeling amazing—at least I hope so. In the next few chapters, we are going to take your regimen even further and think through everything from color to space, food, and beauty. These chapters are meant to give your Power Type sustainable, long-lasting results, not just results for 3 weeks. Check out the great recipes—conjured up in my kitchen—exercises for your Power Type, and secrets to preserving your super powers.

CHAPTER 10

SUPER SUSTAINING NUTRITION

MY OWN HEALTH transformation started in the kitchen, and I still believe that food is the best place to start super charging your health. You won't see any hard-to-find ingredients or gourmet-length cooking instructions among my recipes. I'm a super woman just like you—I value healthy eating, but I don't have hours on end to plan and cook long, leisurely meals. What you will find here are recipes, strategies, and tips for making fast and simple, but delicious and always healthful snacks and meals. This is the way I eat and feed my family and myself, and these are the methods and recipes I suggest to my patients. My critics are real people, little and big, and they don't put up with anything that doesn't delight their tastebuds.

Food is medicine and fuel. It empowers us, transforms us, and sets the tone and rhythm of our health. We cannot skip this piece. I have watched so many women—patients, friends, colleagues—do everything else right, but struggle to master healthy, empowered eating for themselves or their families. Without the nutrition piece of the puzzle in place, I see many women become disheartened or frustrated, and often they give up on goals of health altogether.

I don't blame them. Navigating food and meal planning today can feel like traversing a field full of land mines. *It feels like a full-time job.* First, all of us struggle with a lack of time—too much on our to-do lists and jam-packed schedules put healthy meal planning and eating in last place, or squeezed out altogether. If we're lucky, it's an afterthought, but in many cases we miss it completely. "What? It's 3 p.m. and I haven't eaten lunch?" Or, "I'm already late getting the kids to school and myself to work; I don't have time for breakfast—again!" The running, the doing, the giving, the carpooling—who has time for healthy shopping, meal prep, and sit-down meals?

If you at least think about food to nurture and nourish you, you're a step ahead of many women. Then come the next challenges—knowing which ingredients are okay, if you should be buying organic, if it's okay to eat a breakfast bar when you're feeling rushed (what if sugar's the first ingredient?), and so on.

Exhausting.

Mastering food, let alone the best food for you, is daunting. There is an overload of information available to all of us, and a cacophony of diets from which to choose—paleo, vegan, gluten-free, The Whole 30, Weight Watchers, the list goes on and on. I applaud many of them to some extent—most at least fundamentally attempt to help us to eat better, prescribe a plan or road map for healthy eating, and improve or promote our health. Unfortunately, many of these eating plans are one-size-fits-all, too difficult to figure out or implement on your own, and/ or the wrong fit for your Power Type. That's why *Super Woman Rx* provides five easy-to-follow individualized plans that incorporate the best from all diets and nutritional plans *to fuel your specific super powers!*

I learned this lesson the hard way in my twenties, when my own health suffered. I thought popcorn for dinner was healthy and Diet Coke was the elixir of champions. My entire health story would eventually be traced back to one central theme: I needed to be gluten-free. Gluten was affecting my thyroid and other hormones, which in turn was triggering inflammation—but reaching this conclusion took a lot of detective work and trial and error on my part (and I'm a medical doctor!). After an 8-year search for answers that included multiple frustrating visits with doctors and specialists, I finally came back to food as the answer and got inspired to get in the kitchen. Don't laugh, but I had to learn to master the little things—like turning the stove on, or setting the right oven temperature. That's how disconnected I was, and how many of us are today, from food and nutrition *and our bodies*. Sure, there is the prepped food you can grab quickly at stores, convenience foods, packaged foods—food is everywhere, 24/7—but it isn't exactly nourishing and healthy.

Food, as you may have noticed, is a central theme throughout each of the Five Power Plans covered in Chapters 5 through 9. Different super women have different needs: Gypsy Girls need fat and protein, while Savvy Chicks struggle with foods to enhance their thyroid and the adrenals. Boss Ladies need foods to balance sensitive digestive systems, and Earth Mamas and Nightingales need portion control and have to watch other food sensitivities. You get it—you have seen the plans.

HOW TO USE THIS CHAPTER

In this chapter, you'll find my favorite recipes. If you turn back to the end of each of Chapters 5 through 9, you'll find menus for your Power Type that include these recipes. These recipes will work for you as long as you use them with your personal Power Plan, in the sequence prescribed. I hope these recipes inspire you to get back in the kitchen and have some fun with food. In my YouTube.com channel, Kitchen Cures (see https://doctortaz.com/category/kitchen-cures/), I show fun ways to get food together quickly and efficiently. Remember, I am no master chef—I am a real-life multitasker just like you—and I don't need chef-quality food, just delicious food to nurture me and my family.

FOOD PREP

Typically, I get in the kitchen a few nights per week or on a Sunday, and I prep food for at least 3 days ahead. That way, I don't have the worry or the hassle of daily meal prep. Cooking is also a whole family venture—the kids get in there, my husband helps, and my mother-in-law often joins in trying to make sure we are all well fed. I am grateful for the support and encourage you to get your whole family in the kitchen and make it a family affair. If you don't have the responsibility of feeding a family, make it a neighborhood or community affair by involving your friends or neighbors and getting cooked up for the week ahead— and it's more fun that way!

Treat this chapter as a recipe book, or use the menu charts to follow a prescribed plan. Most important, *enjoy!* Remember that food is meant to be enjoyed! Savor the flavors, experiment with new ingredients, and find ways to reconnect to the primal need to find, prepare, and serve food to yourself and those you love.

THE SUPER POWERED KITCHEN

Here are the basic items you'll want to stock, along with some of my favorite kitchen products. When choosing products, make sure that they are as natural, local, and organic as possible. Double-check that nut butters, sauces, and other products have no added sugars. Note that this is not a complete list; you'll still need to check your recipes and add items as needed, but the suggestions will give you a good head start on the basics.

KITCHEN TOOLS/ITEMS		
NutriBullet or Vitamix	Food processor	16-ounce mason jars
Frother	Pressure cooker/Instant Pot	Spiralizer
Immersion blender		
IN YOUR HERB AND SPICE CABINET		
Cinnamon	Cumin seeds	Italian seasoning
Salt and pepper	Cumin, ground	Ground red pepper
Turmeric	Coriander, ground	Arrowroot powder
Garam masala	Curry powder	
Real vanilla extract	Paprika	
IN YOUR PANTRY		
Chicken and/or veggie broth	Honey	Safflower oil
Rice noodles	Unsweetened cocoa powder	Red wine vinegar
Spaghetti noodles	Gluten-free baking mix	Baking soda
Protein powder (see page 196)	Salt-free brown rice cakes	Baking powder
Brown and/or white rice	Chickpeas, canned	
Quinoa	Chopped tomatoes, canned	
Dried mung beans, split peas, and lentils	Tomato paste, canned	
IN THE BREADBOX		
Gluten-free bread and/or whole grain bread		
IN THE FRUIT AND VEGGIE BOWL		
Bananas	Lemons	Garlic
Tomatoes	Onions	Avocados

IN YOUR FREEZER		
Chopped spinach	Mixed veggies	Chicken thighs, bone-less, skinless
Mixed berries	Walnuts	Chicken breasts, bone-less, skinless
Strawberries	Almonds	
Blueberries		Sea bass
		Salmon

IN THE FRIDGE					
HEALTHY FATS	CONDIMENTS	FOOD AS MEDICINE	IN THE PRODUCE DRAWER	DAIRY AND ALTERNATIVES	MISC
Peanut butter	Dijon mustard	Apple cider vinegar	Spinach and/or kale	Unsweet-ened almond, coconut, cashew, soy, or dairy milk	Chia seeds
Almond butter	Yellow mustard		Romaine lettuce		Maple syrup
Cashew butter	Balsamic vinegar		Ginger		Coconut flour
Extra-virgin olive oil	Soy sauce		Parsley	0% plain Greek yogurt	Almond Flour
Ghee	Tamari sauce		Carrots		Eggs
Coconut oil			Celery		Hummus
Grass-fed butter			Cucum-bers		
			Sweet potatoes		

WHEN TO GO ORGANIC AND HOW TO AVOID ADDITIVES

Understanding what and when to buy organic can be overwhelming. Buying everything organic can be expensive, so it is important to know the most critical foods to always buy organic.

The Environmental Working Group (EWG) is a nonprofit organization that works to protect the environment (for more information, visit ewg.org). The EWG provides two lists for the public. The first lists those fruits and veggies that are more likely to have higher amounts of pesticides, even after washing. This "Dirty Dozen" should be purchased and used only if they are certified organic and are pesticide-free. The second list is the "Clean 15," which tells you the fruits and veggies that have the least amounts of pesticides. Find both lists at ewg.org.

Buy Only Certified Organic

In a consumer market where we all desire healthier, less toxic foods, labels can be confusing. Packaging and labels can boast that foods are "natural" or "fresh," without being certified organic. The safest way to make sure that a food is organic and pesticide-free is to look for the USDA-certified organic label (see the picture at right).

Common Chemicals and Additives to Avoid

The best way to avoid chemicals and additives is to eat real, whole USDA-certified organic foods, and to avoid anything that comes in a package, bag, or box. That said, I live in the same world you do, and I can't always go 100 percent package-free, but I do try to avoid foods with the biggest chemical and additive offenders, which include MSG, nitrates, BHA, BHT, sodium benzoate, FD&C dyes, and many more. You can find an extensive list of foods that are safe and foods with toxins and additives to avoid at https://cspinet.org/eating-healthy/chemical-cuisine.

RECIPES

Regardless of your Super Woman Power Type, getting into the kitchen can be a matter of time and energy—we are all busy women juggling multiple roles, responsibilities, and obligations! Here is where you'll find all the recipes for all the Power Types (save for some simple snacks). You'll see some recipes here that aren't included in the first 3 weeks of your meal plan. Use these extra recipes for added variety and sustained super powers as you move beyond your first 3 weeks. Just make sure to check that the numbers are comparable for calories, protein, and fat, especially if weight loss is one of your goals. Most of the recipes I have included are my own or those of my talented sister, Shireen, a busy mom who happens to be an anesthesiologist. We both love to cook and create, and while we are different Power Types (I'm a Savvy Chick, she's an Earth Mama), we are both the same when it comes to being short on time. With that in mind, the recipes you'll find included are quick and easy.

Secondly, many of the following recipes already are or can be made gluten free, lactose free, paleo, vegan, and so on. Depending on your Power Type and 3-week plan, you'll want to choose appropriate recipes or modify them to make them work for you.

- Vegetarian (V)

- Vegan (Vg)

- Paleo (P)

- Gluten-Free (GF)

- Lactose-Free (LF)

Remember, you have a sample menu you can choose from in the 3-Week Rx you are following (Chapters 6 through 10), or you can read through the recipes and look for the symbols that match your dietary requirements.

SUPER POWERED SMOOTHIES

Smoothies are my go-to Super Woman Rx meal or snack. They are power-packed full of nutrients and are great for breakfast, lunch, snacks, and dinners. You'll see them in each and every 3-Week Rx—and because they serve multiple purposes, they get priority and their own special stand-alone category.

Chocolate Protein Smoothie

(V, Vg, P, GF, LF)   Makes 1 serving

1 cup rice, coconut, or almond milk

1 frozen banana (or 1 regular banana and ¼ cup crushed ice or 8 ice cubes)

2 scoops chocolate protein powder (see "Dr. Taz's Favorite Protein Powders" on page 196)

1 tablespoon almond butter

10 chocolate chips (optional)

1 teaspoon instant coffee (optional)

In a blender, combine the milk, banana, protein powder, and almond butter. If desired, add the chocolate chips or coffee. Blend until smooth. Pour into a glass and enjoy.

Nutrition per Serving

410 calories, 11 g fat, 1 g saturated fat, 600 mg sodium, 39 g carbohydrates, 16 g sugars, 12 g fiber, 42 g protein

CANNED VERSUS COLD COCONUT MILK

Please note that some of the recipes call for canned coconut milk while others simply call for coconut milk. In the latter I am referring to the cartons of coconut milk that you find in the dairy section of your grocery store. This refrigerated version of coconut milk has been more diluted to make it less fatty and more drinkable, while canned coconut milk is higher in fat and creamier. The canned version is traditionally used for cooking. Coconut water often has added sugars and is often used as a sports drink. It isn't used in any of the recipes in this book.

Tropical Delight

(V, Vg, P, GF, LF)   Makes 1 serving

1 cup coconut, rice, or almond milk

¼ cup frozen chopped pineapple

¼ cup frozen chopped mango

2 teaspoons coconut oil

1 banana

2 scoops vanilla protein powder (see "Dr. Taz's Favorite Protein Powders" on page 196)

In a blender, combine the milk, pineapple, mango, oil, banana, and protein powder. Blend until smooth. Pour into a glass and enjoy.

Nutrition per Serving

With Almond Milk:

530 calories, 21 g fat, 9 g saturated fat, 600 mg sodium, 52 g carbohydrates, 28 g sugars, 14 g fiber, 43 g protein

With Coconut Milk:

610 calories, 20 g fat, 9 g saturated fat, 540 mg sodium, 75 g carbohydrates, 41 g sugars, 13 g fiber, 42 g protein

With Rice Milk:

610 calories, 20 g fat, 9 g saturated fat, 540 mg sodium, 75 g carbohydrates, 41 g sugars, 13 g fiber, 42 g protein

NOTE: For Savvy Chicks, substitute coconut kefir.

Berry Bomb

(V, Vg, P, GF, LF)   Makes 1 serving

1 cup coconut or almond milk

2 scoops vanilla or plain protein powder (see "Dr. Taz's Favorite Protein Powders" on page 196)

2 teaspoons coconut oil

½ cup frozen blueberries

½ cup frozen strawberries

1–2 mint leaves (optional)

½ cup spinach or kale (optional)

In a blender, combine the milk, protein powder, oil, blueberries, and strawberries. If desired, add the mint or spinach or kale. Blend until smooth. Pour into a glass and enjoy.

Nutrition per Serving

510 calories, 27 g fat, 13 g saturated fat, 440 mg sodium, 39 g carbohydrates, 13 g sugars, 18 g fiber, 41 g protein

DR. TAZ'S FAVORITE PROTEIN POWDERS

With a ton of available protein powders on the market, picking the right one can be tough. The protein in most powders comes from whey, whey isolate, soy, egg, rice, pea, or hemp protein, or some combination of these proteins. Some general rules to observe when picking a protein powder include:

1. Don't pick a protein powder that has sugar listed as one of the first three ingredients. If you are trying to lose weight, don't pick protein powders with other sweeteners like dextrin or maltodextrin.

2. Skip soy, whey, and branched chain amino acid protein powders. These powders are designed for bulking or building muscle and aren't as sensitive to super women digestive systems.

3. For people with delicate digestive systems, which includes just about all super women, rice, pea, and hemp protein are your best choices.

Here are the brands I recommend.

- ◆ Metagenics: UltraMeal Advanced Protein, Ultra Glucose Control
- ◆ Vega: Chocolate
- ◆ Garden of Life: Vanilla
- ◆ Dr. Taz Protein Powder

Note: See Resources, page 316, for ordering information.

Cinnamon Banana Smoothie

(V, P, GF)   Makes 1 serving

1 medium banana

⅔ cup plain Greek yogurt

1 teaspoon maple syrup

Pinch of ground cinnamon

1 scoop vanilla protein powder

In a blender, combine the banana, yogurt, maple syrup, cinnamon, and protein powder. Blend until smooth.

Nutrition per Serving

360 calories, 5 g fat, 1 g saturated fat, 360 mg sodium, 52 g carbohydrates, 34 g sugars, 7 g fiber, 32 g protein

Mocha Banana Jump Start

(V, Vg, P, GF, LF)

This is one of my favorites.   Makes 1 serving

2 scoops chocolate protein powder

1 frozen banana

½ teaspoon instant coffee

1 cup rice or coconut milk

In a blender, combine the protein powder, banana, coffee, and milk. Blend until smooth.

Nutrition per Serving

410 calories, 13 g fat, 5 g saturated fat, 440 mg sodium, 41 g carbohydrates, 16 g sugars, 12 g fiber, 41 g protein

Grocer's Choice Green Drink

(V, Vg, GF, LF)   Makes 1 serving

This is a simple smoothie that uses whatever is in your produce drawer and freezer.

2 cups assorted greens, such as kale, spinach, beet greens, arugula, and/or Swiss chard

1 cup chopped frozen fruit, such as mango, blueberries, strawberries, or peaches

1 banana, ½ avocado, or 1 tablespoon cashew butter

1 cup water

1 teaspoon chia seeds, finely chopped dates, or coconut flakes (optional)

In a blender, combine the greens; fruit; banana, avocado, or cashew butter; water; and chia seeds, dates, or coconut (if desired). Blend until smooth.

Nutrition per Serving

270 calories, 3 g fat, 0 g saturated fat, 55 mg sodium, 60 g carbohydrates, 37 g sugars, 11 g fiber, 8 g protein (*Note:* Nutrition information will change depending on ingredients used.)

Dr. Taz's Liver Lover Smoothie

(V, Vg, GF, LF)   Makes 1 serving

Greens flush and cleanse your liver, especially those greens packed with antioxidants, such as dandelion, parsley, and cilantro. This smoothie is crammed with all three, and you'll see it on many of the 3-Week Power Plans.

1 cup chopped raw or steamed beets

1 carrot, coarsely chopped

1 rib celery, coarsely chopped

½ cup dandelion greens

¼ cup parsley

¼ cup cilantro

¾–1 cup water

In a blender, combine the beets, carrot, celery, dandelion greens, parsley, cilantro, and water. If desired, add 4 ice cubes for a thicker consistency.

Nutrition per Serving

90 calories, 1 g fat, 0 g saturated fat, 190 mg sodium, 20 g carbohydrates, 10 g sugars, 7 g fiber, 4 g protein

DRINKS, TONICS, AND TEAS

These gut-building, immunity-strengthening, digestion-boosting beverages offer a powerful punch.

Ginger Tea

Makes 1 serving

Ginger is a warming agent in both Chinese and Ayurvedic medicine. It helps to wake up the digestive system, making it a perfect morning beverage. Numerous studies point to the health benefits of ginger.

½ teaspoon peeled and finely sliced fresh ginger

½ teaspoon honey

1 cup boiling water

Add the ginger to the boiling water and allow to simmer for 1 to 3 minutes. Stir in the honey. Strain into a mug and enjoy!

Honey Lemon Tea

Makes 1 serving

Lemon juice helps to activate the gut and digestive system.

Juice of ½ lemon

½ teaspoon honey

1 cup boiling water

Stir the lemon juice into the boiling water. Add the honey and stir, or froth for 1 minute.

Honey Turmeric Tea

Makes 1 serving

Turmeric is one of the most powerful natural anti-inflammatories. It helps to ease inflammation, wake up the gut, and boost the immune system.

1 cup boiling water   1–2 teaspoons honey
1 teaspoon ground turmeric

Combine the boiling water, turmeric, and honey and stir well.

Turmeric Pepper Honey Tea

Makes 1 serving

This is a great daily drink that reduces inflammation and keeps your hormones in check. Plus, this simple home remedy is easy to make. Turmeric, with its active ingredient curcumin, is known to fight inflammation and balance hormones. This recipe adds black pepper, another anti-inflammatory, which helps boost turmeric's bioavailability in the body. When you mix these two immunity boosters with two more, black or green tea (known to help the body fight viruses) and honey, another of nature's immune-building agents, you have a soothing powerhouse in one little cup.

2 teaspoons ground turmeric   1 cup boiling water
½ teaspoon ground black   1 tea bag (your favorite variety)
  pepper   1 teaspoon honey

Add the turmeric and pepper to the boiling water and stir well. Add the tea bag and honey. Steep for 5 minutes.

ACV Shot

Makes 1 serving

While this combo is easy to make, I can't promise that it's tasty. If you can tolerate larger amounts, try 2 tablespoons of vinegar in 4 ounces of water.

1 tablespoon apple cider vinegar

3 tablespoons water

In a cup, combine the vinegar with the water and drink quickly.

Lemon Water

Makes 1 serving

Juice of ½ lemon

¾ cup warm water

½ teaspoon honey (optional)

Combine the lemon juice with the water and stir. If desired, stir in the honey. For even more fun, try frothing this concoction. *Yum!* I crave this in the winter.

Pomegranate Juice

Makes 1 serving

This is a bit of work to make on your own, but it's worth it. Not only is the juice tasty, but it's also absolutely beautiful. Make extra and store it in the fridge for up to 3 days.

½ pomegranate

1 cup water

Scoop out the seeds from the pomegranate half, discarding the membrane and peel. In a blender, combine the pomegranate seeds with the water. Blend until smooth.

Two Green Power Drinks

These blends give you an instant burst of oxygen—in fact, we know that when we blend greens, an important antioxidant called glutathione is released. This antioxidant helps protects the cells in your body—especially the mitochondria (the powerhouses of the cells). Cherries and berries have a high antioxidant load as well. *Tip:* You can add a scoop or two of vanilla or strawberry protein powder to make this drink into a full smoothie meal.

Kale-Cherry-Berry Super Juice

Makes 1 serving

1 cup fresh kale

½ cup frozen cherries

¼ cup frozen blueberries

1 cup water

In a blender, combine the kale, cherries, blueberries, and water. Blend until smooth, pour, and enjoy.

Nutrition per Serving

130 calories, 2 g fat, 0 g saturated fat, 25 mg sodium, 29 g carbohydrates, 17 g sugars, 7 g fiber, 4 g protein

Berry-Spinach Power Punch

Makes 1 serving

1 cup fresh spinach

½ cup frozen strawberries

1 banana

1 cup water

In a blender, combine the spinach, strawberries, banana, and water. Blend until smooth, pour, and enjoy.

Nutrition per Serving

135 calories, 0 g fat, 0 g saturated fat, 25 mg sodium, 8 g carbohydrates, 4 g sugars, 2 g fiber, 1 g protein

SUPER WOMEN BREAKFASTS

Here is the Super Woman Rx secret to a healthy breakfast: Make it or prep it ahead of time. The morning can be chaotic, so many of these recipes were intended for you to prepare them the night before. What is even more efficient is that these recipes can also function as a midmorning snack or afternoon pick-me-up. Just make a bit extra or use the leftovers later in the day!

SAVORY DISHES

Paleo Quiche

(P, GF, LF) — Makes 3 servings

If you'd like to make this quiche with a crust for a meal that's a bit more substantial, try the Sweet Potato Crust (page 204).

6 large eggs

½ cup coconut milk

½ teaspoon sea salt

Pinch of ground nutmeg

1 teaspoon coconut oil

½ medium onion or leek, chopped

1 clove garlic, minced

½ cup chopped mushrooms

1-½ cups chopped fresh spinach

½ cup cooked and crumbled turkey, chicken, or vegetarian sausage

1. Preheat the oven to 300°F.

2. In a blender, combine the eggs, coconut milk, salt, and nutmeg. Blend until smooth. Set aside.

3. In a wide skillet, heat the oil over medium heat. Cook the onion or leek and the garlic, stirring frequently, until nearly tender. Add the mushrooms and cook until most of the liquid has been released.

4. Transfer the onion mixture to a glass bowl and let cool slightly. Add the reserved egg mixture, spinach, and sausage and stir to combine.

5. Pour into a 9" pie pan coated with a small amount of coconut oil.

6. Bake for 50 to 55 minutes, or until the center is set.

Nutrition per Serving

460 calories, 28 g fat, 10 g saturated fat, 300 mg sodium, 6 g carbohydrates, 1 g sugars, 1 g fiber, 22 g protein

Sweet Potato Crust

Makes 8 servings

2 cups shredded sweet
potatoes

2 tablespoons arrowroot
powder

2 tablespoons ghee

1. Preheat the oven to 425°F.

2. In a food processor, combine the sweet potatoes, arrowroot powder, and ghee. Process until a dough begins to form.

3. Transfer to a clean work surface and roll out into about a 10" circle. Press into a 9" pie pan.

4. Bake for 15 minutes. Remove from the oven and add the filling. Proceed with the recipe as directed.

Nutrition per Serving

70 calories, 4 g fat, 2.5 g saturated fat, 25 mg sodium, 8 g carbohydrates, 1 g sugars, 1 g fiber, <1 g protein

Greek Omelet

(V, P, GF)   Makes 1 serving

1 teaspoon olive oil

½ cup chopped tomato

2 teaspoons chopped sun-
dried tomatoes

1 tablespoon chopped onion

½ cup chopped spinach

½ cup kalamata olives, chopped

1 tablespoon crumbled feta
cheese (omit if dairy or
lactose sensitive)

1 teaspoon finely chopped
fresh dill

1 teaspoon chopped fresh
oregano or ½ teaspoon dried

3 large eggs, beaten

Pinch of salt and ground
black pepper

1. In a nonstick skillet, heat the oil over medium-high heat. Cook the tomato, sun-dried tomatoes, onion, and spinach until the juice of the tomato has evaporated. Add the olives, feta, dill, and oregano and stir to combine.

2. Pour in the eggs, reduce the heat to medium, and cook for 3 minutes, or until the eggs are nearly cooked through.

3. Turn off the heat, cover the skillet, and let sit until the eggs have set.

4. Fold the omelet in half and serve.

Nutrition per Serving

360 calories, 24 g fat, 6 g saturated fat, 440 mg sodium, 10 g carbohydrates, 5 g sugars, 3 g fiber, 20 g protein

NOTE: For Savvy Chicks, please omit cheese.

Breakfast Skillet

(V, P, GF, LF)   Makes 2 servings

½ tablespoon coconut, safflower, or sunflower oil

½ cup finely chopped potato (you can steam the potato ahead of time for faster cooking)

1 tablespoon finely chopped onion

½ cup chopped sausage (chicken, beef, turkey, or vegetarian) (you can cook it ahead for faster assembly)

½–1 teaspoon ground red pepper (depending on your desire for spiciness)

½ teaspoon salt

1 teaspoon ground cumin

1 teaspoon garlic powder

1 cup chopped kale

½ cup finely chopped Brussels sprouts

1 teaspoon honey

2 eggs

1. In an 8" skillet, heat the oil over medium-high heat. Cook the potato and onion, stirring frequently, for 5 to 10 minutes, or until tender.

2. Add the sausage and cook, stirring frequently, for 5 minutes, or until no longer pink. Add the red pepper, salt, cumin, and garlic powder and stir to combine. Add the kale and Brussels sprouts and cook, stirring frequently, for 3 minutes, or until browned. Add the honey and stir to combine.

3. Crack the eggs over the skillet mixture and cook, stirring, until the eggs have cooked through. Divide between 2 plates and serve.

Nutrition per Serving

430 calories, 27 g fat, 13 g saturated fat, 575 mg sodium, 24 g carbohydrates, 6 g sugars, 3 g fiber, 24 g protein

Festive Italian Frittata

(V, P, GF)   Makes 4 or 6 servings

12 eggs

¼ cup shredded mozzarella or crumbled goat cheese

1 tablespoon coconut oil or ghee, divided

¼ cup chopped onion

1 tomato, chopped

1 cup arugula

1 tablespoon chopped fresh basil

8 mushrooms, chopped

½ bell pepper, chopped

¼ cup green olives, chopped

1 teaspoon salt

1 teaspoon paprika

¼ teaspoon ground red pepper

Pinch of ground black pepper

1. Preheat the oven to 325°F.

2. In a medium bowl, mix together the eggs, cheese, and ½ tablespoon of the coconut oil or ghee. Set aside.

3. In an ovenproof skillet, heat the remaining ½ tablespoon coconut oil or ghee over medium-high heat. Cook the onion, stirring, for 1 minute. Add the tomato, arugula, basil, mushrooms, bell pepper, olives, salt, paprika, red pepper, and black pepper. Cook, stirring, for 2 minutes, or until the vegetables are tender.

4. Pour the reserved egg mixture into the skillet, reduce the heat to medium, and cook until the edges are set, about 30 seconds.

5. Transfer the skillet to the oven and bake for 10 minutes, or until the center of the frittata is firm. Allow to cool slightly before serving.

Nutrition per Serving

Serving size = ¼ frittata: 300 calories, 20 g fat, 9 g saturated fat, 920 mg sodium, 7 g carbohydrates, 3 g sugars, 4 g fiber, 23 g protein

Serving size = ⅙ frittata: 200 calories, 14 g fat, 6 g saturated fat, 610 mg sodium, 7 g carbohydrates, 2 g sugars, 1 g fiber, 15 g protein

NOTE: For Savvy Chicks and Earth Mamas, omit cheese in this recipe.

Egg-Veggie Roll-Up

(V, P, GF, LF)

Makes 3 servings

8 eggs

¼ cup baking mix (any gluten-free or whole grain variety)

2 teaspoons coconut oil

1 teaspoon chopped red onion

1 teaspoon chopped tomato

½ bell pepper, cut in strips

1 teaspoon salt

½ teaspoon paprika

½ teaspoon ground red pepper (optional)

¼–½ cup chopped kale, spinach, or arugula

1. In a medium bowl, mix together the eggs and baking mix until a clear, thin batter forms.

2. In a large skillet, heat the oil over medium heat. Cook the egg mixture for 1 minute, or until bubbles form on the surface. Turn and cook until the bottom is golden. Slide onto a large plate or tray.

3. In a small bowl, mix together the onion, tomato, bell pepper, salt, paprika, and red pepper (if using).

4. Sprinkle the greens in a line down the center of the egg fritter. Sprinkle the onion mixture over the greens. Starting at one side, roll the egg fritter over the veggies into a log shape. Cut into 3 equal pieces and serve.

Nutrition per Serving

210 calories, 13 g fat, 4g saturated fat, 300 mg sodium, 6 g carbohydrates, 3 g sugars, 2 g fiber, 18 g protein

Huevos Rancheros

(V, P, GF, LF)   Makes 2 servings

1-½ teaspoons coconut oil, divided

1 small yellow onion, thinly sliced

2 medium cloves garlic, thinly sliced

14 ounces (½ of a 28-ounce can) crushed tomatoes

7-½ ounces (½ of a 15-ounce can) red enchilada sauce

½ teaspoon dried oregano (preferably Mexican)

½ teaspoon ground cumin

2 eggs

Kosher salt and ground black pepper, if desired

½ avocado, sliced

1 tablespoon crumbled Cotija cheese, for serving (omit if avoiding lactose)

¼ cup finely chopped cilantro leaves and fine stems, plus more for serving

Lime wedge

1. In a skillet at least 2" deep, heat ¾ teaspoon of the oil over medium heat. Cook the onion and garlic, stirring frequently, until lightly browned and aromatic.

2. In a medium bowl, combine the tomatoes and enchilada sauce. Add to the onion mixture. Stir in the oregano and cumin. Reduce the heat to low and simmer for 5 to 10 minutes.

3. In another skillet, heat the remaining ¾ teaspoon oil over medium heat. Cook the eggs as you like them (over easy is traditional). Add salt and pepper, if desired.

4. Spoon the sauce onto 2 plates. Top each with an egg, half of the avocado slices, and cheese (if using). Garnish with cilantro and squeeze the lime over both plates for a finishing dash of flavor.

Nutrition per Serving

330 calories, 26 g fat, 6 g saturated fat, 250 mg sodium, 19 g carbohydrates, 1 g sugars, 6 g fiber, 9 g protein

NOTE: For Savvy Chicks and Earth Mamas, omit cheese.

Avocado Toast

(V, Vg, GF, LF)Makes 2 servings

This also makes a great snack.

1 small avocado, halved, pitted, peeled, and mashed

1 teaspoon salt

½ teaspoon ground black pepper

½ teaspoon paprika

¼ tomato, chopped

2 slices gluten-free or Ezekiel bread (or other sprouted bread)

1 tablespoon olive oil

1 hard-cooked egg or ¼ cup mashed tofu (if you are vegan)

1. In a small bowl, mix the avocado with the salt, pepper, paprika, and tomato.

2. Lightly toast the bread.

3. Brush the toast with the oil. Spread the avocado mixture over the toast. Cut the egg into thin slices and place on top of the avocado (if using tofu, mash and mix it with the avocado).

Nutrition per Serving

290 calories, 20 g fat, 3 g saturated fat, 170 mg sodium, 23 g carbohydrates, 4 g sugars, 9 g fiber, 8 g protein

Tofu Scramble

(V, Vg, P, GF, LF)Makes 2 servings

1 tablespoon coconut oil or ghee

1 tablespoon chopped red onion

1 package (14 ounces) extra-firm tofu, cut into small squares

1 cup chopped kale, spinach, or Swiss chard

1 tomato, chopped

½ teaspoon Himalayan or regular salt

½ teaspoon paprika

Pinch of ground black pepper

2 tablespoons crumbled feta or goat cheese

In a skillet, melt the oil or ghee over medium-high heat. Cook the onion, stirring frequently, for 2 minutes, or until tender. Add the tofu and cook, stirring frequently, until tender. Add the greens and tomato and cook, stirring, for 1 to 2 minutes, or until tender. Stir in the salt, paprika, and pepper. Divide between 2 plates. Sprinkle with the cheese.

Nutrition per Serving

250 calories, 15 g fat, 6 g saturated fat, 80 mg sodium, 13 g carbohydrates, 3 g sugars, 4 g fiber, 20 g protein

Pancake Imposters

(V, P, GF, LF)   Makes 2 servings

My kids love these so much that they are practically a staple in our home.
They also make a great snack.

½ cup pancake mix (paleo,
gluten free, or regular)

4 eggs

1 tablespoon coconut oil

1 tablespoon chocolate chips
(omit on Earth Mama and
Nightingale plans)

1 tablespoon chopped walnuts
(toasted, if desired)

1 teaspoon unsweetened
coconut flakes

½ teaspoon honey

1. In a medium bowl, mix the pancake mix with the eggs, oil, and chocolate
   chips.

2. Grease a nonstick skillet or griddle and heat over medium heat. Pour the
   batter into the skillet in 3" to 4" circles. Sprinkle with the walnuts and coconut. Cook for 30 to 45 seconds, or until bubbles form on the surface. Turn
   and cook until the bottoms are brown. Divide between 2 plates and drizzle
   with the honey or eat plain.

Nutrition per Serving

240 calories, 16 g fat, 6 g saturated fat, 350 mg sodium, 5 g carbohydrates, 4.5 g
sugars, 1 g fiber, 17 g protein

It's Not Really French Toast

(V, GF, LF)   Makes 4 servings

1 tablespoon melted grass-fed
butter or ghee, divided

4 slices bread (gluten-free,
wheat, sprouted, or fermented)

6 eggs

1 cup unsweetened vanilla
coconut, almond, or cashew
milk

2 teaspoons vanilla extract

½ cup sliced bananas or
peaches

¼ cup maple syrup

1. Preheat the oven to 350°F.

2. Pour half of the butter or ghee in an 8" x 8" or 9" x 9" shallow baking pan and tip the pan to distribute evenly. Layer the bread evenly in the pan and brush the remaining butter evenly over the tops.

3. In a medium bowl, whisk together the eggs, milk, and vanilla. Pour over the bread. Layer the bananas or peaches evenly over the bread. Pour the maple syrup evenly over the top.

4. Place in the center of the oven and bake for 20 to 30 minutes, or until firm and slightly browned. Cool for 10 minutes before serving.

Nutrition per Serving

350 calories, 14 g fat, 5 g saturated fat, 230 mg sodium, 45 g carbohydrates, 30 g sugars, 2 g fiber, 11 g protein

NOTE: For Savvy Chicks, please use coconut oil instead of butter or ghee.

PARFAITS AND PUDDING

Granola-Berry Parfait

(V, GF)   Makes 1 serving

This is another easy one that your kids (and you) will love.

1 cup plain Greek yogurt

1 cup berries (your favorite variety)

¼ cup sliced almonds

½ cup granola (I like Nature's Path Sunrise Crunchy Vanilla and Bob's Red Mill Gluten-Free Granola)

1 teaspoon honey

In a large cup or a Mason jar (if you're making the parfait to go), layer ¼ cup of the yogurt, ¼ cup of the berries, 1 tablespoon of the nuts, and 2 tablespoons of the granola. Repeat the layers 3 times. Drizzle the top with the honey and enjoy immediately or put the lid on the Mason jar and store in the refrigerator for later.

Nutrition per Serving

410 calories, 13 g fat, 2 g saturated fat, 280 mg sodium, 55 g carbohydrates, 31 g sugars, 8 g fiber, 22 g protein

NOTE: For Savvy Chicks, please use dairy-free yogurt.

Walnut-Berry-Yogurt Parfait

(V, P, GF)   Makes 1 serving

Even faster to make than a smoothie, this quick cup of high-powered protein, omega-3 healthy fats, and antioxidant-packed berries will get you out the door, ready for your day.

⅔ cup plain Greek yogurt   5 walnut halves, chopped

½ cup thawed frozen berries

In a small bowl, mix the yogurt and berries. Sprinkle the walnuts on top.

Nutrition per Serving

340 calories, 25 g fat, 2 g saturated fat, 280 mg sodium, 60 g carbohydrates, 13 g sugars, 11 g fiber, 27 g protein

Coconut Chia Seed Pudding

(V, Vg, GF, LF)   Makes 4 servings

This is one of my family's favorites—and once your family discovers this pudding, you may want to double or even triple the recipe (it disappears fast). This reminds me of the famous Pomegranate Chia Pudding at the Le Pain Quotidien restaurants I've dined at in New York City and Los Angeles. Make it the night before and have a delicious breakfast waiting for you when you wake up.

½ cup chia seeds   1 tablespoon canned coconut
                                             cream (can freeze extra)
2 cups coconut, almond,
cashew, or soy milk   1 tablespoon honey

2 teaspoons vanilla extract

In a medium bowl, mix together the chia seeds, milk, vanilla, coconut cream, and honey. Pour into 4 ramekins or small dishes. Cover with plastic wrap and refrigerate overnight to set.

Nutrition per Serving

185 calories, 12 g fat, 4 g saturated fat, 8 mg sodium, 16 g carbohydrates, 3 g sugars, 11 g fiber, 5 g protein

Nut Butter Sandwich

(V, GF, LF) Makes 1 serving

So easy—and great for when you're on the go.

2 slices whole grain or gluten-free bread

1 tablespoon almond butter

1 teaspoon honey

Place 1 slice of bread on a clean work surface. Spread the almond butter over the bread. Drizzle with the honey. Top with the second slice of bread.

Nutrition per Serving

240 calories, 11 g fat, 1.5 g saturated fat, 290 mg sodium, 28 g carbohydrates, 4 g sugars, 5 g fiber, 10 g protein

Nut Butter Dream Bars

(V, Vg, P, GF, LF) Makes 12

This recipe is equally good for breakfast and snacks.

2 cups almond butter

1 cup cashew butter

1 cup pumpkin puree or applesauce

½ cup chocolate chips or 1 tablespoon maple syrup

1 tablespoon coconut oil or grass-fed butter, melted

2 scoops chocolate protein powder

In a large bowl, combine the almond butter, cashew butter, pumpkin puree or applesauce, chocolate chips or maple syrup, oil or butter, and protein powder. Stir well. Pour into an 8" x 8" baking dish. Cover with plastic wrap and refrigerate overnight. Cut into 12 bars.

Nutrition per Bar

430 calories, 36 g fat, 6 g saturated fat, 190 mg sodium, 19 g carbohydrates, 8 g sugars, 6 g fiber, 15 g protein

Mini Protein Muffins

(V, P, GF, LF)   Makes 12

These muffins are another great recipe option for breakfast or a snack.

6 eggs, beaten

1 cup gluten-free cornmeal

1 tablespoon chopped tomato

1 tablespoon chopped onion

1 tablespoon chopped mushroom

1 teaspoon baking soda

2 teaspoons coconut sugar

1. Preheat the oven to 350°F. Place paper liners in a 12-cup muffin pan or coat with cooking spray.

2. In a medium bowl, combine the eggs, cornmeal flour, tomato, onion, mushroom, baking soda, and coconut sugar. Use a fork to mix.

3. Divide among the muffin cups. Bake for 20 to 25 minutes, or until an inserted toothpick comes out clean. Cool on a rack.

Nutrition per Muffin

80 calories, 3 g fat, 1 g saturated fat, 0 mg sodium, 9 g carbohydrates, <1 g sugars, 1 g fiber, 4 g protein

Protein Banana Bread

(V, P, GF, LF)   Makes 10 servings

2 tablespoons grass-fed butter or coconut oil, melted

½ cup almond or cashew butter

½ cup brown sugar

1 teaspoon vanilla extract

¾ teaspoon baking soda

½ teaspoon salt

3 medium bananas, mashed

2 tablespoons honey

2 eggs, beaten

1-½ cups buckwheat flour (or gluten-free flour blend)

⅓ cup dark chocolate chips (optional)

1. Preheat the oven to 350°F. Coat an 8" x 4" or 9" x 5" loaf pan with a small amount of coconut oil.

2. In a large bowl, combine the butter or oil, nut butter, sugar, vanilla, baking soda, salt, bananas, honey, eggs, flour, and chocolate chips (if using). Stir until mixed.

3. Pour into the loaf pan and bake for 45 minutes, or until an inserted toothpick comes out clean. Cool on a rack.

Nutrition per Serving

310 calories, 11 g fat, 3.5 g saturated fat, 260 mg sodium, 50 g carbohydrates, 23 g sugars, 4 g fiber, 5 g protein

WHAT ABOUT MY MORNING COFFEE?

There was a time when I used to think I couldn't live without my morning coffee and afternoon sodas. Coffee does have antioxidants and some beneficial effects, so 4 to 6 ounces of coffee daily is okay, but more than that and it spikes insulin and can keep you awake. So stick to one small cup and replace subsequent servings with black or green tea.

SUPER WOMAN LUNCHES AND DINNERS

I grouped the Super Woman Rx lunches and dinners together, since these recipes are interchangeable, and depending on your type, you may need to eat more through the early part of your day than you do at dinner. My secret? Prep three meals at the start of every week, make it to hump day (Wednesday) and prep one more, and then the kitchen—as I joke with my family—is closed on Friday. Between leftovers and hopefully a few fun events, I give myself a break on Friday and Saturday.

SALADS

Mason Jar Salads

(V, P, GF)   Makes 1 serving

These are fun, easy ways to create salads for work or on the go anywhere. Find medium-size (16-ounce) Mason jars if you want to prep several salads for the week. Just line them up and play with the following variations.

Chicken or Turkey Mason Jar Salad

1 tablespoon any dressing or just olive oil and balsamic vinegar

¼ cup chopped cooked chicken breast or turkey (omit if vegetarian)

1 cup salad greens

2 tablespoons chopped walnuts

½ cup chopped apple or pear

½ cup crumbled goat cheese

Pour the dressing in the bottom of the jar. Over the dressing, layer the greens, apple or pear, chicken or turkey (if using), walnuts, and goat cheese. Seal the jar and refrigerate. Stays fresh for days! Shake before serving, or dump into a bowl and toss.

Nutrition per Serving

630 calories, 30 g fat, 9 g saturated fat, 105 mg sodium, 20 g carbohydrates, 9 g sugars, 6 g fiber, 27 g protein

Vegetarian or Vegan Mason Jar Salad

1 tablespoon any dressing or just olive oil and balsamic vinegar

1 cup salad greens

½ cup chopped cucumber

½ cup chopped tomato

¼ cup chopped olives

¼ cup crumbled feta cheese (omit for vegan)

1 hard-cooked egg, sliced (use ½ cup chickpeas for vegan)

Pour the dressing in the bottom of the jar. Over the dressing, layer the greens, cucumber, tomato, olives, feta (if using), and egg or chickpeas. Seal the jar and refrigerate. Shake before serving.

Nutrition per Serving

370 calories, 30 g fat, 10 g saturated fat, 660 mg sodium, 10 g carbohydrates, 5 g sugars, 4 g fiber, 13 g protein

BBQ Chicken Salad

(P, GF, LF)   Makes 4 servings

2 boneless, skinless chicken breasts (about 5 ounces each)

1 tablespoon olive oil

1 teaspoon salt

½ cup barbecue sauce, divided

1 head romaine lettuce

1 can (15 ounces) corn, drained

1 cucumber, chopped

1 tablespoon crumbled goat cheese

1. Preheat the grill or broiler.

2. Coat the chicken breasts with the oil and sprinkle with the salt. Brush on ¼ cup of the barbecue sauce. Grill or broil the chicken for 10 to 20 minutes, turning once, or until a thermometer inserted in the thickest portion registers 165°F and the juices run clear. Allow to cool slightly. Chop into cubes.

3. Chop the lettuce and place it in a large bowl. Add the corn, cucumber, and goat cheese and toss to combine. Add the chicken and remaining ¼ cup barbecue sauce. Toss well to combine.

Nutrition per Serving

560 calories, 17 g fat, 7 g saturated fat, 590 mg sodium, 53 g carbohydrates, 10 g sugars, 5 g fiber, 39 g protein

Chickpea Salad

(V, Vg, GF, LF)   Makes 4 servings

This is a great, portable meal that is easy to throw together. Make this dish a day ahead and let it sit in the fridge in a plastic container—the flavors will meld and be wonderful for lunch the next day.

- 1 can (15 ounces) chickpeas, rinsed and drained
- 1 can (15 ounces) navy beans, rinsed and drained
- 1 can (15 ounces) red kidney beans, rinsed and drained
- ¼ onion, chopped
- 1 tablespoon chopped cilantro
- 1 teaspoon chopped parsley
- 1–2 red tomatoes, chopped
- 2 teaspoons salt
- 1 teaspoon ground black pepper
- 1-½ tablespoons fresh lemon juice

In a large bowl, combine the chickpeas, navy beans, kidney beans, onion, cilantro, parsley, tomatoes, salt, and pepper. Refrigerate until serving. Just before serving, pour the lemon juice over the salad and toss. Adjust salt and pepper to taste.

Nutrition per Serving

360 calories, 2 g fat, 0 g saturated fat, 280 mg sodium, 67 g carbohydrates, 4 g sugars, 17 g fiber, 23 g protein

Chicken Salad with Avocado "Mayo"

(P, GF, LF)   Makes 4 servings

- 1 teaspoon chopped fresh thyme
- 1 teaspoon chopped fresh oregano
- 1 teaspoon chopped fresh rosemary
- 2 split bone-in, skin-on chicken breasts
- 1 tablespoon olive oil
- Sea salt
- 1 cup grapes, halved
- ½ cup apple slices
- 2–3 ribs celery, chopped
- 3 scallions, chopped
- ½ cup slivered almonds
- Romaine lettuce leaves

Avocado "Mayo"

- ½ cup plain Greek yogurt
- 1 medium avocado, halved, pitted, and peeled
- ½ clove garlic
- ¼ cup parsley
- ¼ cup fresh dill
- 3 tablespoons fresh lemon juice
- Kosher salt
- Ground black pepper

1. *To make the salad:* Preheat the oven to 425°F. Line a broiler pan with foil.

2. In a small bowl, combine the thyme, oregano, and rosemary. Stir to mix well.

3. Brush the skin of each chicken breast with the oil. Using a finger, carefully loosen the skin from the meat and spread the herb mixture underneath it. Season both sides of the chicken liberally with sea salt.

4. Place the breasts on the broiler pan, skin side up, and roast for 40 to 45 minutes, or until a thermometer inserted in the thickest portion registers 170°F, the juices run clear, and the skin is golden brown. Transfer to a cutting board to rest for 5 minutes.

5. Remove the skin and bones and discard. Shred the chicken by hand or pulse briefly in a food processor. Be careful not to overprocess. Transfer to a bowl and add the grapes, apple, celery, scallions, and almonds. Toss to combine.

6. *To make the avocado "mayo":* In a food processor, combine the yogurt, avocado, garlic, parsley, dill, and lemon juice. Process until smooth. Add kosher salt and pepper to taste.

7. Pour the avocado "mayo" over the chicken mixture. Divide into four equal portions and serve in the lettuce leaves.

Nutrition per Serving

390 calories, 24 g fat, 4 g saturated fat, 150 mg sodium, 15 g carbohydrates, 7 g sugars, 6 g fiber, 22 g protein

Super Woman Cobb Salad

(V, Vg, P, GF, LF)   Makes 2 servings

3 cups kale leaves

1 cup chopped romaine lettuce

2 slices turkey or veggie bacon, cooked and chopped

8 –10 red grape tomatoes, halved

3 hard-cooked eggs, peeled and sliced (or 3 ounces lightly fried tofu if vegan)

2 avocados, halved, pitted, peeled, and chopped

3 scallions, chopped

½ cup chopped cooked sweet potato

Sea salt

Dressing

2 tablespoons olive oil

2 tablespoons fresh lemon juice

1 clove garlic

⅓ cup parsley

⅓ cup basil

1. *To make the salad:* In a large bowl, combine the kale, romaine, bacon, tomatoes, eggs or tofu, avocados, scallions, sweet potato, and salt to taste.

2. *To make the dressing:* In a food processor or blender, combine the oil, lemon juice, garlic, parsley, and basil. Process or blend until smooth.

3. Add the dressing to the salad and toss to combine. Split into two equal portions.

Nutrition per Serving

600 calories, 44 g fat, 6 g saturated fat, 220 mg sodium, 46 g carbohydrates, 9 g sugars, 21 g fiber, 19 g protein

Salmon-Kale Caesar Salad

(P, GF, LF)   Makes 4 servings

1 tablespoon extra-virgin olive oil

2 cloves garlic, minced, divided

2 salmon fillets (4 ounces each)

4 cashews

½ tablespoon nutritional yeast

2 bunches kale or 1 package (5 ounces) baby kale leaves

8 –10 grape tomatoes

Turkey or veggie bacon crumbles (optional)

Caesar Dressing

1 avocado, halved, pitted, and peeled

¼ cup fresh lemon juice

1 small clove garlic

½ tablespoon Dijon mustard

2 anchovy fillets (can substitute capers)

1. *To make the salad:* In a skillet, heat the oil over medium-high heat. Cook half of the garlic, stirring, until aromatic. Add the salmon and sear on both sides. Reduce the heat to medium and cook for 5 minutes, or until opaque. Set aside.

2. Meanwhile, in a food processor, combine the cashews, yeast, and remaining garlic. Process until smooth. Transfer to a small bowl and set aside.

3. *To make the dressing:* In the food processor, combine the avocado, lemon juice, garlic, mustard, and anchovies. Process until smooth.

4. In a large bowl, combine the kale, tomatoes, bacon (if using), and processed cashew mixture. Toss to mix. Top with the warm salmon and 2 tablespoons of dressing per serving.

Nutrition per Serving

340 calories, 14 g fat, 2 g saturated fat, 130 mg sodium, 5 g carbohydrates, 1 g sugars, 2 g fiber, 42 g protein

NOTE: 2 tablespoons of dressing was used in this calculation.

Greek Salad with Chicken or Chickpeas

(V, P, GF, LF)   Makes 1 serving

2 tablespoons extra-virgin olive oil

1 clove garlic, minced

2 chicken cutlets or ½ cup chickpeas, rinsed and drained

2 cups chopped romaine lettuce

2 tomatoes, chopped

1 cucumber, chopped

1 red or green bell pepper, chopped

½ cup pitted kalamata olives

1 tablespoon chopped fresh oregano

Mixture of fresh chopped herbs (1 teaspoon each dill, oregano, and mint)

Dressing

2 tablespoons fresh lemon juice

1 teaspoon dried oregano

½ tablespoon olive tapenade or capers

4 cashews or blanched almonds

1 clove garlic, halved

Salt

1. *To make the salad:* In a skillet, heat the oil over medium-high heat. Cook the garlic until aromatic. Add the chicken cutlets and sear on both sides. Reduce the heat to medium and cook for 3 to 5 minutes, or until no longer pink and the juices run clear. If using chickpeas, add to the garlic and toss until warm. Transfer the chicken to a cutting board to cool slightly. Slice. Transfer the chickpeas to a plate.

2. *To make the dressing:* In a food processor, combine the lemon juice, oregano, tapenade or capers, nuts, garlic, and salt to taste. Process until smooth.

3. In a bowl, combine the lettuce, tomatoes, cucumber, pepper, olives, oregano, and herbs. Toss to mix. Top with the warm chicken or chickpeas and 2 teaspoons of the dressing.

Nutrition per Serving

With chicken: 570 calories, 13 g fat, 2 g saturated fat, 400 mg sodium, 34 g carbohydrates, 16 g sugars, 12 g fiber, 60 g protein

Nutrition per Serving

With chickpeas: 490 calories, 10 g fat, <1 g saturated fat, 600 mg sodium, 50 g carbohydrates, 17 g sugars, 17 g fiber, 13 g protein

Warm Quinoa and Green Bean Salad

(V)   Makes 2 servings

½ teaspoon olive oil

1 small onion, chopped

1 cup quinoa, cooked

½ teaspoon salt

1 teaspoon ground black pepper

2 cups green beans

1 tablespoon red wine vinegar

1. In a skillet, heat the oil over medium heat. Cook the onion for 3 minutes, or until tender. Add the quinoa, salt, and pepper and stir to combine. Cook until heated through.

2. Meanwhile, in a separate pot, steam or boil the green beans for 5 minutes, or until slightly crisp. Drain.

3. Fold the beans into the quinoa mixture. Top with the vinegar.

Nutrition per Serving

380 calories, 7 g fat, 1 g saturated fat, 600 mg sodium, 67 g carbohydrates, 5 g sugars, 9 g fiber, 14 g protein

FINGER FOODS

Lettuce Roll-Ups

(V, Vg, P, GF, LF)   Makes 1 serving

There are so many variations—shrimp, turkey, beef, chicken, or vegetarian.

4–6 large romaine lettuce leaves

1 medium avocado, halved, pitted, and peeled

¼ teaspoon salt

1 teaspoon garlic powder or 1 clove garlic, minced

Pinch of ground black pepper

¼ cup grated carrots

¼ cup chopped cucumber

1–2 radishes, sliced

4–6 steamed shrimp, ½ cup cooked ground turkey or ground grass-fed beef, ½ cup chicken salad, 3 tablespoons hummus, or 3 ounces lightly browned tofu

1. Spread out the lettuce leaves on a platter.

2. In a bowl, mash the avocado. Add the salt, garlic, and pepper. Stir to combine.

3. Place equal amounts of the avocado mixture 1" above the bottom edge of each leaf. Top each with equal amounts of carrots, cucumber, and radishes. Add your protein of choice and roll up. Use a wooden pick to hold, if desired.

Nutrition per Serving

With shrimp: 420 calories, 31 g fat, 4.5 g saturated fat, 575 mg sodium, 30 g carbohydrates, 6 g sugars, 19 g fiber, 15 g protein

With ground turkey: 520 calories, 39 g fat, 7 g saturated fat, 575 mg sodium, 29 g carbohydrates, 6 g sugars, 19 g fiber, 29 g protein

With ground beef: 600 calories, 35 g fat, 8 g saturated fat, 575 mg sodium, 29 g carbohydrates, 6 g sugars, 19 g fiber, 40 g protein

With chicken salad: 450 calories, 30 g fat, 8 g saturated fat, 575 mg sodium, 29 g carbohydrates, 6 g sugars, 15 g fiber, 38 g protein

With hummus: 460 calories, 35 g fat, 5 g saturated fat, 590 mg sodium, 36 g carbohydrates, 6 g sugars, 22 g fiber, 11 g protein

With tofu: 520 calories, 39 g fat, 4.5 g saturated fat, 575 mg sodium, 35 g carbohydrates, 6 g sugars, 20 g fiber, 29 g protein

Kale Pesto and Eggplant Lettuce Wraps

(V, Vg, P, GF, LF)   Makes 2 servings

Kale Pesto

2 cups baby kale leaves or chopped regular kale

⅓ cup toasted pine nuts (can substitute walnuts or almonds)

¼ cup olive oil

2 large cloves garlic, roughly chopped

2–3 teaspoons freshly grated lemon peel

Freshly squeezed lemon juice

6–10 blanched almonds or cashews

¼ teaspoon garlic salt

2 chicken cutlets or 2 squares tofu (each about the size of a deck of cards)

1 eggplant, cut into large sandwich-bread-size slices

¼ cup olive oil

2 large romaine lettuce leaves

1 red onion, chopped

1 tomato, sliced

1. *For the kale pesto:* In a food processor, combine the kale, nuts, olive oil (reserving 1 teaspoon), garlic, lemon peel and juice, almonds, and garlic salt. Process until smooth.

2. Sprinkle the garlic salt on the chicken or tofu and the eggplant. Heat a skillet or electric grill over high heat. Drizzle the reserved teaspoon olive oil into the pan and sear the chicken or tofu and the eggplant on both sides. Cook until the eggplant is tender and the chicken is no longer pink and the juices run clear or the tofu is heated through.

3. To assemble, place the lettuce leaves horizontally on a clean work surface and spread each with 1 tablespoon of the pesto. Sprinkle with equal amounts of the red onion. For each wrap, layer half of the eggplant, chicken or tofu, and tomato on top of the lettuce and spread an additional 1 tablespoon of the pesto in between the layers. Fold the ends of the lettuce leaves around both sides to complete the wraps.

Nutrition per Serving

With tofu: 290 calories, 17 g fat, 0 g saturated fat, 20 mg sodium, 26 g carbohydrates, 7 g sugars, 5 g fiber, 16 g protein

With chicken: 350 calories, 19 g fat, 1 g saturated fat, 90 mg sodium, 23 g carbohydrates, 7 g sugars, 5 g fiber, 32 g protein

Basil Rolls

(P, GF, LF)   Makes 4 servings

1 tablespoon safflower oil

½ pound boneless, skinless chicken breasts, cut into bite-size pieces

16 medium shrimp, peeled and deveined, steamed

2 cups finely chopped dark leafy greens, such as romaine, kale, spinach, or seaweed

½ cup bean sprouts

½ cup chopped fresh mint

½ cup chopped fresh cilantro

8 round rice paper wrappers

24 fresh leaves basil

½ cup hoisin sauce

¼ cup low-sodium soy sauce

1. In a 12" skillet, heat the oil over medium heat. Cook the chicken, stirring frequently, for 3 to 5 minutes, or until no longer pink. Stir in the shrimp and remove the skillet from the heat.

2. In a medium bowl, combine the greens, sprouts, mint, and cilantro. Toss to mix.

3. Fill a shallow dish with warm water. Dip each wrapper in the water for 30 seconds, or until it softens and becomes pliable.

4. Divide the chicken and shrimp mixture among the wrappers. Top with equal amounts of the greens mixture, followed by 3 basil leaves each. Wrap into a tight roll, burrito-style.

5. In a small bowl, mix the hoisin and soy sauces together. Serve along with the rolls as a dipping sauce to share.

Nutrition per Serving

210 calories, 2 g fat, 0.5 g saturated fat, 60 mg sodium, 23 g carbohydrates, 0 g sugars, 0 g fiber, 22 g protein

Portobello BLT

(V, Vg, P, GF, LF)   Makes 1 serving

This decadent sandwich can be a little messy, but the flavor makes it well worth it.

1 teaspoon olive oil

1 large portobello mushroom cap

3–4 thick slices double-smoked bacon (turkey or vegan)

2 thin slices from a large tomato

1 handful baby romaine or baby spinach

2 large romaine lettuce leaves

1 teaspoon Avocado "Mayo" (recipe on page 218)

1 handful sprouts

1. Heat a skillet or electric grill over high heat. Drizzle the oil over both sides of the mushroom and sear on both sides. Add the bacon and cook through.

2. Layer the tomato, baby romaine or spinach, and bacon on 1 romaine lettuce leaf. Top with the mushroom. Drizzle with 1 teaspoon of the Avocado "Mayo" on page 218. Top with the sprouts and the remaining romaine lettuce leaf.

Nutrition per Serving

430 calories, 33 g fat, 4 g saturated fat, 790 mg sodium, 6 g carbohydrates, 2 g fiber, 3 g sugars, 13 g protein

Dr. Taz's Spicy Bone Broth

(P, GF, LF)   Makes 16 servings

Rich in minerals, gelatin, and probiotics that support the immune system
and gut, this healing broth is something I like to have on hand at all times.

3 pounds chicken, goat, or beef bones

1 onion, chopped

4 cloves garlic, minced

1 tablespoon chopped fresh ginger

1 tomato, chopped

1 teaspoon cumin seeds

2–3 teaspoons kosher salt

1 tablespoon coconut oil, ghee, or grass-fed butter

1 rib celery, chopped (optional)

1 carrot, chopped (optional)

4 quarts water

1. In a medium pressure cooker, slow cooker, or stockpot over medium heat, combine the bones, onion, garlic, ginger, tomato, cumin seeds, salt, and oil, ghee, or butter. If using, also add the celery and carrot. Cook, stirring occasionally, until the cumin seeds brown.

2. Add the water. If using a pressure cooker, cook under pressure for 8 to 10 minutes. If using a slow cooker or cooking on the stove, bring to a boil, reduce the heat to low, and simmer for 1 to 2 hours. (I know some recipes suggest longer cooking times, but this is designed for the fast pace of a super woman lifestyle.)

3. Strain the broth and discard the solids. Cool. The broth can be stored in the refrigerator for 5 to 7 days.

Nutrition per Serving

1 cup: 15 calories, 1 g fat, 1 g saturated fat, 300 mg sodium, 2 g carbohydrates, <1 g sugars, 0 g fiber, 9 g protein

Black Bean Soup and Portable Tacos

(V, Vg, P, GF, LF)   Makes 4 servings

I love this meal because it can be lunch and dinner for a few days.

1–1¼ cups unsweetened coconut or almond milk

½ cup water

1 tablespoon coconut or safflower oil

2 cans (15 ounces each) black beans, rinsed and drained

1 onion, chopped

1 tomato, chopped

4 teaspoons cumin powder

3–4 cloves garlic, minced

⅛ cup water

1 avocado, halved, pitted, peeled, and sliced

Tacos

8 small corn tortillas or lettuce leaves

1 cup chopped grilled chicken, steak, shrimp, tofu, or portobello mushrooms

¼ cup salsa

1. *To make the soup:* Place 1 cup of the milk and ½ cup of water in a pot or a Vitamix blender.

2. In a medium skillet, heat the oil over medium-high heat. Cook the black beans, onion, tomato, cumin, and garlic for 5 minutes. Reduce the heat to low, add ⅛ cup of water, and simmer for 15 minutes.

3. Add the bean mixture to the milk mixture. Run the Vitamix on the soup cycle (it will heat the soup) or blend the mixture together in the pot using a hand-held immersion blender. If using the stovetop, bring the soup to a boil, reduce the heat to medium-low, and simmer for 10 to 15 minutes. Check the consistency and thin the soup if desired with the extra ¼ cup milk. Pour into bowls and top with a few avocado slices.

4. *To make the tacos:* Heat the tortillas according to package directions. Divide the protein of your choice among the tortillas or lettuce leaves. Top with any leftover avocado slices and a few teaspoons of salsa. Serve 2 tacos with each bowl of soup.

With chicken: 580 calories, 16 g fat, 6 g saturated fat, 570 mg sodium, 76 g carbohydrates, 4 g sugars, 25 g fiber, 37 g protein

With steak: 620 calories, 20 g fat, 8 g saturated fat, 580 mg sodium, 76 g carbohydrates, 4 g sugars, 25 g fiber, 39 g protein

With shrimp: 590 calories, 17 g fat, 5 g saturated fat, 550 mg sodium, 78 g carbohydrates, 4 g sugars, 25 g fiber, 38 g protein

With tofu: 560 calories, 17 g fat, 5 g saturated fat, 570 mg sodium, 78 g carbohydrates, 4 g sugars, 26 g fiber, 29 g protein

With mushrooms: 520 calories, 14 g fat, 5 g saturated fat, 570 mg sodium, 78 g carbohydrates, 4 g sugars, 25 g fiber, 24 g protein

Chicken Soup

(P, GF, LF)   Makes 4 servings

I like using a pressure cooker since it is quick and easy, but you can also use a Dutch oven or large stockpot.

1 tablespoon safflower or coconut oil

1 chicken leg quarter, cut into 4 pieces

½ onion, chopped

3–4 cloves garlic, minced

2 cups frozen vegetables (any variety)

2 teaspoons cumin powder

2–3 teaspoons salt

1 teaspoon ground black pepper

1 tablespoon ground turmeric

2 teaspoons ground red pepper

2 teaspoons Italian seasoning (or a mixture of dried basil, parsley, and oregano)

2–3 carrots, sliced

2 cups chicken broth

2 quarts water

1 package (8 ounces) rice noodles (or any other noodles)

1. In a pressure cooker, heat the oil over medium-high heat. Cook the chicken, onion, and garlic, stirring frequently, until the chicken browns slightly.

2. Add the frozen vegetables, cumin, salt, black pepper, turmeric, red pepper, Italian seasoning, and carrots. Stir together for 1 to 2 minutes. Pour in the broth and water. Close the lid to the pressure cooker and seal properly. Reduce the heat to medium and cook under pressure for 7 to 10 minutes, or until the chicken is no longer pink and the vegetables are tender.

3. Remove the pressure cooker from the stove. Release the pressure, add the noodles, and return to the stove. Simmer for 10 to 15 minutes, or until the noodles are cooked.

Nutrition per Serving

280 calories, 6 g fat, 3 g saturated fat, 730 mg sodium, 41 g carbohydrates, 5 g sugars, 7 g fiber, 14 g protein

Immunity-Boosting Chicken Soup

(P, LF)   Makes 8 servings

This is my variation of the chicken soup mentioned for Nightingales on page 176. Have some any time you are feeling out of balance. Add some sliced ginger for an extra kick, especially if you feel any signs of a cold or flu coming on.

1 pound chicken drumsticks, beef bones, or goat bones (or a mixture of all 3)

1 tablespoon chopped onion

3 cloves garlic, minced

1 teaspoon chopped fresh dill

1 teaspoon chopped parsley

1 cup frozen vegetables (any variety)

1 tablespoon ghee or coconut oil

2 teaspoons salt

2 teaspoons ground black pepper or red pepper

2 teaspoons ground turmeric

8–10 cups water

2 cups chicken broth

6 ounces rice, egg, or spaghetti noodles

1. In a pressure cooker, combine the bones, onion, garlic, dill, parsley, frozen vegetables, ghee or oil, salt, pepper, and turmeric. Cook over medium heat, stirring frequently, until the meat changes color slightly.

2. Add the water and broth and close the lid. Cook under pressure for 8 to 10 minutes. (Alternatively, you can combine all of the ingredients in a soup pot and bring to a boil on the stove, and then simmer for 20 minutes.)

3. Open the lid slowly and add the noodles. Simmer for 3 to 5 minutes, or until the noodles are tender and the meat is falling off the bones.

Nutrition per Serving

250 calories, 8 g fat, 3.5 g saturated fat, 810 mg sodium, 16 g carbohydrates, <1 g sugars, 2 g fiber, 18 g protein

Dairy-Free Tomato Soup

(V, Vg, GF, LF)   Makes 2 servings

I love using my Vitamix blender for this recipe, but if you don't have one, you can easily make it on the stovetop.

1 tablespoon safflower or coconut oil

1 can (15 ounces) diced tomatoes

4–5 medium tomatoes, chopped

2–3 cloves garlic, minced

1 tablespoon chopped onion

1 tablespoon dried Italian seasoning + additional for garnish

1 teaspoon salt

1 teaspoon ground black pepper

1 cup unsweetened coconut or almond milk

½ cup water

1. In a medium skillet, heat the oil over medium-high heat. Cook the canned tomatoes, fresh tomatoes, garlic, onion, Italian seasoning, salt, and pepper, stirring frequently, for 3 to 5 minutes, or until tender.

2. In a pot or a Vitamix, combine the milk and water. If not using a Vitamix, add the tomato mixture to the milk mixture and use a handheld immersion blender to blend the soup into a smooth consistency. Heat to a boil and boil for 1 to 2 minutes. Reduce the heat to low and simmer for 30 minutes. If using a Vitamix, add the tomato mixture. Run the Vitamix on the soup cycle (it will heat the soup). Top the finished soup with additional Italian seasoning.

Nutrition per Serving

150 calories, 10 g fat, 8 g saturated fat, 610 mg sodium, 14 g carbohydrates, 8 g sugars, 3 g fiber, 3 g protein

Bissara (Moroccan Lentil Soup)

(V, Vg, P, GF, LF)   Makes 6 servings

Set aside time on the Saturday or Sunday before a busy week and make this soup for an easy weekday grab-and-go hot lunch.

4 tablespoons olive oil, divided + additional for serving

1 large onion, chopped

4–5 cloves garlic, minced

3 teaspoons paprika, divided

2 teaspoons ground cumin, divided

6 cups chicken broth, vegetable broth, or Dr. Taz's Spicy Bone Broth (page 226)

4 cups water

3 cups dried split peas or lentils

¼ cup chopped parsley

½ teaspoon salt, or to taste

⅛ teaspoon ground red pepper, or to taste

Dash of sea salt

Sumac, in your spice aisle, for garnish (optional)

1. In a large pot, heat 1 tablespoon of the oil over low heat. Cook the onion and garlic until lightly browned. Add 1½ teaspoons of the paprika and 1 teaspoon of the cumin and stir to combine.

2. Pour in the broth and water and remaining 3 tablespoons oil. Stir in the split peas or lentils.

3. Bring to a boil, reduce the heat to low, and simmer for 45 minutes, stirring occasionally so that the peas or lentils don't stick to the bottom of the pot.

4. When the peas or lentils are tender, mash them with a wooden spoon until smooth. Stir in a little water, if needed, to reach desired consistency.

5. Add the parsley, remaining 1½ teaspoons paprika, remaining 1 teaspoon cumin, ½ teaspoon salt, and red pepper. Stir to combine. Serve with a dash of olive oil and sea salt, plus some sumac for garnish, if using. Or cool and store in 6 small containers. If you don't think you'll use all of the soup this week, it freezes well.

Nutrition per Serving

290 calories, 10 g fat, 1.5 g saturated fat, 220 mg sodium, 65 g carbohydrates, 8 g sugars, 26 g fiber, 24 g protein

Kabocha Squash Soup with Cauliflower-Quinoa Meatballs

(V, P, GF)   Makes 3 servings

1 kabocha squash (2–3 pounds) or butternut squash or pumpkin

1 tablespoon coconut oil

1 shallot, chopped

1 piece (1") fresh ginger, peeled and grated

2 cloves garlic, minced

3 cups Dr. Taz's Spicy Bone Broth (page 226) or vegetable broth

1 cup full-fat coconut milk

½ tablespoon curry powder

Ground red pepper

Salt and ground black pepper

1 recipe Cauliflower-Quinoa Meatballs (page 243)

1. Preheat the oven to 425°F. Line a baking sheet with parchment paper.

2. Cut the squash in half, scoop out the seeds, and place skin side down on the parchment paper. Roast for 25 minutes, or until fork-tender. Let cool.

3. Meanwhile, in a stockpot, heat the oil over medium-low heat. Cook the shallot, ginger, and garlic until the shallot is tender and somewhat translucent.

4. Add the broth, squash meat (discard the skin), coconut milk, and curry powder. Puree with a handheld immersion blender. Increase the heat to medium and bring to a low simmer. Add the red pepper and salt and black pepper to taste. Pour the soup into bowls, add the meatballs, and serve.

Nutrition per Serving

480 calories, 23 g fat, 0 g saturated fat, 640 mg sodium, 70 g carbohydrates, 12 g sugars, 11 g fiber, 9 g protein

Tandoori-Spiced Salmon with Yogurt Cucumber Sauce

(P, GF)   Makes 1 serving

1 medium salmon fillet (about the size of a deck of cards or 4 ounces)

½ lemon

½ cup plain Greek yogurt

2 teaspoons tandoori spice mix or ground red pepper

1 teaspoon ground turmeric

1 teaspoon curry powder

¼ teaspoon salt

1 teaspoon ginger paste (or grind 1 teaspoon fresh ginger with water to create a paste)

4 cloves garlic mashed with a little water to make a paste

1 tablespoon olive oil

Yogurt Cucumber Sauce (recipe on page 234)

1. Preheat the oven to 350°F.

2. Rinse the fish and pat it dry with paper towels. Place in a small baking pan coated with cooking spray, or coat the pan with a small amount of coconut oil, ghee, or butter. Squeeze the lemon half on top of the fish. Set aside.

3. In a small bowl, combine the yogurt, tandoori spice mix or red pepper, turmeric, curry powder, salt, garlic paste, and ginger paste. Mix well to make a paste.

4. Brush the salmon with the oil. Add the paste liberally to both sides of the fillet. Return to the pan. Cover with foil.

5. Bake for 15 minutes. (Meanwhile, make the yogurt sauce.) Remove the foil and turn the oven to broil. Broil the fish for 2 to 3 minutes, or until opaque. Serve with the yogurt sauce.

Nutrition per Serving

750 calories, 39 g fat, 6 g saturated fat, 575 mg sodium, 8 g carbohydrates, 4 g sugars, <1 g fiber, 90 g protein

NOTE: Earth Mamas, either skip the yogurt sauce or make with dairy-free yogurt.

Yogurt Cucumber Sauce   Makes 4 servings

This sauce also makes a great dip for veggie sticks.

1 cup plain Greek yogurt	½ teaspoon chopped parsley
1 small cucumber, finely chopped	½ teaspoon chopped fresh cilantro

In a small bowl, combine the yogurt, cucumber, parsley, and cilantro. Mix well.

Nutrition per Serving

35 calories, 0 g fat, 0 g saturated fat, 25 mg sodium, 3 g carbohydrates, 2 g sugars, 0 g fiber, 6 g protein

Oven "Grilled" Sea Bass with Wilted Spinach

(P, GF, LF)   Makes 2 servings

This is another easy dinner for a busy evening that tastes as if you'd fired up the outdoor grill.

2 sea bass fillets (6 ounces each)	½ teaspoon salt, divided
1 tablespoon tamari sauce whisked with 1 tablespoon olive oil	1 tablespoon coconut or safflower oil
	4 cups fresh spinach
1 teaspoon crushed peppercorns	1 tablespoon minced garlic

1. Preheat the oven to 400°F.

2. Coat the fish fillets in the tamari sauce mixture. Rub the peppercorns and ¼ teaspoon of the salt onto both sides of the fillets. Place in a baking pan and cover with foil.

3. Bake for 10 to 15 minutes. Remove the foil and turn the oven to broil. Broil for 1 to 2 minutes, or until the fish flakes easily. Set aside and keep warm.

4. In a skillet, heat the oil over medium-high heat. Cook the spinach, garlic, and remaining ¼ teaspoon salt, stirring frequently, until the spinach is just wilted.

5. Place the fillets on 2 plates and top with the spinach, or place 1 fillet in a container for lunch tomorrow.

Nutrition per Serving

270 calories, 17 g fat, 8 g saturated fat, 575 mg sodium, 3 g carbohydrates, 0 g sugars, 1 g fiber, 26 g protein

Middle Eastern Chicken Skewers with Quinoa Tabbouleh

(P, GF)   Makes 4 servings

1½ cups plain yogurt

2 teaspoons ground cumin

2 teaspoons ground coriander

2 teaspoons ground cardamom

2 teaspoons paprika

2 teaspoons garlic salt

½ tablespoon ground turmeric

4 cloves garlic, minced

2 tablespoons dried thyme

3 tablespoons fresh lemon juice

1 pound boneless, skinless chicken thighs

Quinoa Tabbouleh

½ cup uncooked quinoa

2 cups parsley leaves

8–10 fresh mint leaves

¼ cup olive oil

3 tablespoons fresh lemon juice

Salt

3 medium tomatoes, chopped

½ large cucumber, chopped

1. *To make the skewers:* In a large bowl, combine the yogurt, cumin, coriander, cardamom, paprika, garlic salt, turmeric, garlic, thyme, and lemon juice. Mix well. Add the chicken and toss to coat. Cover and marinate in the refrigerator overnight.

2. Preheat the grill. Remove the chicken from the marinade and place on metal skewers. Grill over direct heat for 14 to 20 minutes, turning once, or until a thermometer inserted in the thickest portion registers 165°F and the juices run clear.

3. *To make the tabbouleh:* Prepare the quinoa according to package directions and allow to cool.

4. In a food processor, combine the parsley and mint. Process until smooth. With the blade running, add the oil, lemon juice, and salt to taste. Pour into a bowl. Add the cooled quinoa, tomatoes, and cucumber and toss. Season with additional salt as needed. Serve alongside the chicken.

Nutrition per serving

410 calories, 22 g fat, 6 g saturated fat, 320 mg sodium, 21 g carbohydrates, 9 g sugars, 0 g fiber, 34 g protein

Faux Fried Coconut Chicken with Honey Mustard Dipping Sauce

(P, GF, LF)   Makes 4 servings

1-½ cups almond flour

¼ cup arrowroot powder

½ cup shredded unsweetened coconut

2 teaspoons garlic powder

2 teaspoons paprika

1 teaspoon garlic salt

2 large eggs

4 boneless, skinless chicken thighs or legs

Dipping Sauce

¼ cup Dijon mustard

2 tablespoons honey

1. Preheat the oven to 400°F. Line a baking sheet with parchment paper and brush the paper with coconut oil or ghee.

2. In a shallow bowl, combine the almond flour, arrowroot powder, coconut, garlic powder, paprika, and garlic salt. Mix well.

3. In another shallow bowl, whisk the eggs.

4. Dip each chicken piece in the egg wash, then coat evenly with the flour mixture. Place on the baking sheet. Bake for 14 to 20 minutes, turning once, or until a thermometer inserted in the thickest portion registers 165°F and the juices run clear.

5. *To make the dipping sauce:* Meanwhile, in a small bowl, blend together the mustard and honey.

6. Serve the chicken with the dipping sauce or store-bought paleo barbecue sauce.

Nutrition per Serving

540 calories, 37 g fat, 9 g saturated fat, 870 mg sodium, 29 g carbohydrates, 11 g sugars, 7 g fiber, 31 g protein

Chicken Saag

(P, GF, LF)   Makes 4 servings

You can make this dish vegetarian and vegan by using vegetable broth and substituting one (15-ounce) can of chickpeas or 2 cups of pan-fried tofu cubes for the chicken. If so, reduce the cooking time to 15 minutes.

3 cloves garlic, minced

1 piece (1") fresh ginger, peeled and grated

1 tablespoon water

1-½ teaspoons ghee or coconut oil, divided

1 onion, chopped

Pinch of sea salt

1 teaspoon garam masala

1 teaspoon paprika

1 teaspoon ground cumin

1 teaspoon ground coriander

4 boneless, skinless chicken thighs

½ cup broth (vegetable broth, chicken broth, or Dr. Taz's Spicy Bone Broth, page 226)

1 cup chopped spinach

1 cup chopped kale leaves

1. In a small bowl, blend the garlic, ginger, and water to form a paste. In a large skillet, melt ¾ teaspoon of the ghee or oil over medium heat. Cook the onion and salt for 5 minutes, or until the onion has caramelized and become golden brown. Add the garlic paste and cook until the pan is mostly dry. Add the garam masala, paprika, cumin, coriander, and the remaining ¾ teaspoon ghee or oil. Reduce the heat to medium-low and cook for 2 to 3 minutes to let the flavors combine.

2. Add the chicken and increase the heat to medium-high. Turn the chicken once to coat both sides. Add the broth and reduce the heat to low. Cook, uncovered, for 15 to 20 minutes, or until the liquid has reduced by half and a thermometer inserted in the thickest portion registers 165°F. During the last 5 minutes of cooking time, add the spinach and kale.

Nutrition per Serving

220 calories, 11 g fat, 3 g saturated fat, 110 mg sodium, 10 g carbohydrates, 2 g sugars, 3 g fiber, 23 g protein

Chicken Wings, Three Ways   Makes 8 servings

1 pound chicken wings

1 recipe Teriyaki Marinade, Carolina Marinade, or Hot 'n' Spicy Marinade (see below)

1. Preheat the oven to 425°F. Line a baking sheet or rimmed sheet pan with parchment paper.

2. Place the wings in a bowl and pour your marinade of choice over the top. Toss to combine. Marinate in the refrigerator for 30 minutes.

3. Remove the wings from the marinade and place on the baking sheet. Bake for 15 minutes. Reduce the heat to 400°F and bake for 20 minutes. Turn the broiler on low and broil for 5 minutes, or until the juices run clear.

Teriyaki Marinade

(V, Vg, P, GF, LF)

½ cup tamari or coconut aminos (a gluten- and soy-free alternative to soy sauce)

½ cup honey

2 tablespoons apple cider vinegar

2 tablespoons sesame oil

1 tablespoon almond butter

1 piece (½") fresh ginger, peeled and grated

In a food processor, combine the tamari or coconut aminos, honey, vinegar, oil, almond butter, and ginger. Process until smooth.

Nutrition per Serving

260 calories, 13 g fat, 3 g saturated fat, 1,030 mg sodium, 20 g carbohydrates, 19 g sugars, <1 g fiber, 15 g protein

Carolina Marinade

(V, Vg, P, GF, LF)

¾ cup yellow mustard

½ cup honey

¼ cup apple cider vinegar

2 tablespoons tomato paste

2 teaspoons coconut aminos (a gluten- and soy-free alternative to soy sauce)

2 teaspoons hot-pepper sauce

In a food processor, combine the mustard, honey, vinegar, tomato paste, coconut aminos, and hot-pepper sauce. Process until smooth.

Nutrition per Serving

200 calories, 9 g fat, 2.5 g saturated fat, 650 mg sodium, 21 g carbohydrates, 18 g sugars, 1 g fiber, 22 g protein

Hot 'n' Spicy Marinade

(V, P, GF)

1 cup paleo-friendly hot-pepper sauce (Tabasco, Frank's, Crystal's)

2 tablespoons ghee, melted

1 tablespoon apple cider vinegar

In a food processor, combine the hot-pepper sauce, ghee, and vinegar. Process until smooth.

Nutrition per Serving

160 calories, 12 g fat, 4.5 g saturated fat, 460 mg sodium, 2 g carbohydrates, 0 g sugars, 0 g fiber, 21 g protein

Chicken Curry in a Hurry

(P, GF, LF)   Makes 4 servings

You can make a vegetarian version of this fast dinner by using vegetable broth and swapping out the chicken for one (15-ounce) can of chickpeas and a package of tofu cubes that have been pan-fried. If so, reduce the cooking time to 15 minutes and add the pan-fried tofu cubes for the last 10 minutes of cooking.

1 can (14-½ ounces) organic fire-roasted diced tomatoes

3 cloves garlic, minced

1 piece (1") fresh ginger, peeled and grated

1 tablespoon water

1 -½ teaspoons coconut oil or ghee, divided

1 onion, chopped

Pinch of sea salt

1 teaspoon garam masala

1 teaspoon paprika

2 teaspoons ground turmeric

4 boneless, skinless chicken thighs

½ cup Dr. Taz's Spicy Bone Broth (page 226), vegetable broth, or chicken broth

1. In a small bowl, blend the tomatoes, garlic, ginger, and water to form a paste. In a large skillet, melt ¾ teaspoon of the oil or ghee over medium heat. Cook the onion and salt for 5 minutes, or until the onion has caramelized and become golden brown. Add the garlic paste and cook until the pan is mostly dry. Add the garam masala, paprika, turmeric, and the remaining ¾ teaspoon oil or ghee. Reduce the heat to medium-low and cook for 2 to 3 minutes to let the flavors combine.

2. Add the chicken and increase the heat to medium-high. Turn the chicken once to coat both sides. Add the broth and reduce the heat to low. Cook,

uncovered, for 20 to 25 minutes, or until the liquid has reduced by half and a thermometer inserted in the thickest portion registers 165°F.

Nutrition per Serving

420 calories, 24 g fat, 8 g saturated fat, 190 mg sodium, 12 g carbohydrates, 4 g sugars, 3 g fiber, 42 g protein

Paleo Pad Thai

(P, GF, LF)   Makes 4 servings

Sauce

½ tablespoon Thai red curry paste

½ tablespoon honey

¼ cup almond butter

½ cup coconut milk

¼ cup fresh lime juice (from 2 limes)

½ tablespoon fish sauce, tamari, or coconut aminos (a gluten- and soy-free alternative to soy sauce)

1 piece (1") fresh ginger, peeled and minced

2 cloves garlic, minced

Pad Thai

2 teaspoons sesame or coconut oil

4 boneless, skinless chicken thighs, cut into thin strips

2 medium zucchini, cut into noodles using a spiralizer or food processor

1 cup shredded carrots

4 scallions, chopped

2 tablespoons chopped fresh cilantro

2 eggs, whisked

¼ cup chopped cashews

1. *To make the sauce:* In a food processor, combine the curry paste, honey, almond butter, coconut milk, lime juice, fish sauce or tamari or coconut aminos, ginger, and garlic. Process into a thin paste.

2. *To make the pad Thai:* In a large skillet, heat the oil over medium heat. Cook the chicken and 1 tablespoon of the sauce, stirring occasionally, until the chicken is no longer pink. Transfer to a plate and set aside.

3. Add a few tablespoons of additional sauce to the pan and the zucchini noodles. Cook, stirring occasionally, for 1 to 2 minutes. Stir in the carrots, scallions, and cilantro. Cook for 1 to 2 minutes, or until the vegetables are tender.

4. Return the reserved chicken to the pan, along with the remaining sauce. Move the mixture to one side and add the eggs. Cook the eggs, stirring, until cooked through. Stir to combine the eggs with the chicken mixture. Top with the cashews.

Nutrition per Serving

450 calories, 31 g fat, 7 g saturated fat, 280 mg sodium, 19 g carbohydrates, 8 g sugars, 5 g fiber, 30 g protein

Quick Cumin Chicken with Crunchy Kale Chips

(P, GF)   Makes 4 servings

2 teaspoons olive or coconut oil

¼ cup plain yogurt

4 teaspoons garlic salt

4 teaspoons cumin powder

2 pounds chicken thighs or drumsticks, trimmed of fat

1 cup chopped fresh cilantro

½ cup water

4 cloves garlic, halved

1 teaspoon salt

Crunchy Kale Chips (page 252)

1. In a large bowl, combine the yogurt, garlic salt, and cumin powder. Mix well. Add the chicken, turning to coat on both sides. Cover and marinate in the refrigerator for at least 1 hour, or preferably overnight.

2. Preheat the oven to 400°F. Coat an 8" x 8" baking dish with cooking spray.

3. In a food processor or blender, combine the cilantro, water, garlic, and salt. Process or blend until smooth. Divide into 2 equal portions.

4. Remove the chicken from the marinade and place in the baking dish. Top with half of the cilantro mixture. Cover with foil and bake for 35 minutes. Remove the foil and bake or broil for 5 to 10 minutes, or until a thermometer inserted in the thickest portion registers 170°F and the juices run clear.

5. Serve with kale chips and the remaining cilantro sauce.

Nutrition per Serving

340 calories, 21 g fat, 6 g saturated fat, 760 mg sodium, 3 g carbohydrates, 1 g sugars, <1 g fiber, 40 g protein

BEEF/LAMB

Paleo Shepherd's Pie

(P, GF, LF)   Makes 4 servings

2–3 tablespoons ghee

1 large onion, chopped

3 cloves garlic, minced

1 cup chopped carrots

1 cup chopped celery

1 cup chopped mushrooms

1 pound organic grass-fed ground beef or lamb

½ teaspoon sea salt

1 teaspoon dried thyme

1 teaspoon dried rosemary or 1 sprig fresh rosemary

1 teaspoon ground black pepper

1 teaspoon smoked paprika

2 tablespoons tomato paste

1 cup Dr. Taz's Spicy Bone Broth (page 226)

2 large heads cauliflower, trimmed, chopped, and steamed until very soft

1 tablespoon nutritional yeast flakes

2 tablespoons olive oil

Pinch of garlic salt

1. Preheat the oven to 350°F.

2. In a skillet, heat 2 tablespoons of ghee over medium-high heat. Cook the onion, garlic, carrots, and celery, stirring frequently, for 10 minutes, or until tender. Transfer to a plate and set aside.

3. Add the mushrooms to the skillet and cook until they develop a nice crust and have released their moisture. Add the beef or lamb, reserved cooked vegetables, salt, thyme, rosemary, pepper, and paprika. Cook until the meat is no longer pink.

4. Add the tomato paste and broth and stir to combine. Reduce the heat to medium and simmer for 10 minutes. Reduce the heat to low and simmer for 20 minutes. Transfer the mixture to an ovenproof baking dish and set aside.

5. In a mixing bowl, combine the cauliflower, nutritional yeast, olive oil, garlic salt, and remaining 1 tablespoon ghee (if desired). Mash until smooth.

6. Gently spread the cauliflower mixture over the reserved meat mixture and bake for 20 minutes. Turn on the broiler and broil for 2 to 3 minutes, or until the cauliflower crust is lightly browned.

Nutrition per Serving

440 calories, 9 g fat, 0 g saturated fat, 290 mg sodium, 11 g carbohydrates, 13 g sugars, 11 g fiber, 37 g protein

Cauliflower-Quinoa Meatballs

(V, P, GF, LF)

Makes 8 servings

If you are not a vegetarian, this dish can also be made with beef or lamb; see the variation below.

1 medium head cauliflower, ground in a food processor

½ teaspoon olive oil

¼ cup chopped onion

¼ cup chopped red or green bell pepper

2 cloves garlic, minced

2 cups cooked quinoa (about ⅔ cup dry)

1 cup soft tofu, mashed (If you want animal protein and a paleo option, use ½ pound grass-fed ground beef or lamb and 2 beaten eggs mixed together)

½ cup almond flour

1 tablespoon arrowroot powder

1 tablespoon nutritional yeast

3 tablespoons coconut oil

¼ teaspoon onion powder

½ teaspoon dried oregano leaves

⅛ teaspoon salt (or to taste)

⅓ cup grated Parmesan cheese (if vegetarian and not dairy free)

1. Preheat the oven to 400°F. Line a baking sheet with parchment paper or foil. Brush with coconut oil.

2. In a microwaveable bowl, microwave the cauliflower on high power for 3 to 5 minutes, or until tender, or steam on the stovetop for 10 to 12 minutes, or until tender.

3. In a skillet, heat the olive oil over medium heat. Cook the onion, pepper, and garlic for 5 minutes, or until aromatic.

4. In a large bowl, combine the cauliflower, cooked quinoa, tofu (or meat and egg mixture), pepper mixture, almond flour, arrowroot powder, nutritional yeast, coconut oil, onion powder, oregano, salt, and cheese (if using). Mix well. Roll into 1½" balls.

5. Place the meatballs on the baking sheet and bake for 10 to 15 minutes, turning every 5 minutes. Transfer to a rack to cool. If you are using beef or lamb, bake for 20 to 25 minutes or until no longer pink.

Nutrition per Serving

Vegan option: 290 calories, 7.5 g fat, 5 g saturated fat, 15 mg sodium, 31 g carbohydrates, 1 g sugars, 5 g fiber, 10 g protein

Nutrition per Serving

Paleo option: 330 calories, 16.5 g fat, 6 g saturated fat, 45 mg sodium, 31 g carbohydrates, 4 g sugars, <1 g fiber, 16 g protein

Buckwheat Noodle and Kale Stir-Fry

(V, Vg, GF, LF)   Makes 4 servings

I love buckwheat noodles because they are gluten-free, filling, and delicious.

½ red onion, chopped, divided

3–4 cloves garlic

1 chile pepper, chopped, or 2 teaspoons ground red pepper

1 can (15 ounces) tomato sauce or 3 small tomatoes, chopped

2 teaspoons salt

1 package (8 ounces) buckwheat noodles

1 tablespoon coconut oil

2 cups chopped, stemmed kale

1 cup chopped or sliced shiitake mushrooms

¼ cup roasted pistachios (optional)

1. In a medium mixing bowl, combine half of the onion, the garlic, pepper, tomato sauce or tomatoes, and salt. Blend together using a handheld immersion blender or process in batches in a Nutribullet, Vitamix, or food processor and return to the bowl. This is your spicy sauce. Set aside.

2. Prepare the noodles according to package directions. Drain. Rinse with cold water and set aside.

3. In a skillet or wok, heat the oil over medium heat. Cook the kale, mushrooms, and remaining onion, stirring constantly, until the mushrooms are tender.

4. Add the buckwheat noodles, folding them in with the vegetables. Pour in the spicy sauce and mix thoroughly. Garnish with pistachios, if using.

Nutrition per Serving

260 calories, 4 g fat, <1 g saturated fat, 300 mg sodium, 44 g carbohydrates, 6 g sugars, 6 g fiber, 9 g protein

Persian Eggplant with Yellow Split Peas and Dried Lime

(V, Vg, GF, LF)   Makes 4 servings

3 tablespoons coconut oil, divided

3 onions, finely chopped

2 tablespoons tomato paste

2 teaspoons ground cumin

½ teaspoon ground cinnamon

2 teaspoons ground turmeric

1 teaspoon ground coriander

1 can (15 ounces) diced tomatoes

1-½ cups yellow split peas

¾ cup water

3 dried limes (thinly slice 3 limes and leave out overnight, covered with a paper towel)

1 teaspoon salt + additional for eggplant

½ teaspoon ground black pepper

1 large eggplant

1 cup chopped kale

1. In a pot, heat 1 tablespoon of the oil over low heat. Cook the onions for 10 to 15 minutes, or until tender. Add the tomato paste, cumin, cinnamon, turmeric, coriander, diced tomatoes, and split peas. Mix well. Simmer for 5 minutes. Add the water, limes, 1 teaspoon salt, and pepper, stir, and simmer for 15 minutes, or until the split peas are soft.

2. Meanwhile, cut the eggplant into long slices, salt each slice, and set aside for 15 minutes (this helps eliminate the bitter taste). Rinse and dry the slices. In a skillet, heat the remaining 2 tablespoons oil over medium heat. Cook the eggplant slices in batches of 2 or 3 until all are golden brown on each side.

3. Add the kale to the split pea mixture and simmer for 5 minutes.

4. For each serving, place a slice or two of eggplant on a plate and top with some of the split pea mixture.

Nutrition per Serving

440 calories, 13 g fat, 9 g saturated fat, 730 mg sodium, 66 g carbohydrates, 13 g sugars, 24 g fiber, 21 g protein

Spiced Lentil Cakes with Chickpeas

(V, Vg, GF, LF)   Makes 4 servings

1 cup lentils or green split
peas, soaked overnight

¼ cup coconut flour

2 eggs or 2 vegan flax "eggs"
(2 tablespoons flax meal +
5 tablespoons water, let sit
for 5 minutes)

½ teaspoon salt, divided

2 teaspoons paprika

1 tablespoon coconut or
safflower oil

2 teaspoons olive oil

2 cans (15 ounces each)
chickpeas, drained and
rinsed

1 tomato, chopped

¼ onion, chopped

2–3 teaspoons garam masala

1. Drain and dry the lentils or split peas. In a food processor or blender, combine the lentils or split peas, coconut flour, eggs, ¼ teaspoon of the salt, and
   paprika. Process or blend until you can form into balls (the texture will be
   rough, but the mixture should stick together), adding water if the consistency is too thick. Form into small patties or cakes about ¾" thick.

2. In a large skillet, heat the coconut or safflower oil over medium heat. Cook
   the cakes for 6 to 10 minutes, turning once, or until golden brown on each
   side. Set aside.

3. In a medium skillet, heat the olive oil over medium heat. Cook the chickpeas, tomato, onion, remaining ¼ teaspoon salt, and garam masala, stirring
   frequently, until the onion is tender.

4. Divide the reserved lentil cakes among 4 plates and top with the
   chickpeas.

Nutrition per Serving

490 calories, 14 g fat, 6 g saturated fat, 940 mg sodium, 67 g carbohydrates, 3 g
sugars, 19 g fiber, 27 g protein

Kitchari

(V, Vg, GF, LF)   Makes 4 servings

I use the pressure cooker for this recipe to save time. Soaking mung beans overnight and then cooking them under pressure makes them an easily digestible source of protein. The rice is purposely cooked to an almost mushy consistency so that it is easy on the digestive system.

1 cup mung beans, soaked overnight

1 cup uncooked brown or white rice

1 teaspoon cumin seeds

1 teaspoon salt

1–2 teaspoons garam masala

1 tablespoon ghee, grass-fed butter, or coconut oil

1 quart water

In a pressure cooker, combine the mung beans, rice, cumin seeds, salt, garam masala, and ghee, butter, or oil. Stir to mix. Cook over medium heat for 1 to 2 minutes. Add the water. Cook under pressure for 6 to 8 minutes, or until the water is absorbed and the rice and beans congeal together. (If you don't have a pressure cooker, simmer on the stovetop for 1 hour over medium to medium-low heat.)

Nutrition per Serving

220 calories, 5 g fat, 2.5 g saturated fat, 600 mg sodium, 38 g carbohydrates, 2 g sugars, 3 g fiber, 5 g protein

Vegan Pasta with "Cheese" Sauce

(V, Vg, GF, LF)　　　　　　　　　　　　　　　　　　Makes 4 servings

2 cups lentil or soybean macaroni or rotini noodles

½ tablespoon ghee or coconut oil

1 tablespoon almond flour

½ tablespoon arrowroot powder

½ cup unsweetened cashew milk

¼ cup nutritional yeast flakes

½ teaspoon Dijon mustard

1 clove garlic, minced

Pinch of garlic salt

½ cup white beans

½ zucchini or summer squash, shredded

½ cup chopped spinach

1. Prepare the pasta according to package instructions.

2. Meanwhile, in a saucepan, melt the ghee or oil over medium heat. Reduce the heat to low and cook the flour and arrowroot powder, whisking constantly, for 3 to 5 minutes, or until a smooth mixture forms.

3. Add the cashew milk, nutritional yeast, mustard, garlic, and garlic salt. Whisk for 4 minutes, or until the sauce thickens. Add the white beans, stir, and turn off the heat.

4. Using a handheld immersion blender, blend the sauce until it's smooth. Stir in the squash and spinach and return to low heat. When the vegetables have wilted, add the reserved cooked pasta. Serve warm.

Nutrition per Serving

490 calories, 29 g fat, 1.5 g saturated fat, 60 mg sodium, 82 g carbohydrates, 2 g sugars, 18 g fiber, 33 g protein

Spinach and Kale Lasagna

(V, GF)   Makes 6 servings

1 package (9–10 ounces) gluten-free lasagna noodles

1–2 teaspoons safflower or coconut oil

1 package (10 ounces) frozen spinach, thawed

1 package (10 ounces) frozen kale, thawed

2–3 cloves garlic, minced

¼ teaspoon salt, divided

1 teaspoon ground black pepper

1 cup ricotta cheese or 1 cup tofu, blended using a Vitamix or food processor

2 cups shredded mozzarella cheese, divided

1 egg

2 teaspoons dried parsley

1 jar (24 ounces) marinara sauce

1. Preheat the oven to 400°F. Coat a 13" x 9" baking dish with coconut oil.

2. Prepare the pasta according to package directions, cooking until al dente. Drain and dry the noodles.

3. Meanwhile, in a skillet, heat the oil over medium heat. Cook the spinach, kale, garlic, ⅛ teaspoon of the salt, and the pepper, stirring occasionally, for 3 to 5 minutes, or until cooked through. Set aside. When cool, squeeze out any extra moisture.

4. In a bowl, combine the ricotta or tofu, 1 cup of the mozzarella, the egg, the remaining ⅛ teaspoon salt, and the parsley. Mix well.

5. Spread ¼ cup of the marinara sauce in the bottom of the baking dish. Place half of the lasagna noodles on top of the sauce. Layer the spinach mixture on top of the noodles, and half of the ricotta mixture on top of the spinach. Layer on the remaining noodles, top with the remaining pasta sauce, and finish layering with the remaining mozzarella cheese.

6. Cover the dish with foil and bake for 30 to 40 minutes. Remove the foil and bake for 5 to 10 minutes, or until the cheese is melted and slightly browned and the center is firm (you can use a knife to test). Cool slightly before serving.

Nutrition per Serving

380 calories, 16 g fat, 8 g saturated fat, 930 mg sodium, 39 g carbohydrates, 8 g sugars, 5 g fiber, 22 g protein

NOTE: Earth Mamas, please omit cheese.

Sweet Potato Noodles with Cauliflower-Quinoa Meatballs in Tomato Sauce

(V, P, GF, LF)   Makes 4 servings

2 large sweet potatoes, peeled

½ tablespoon coconut oil

¼ cup chopped onion

3 cloves garlic, minced

1 recipe Cauliflower-Quinoa Meatballs (page 243)

¾ cup jarred marinara sauce, warmed

1. Cut the sweet potatoes into noodles using a spiralizer.

2. In a large skillet, heat the oil over medium heat. Cook the onion and garlic for 3 to 4 minutes, or until soft and fragrant.

3. Add the sweet potato noodles. Cook for 5 to 7 minutes, or until the noodles begin to soften. Cover with a lid and cook until the noodles are cooked through.

4. Plate the cooked noodles with the meatballs and top with the warm marinara sauce.

Nutrition per Serving

With Vegan meatballs: 410 calories, 14.5 g fat, 11 g saturated fat, 50 mg sodium, 46 g carbohydrates, 3 g sugars, 7 g fiber, 11 g protein

With Paleo meatballs: 450 calories, 23.5 g fat, 12 g saturated fat, 80 mg sodium, 46 g carbohydrates, 7 g sugars, 2 g fiber, 17 g protein

Thyroid Trail Mix

(V, P, LF, GF)   Makes 8 servings

Who doesn't love trail mix? This mix is packed with selenium and iodine to support your thyroid.

1 cup roasted, unsalted Brazil nuts

1 cup almonds

½ cup dark chocolate chips

1 cup any gluten- and sugar-free cereal

2 teaspoons pink or iodized salt

1–2 teaspoons dark honey

In a bowl, combine the Brazil nuts, almonds, chocolate chips, cereal, salt, and honey. Mix well. Portion out into ½ cup servings as one of your snacks for the day.

Nutrition per Serving

340 calories, 27 g fat, 7 g saturated fat, 600 mg sodium, 25 g carbohydrates, 15 g sugars, 6 g fiber, 8 g protein

Chia Chocolates

(V, P, LF)   Makes 4 servings

1 cup almond butter

1 tablespoon honey

¼ cup chia seeds

¼ cup cacao powder

2 teaspoons vanilla extract

½ cup rolled oats or granola

¼ cup mini dark chocolate chips

In a medium bowl, stir together the almond butter and honey. Add the chia seeds, cacao powder, vanilla, and rolled oats or granola. Mix well. Roll into small balls. (If desired, use a melon scooper to portion out the dough and form it into 8 balls.) Chill in the refrigerator. Press the chocolate chips into the balls. Yum!

Nutrition per Serving

320 calories, 23 g fat, 3 g saturated fat, 5 mg sodium, 24 g carbohydrates, 5 g sugars, 11 g fiber, 11 g protein

Rice Cakes with Nut Butter

(V, Vg, P, GF, LF)   Makes 1 serving

This is a great go-to when you're hungry. Store these rice cakes in your car or at work to grab when you feel like you're starving!

2 organic unsweetened brown rice cakes

2 tablespoons almond butter

Spread the rice cakes with the almond butter. If desired, first toast the rice cakes for 30 seconds.

Nutrition per Serving

320 calories, 17 g fat, 2 g saturated fat, 30 mg sodium, 16 g carbohydrates, 0 g sugars, 5 g fiber, 10 g protein

Crunchy Kale Chips

(V, Vg, P, GF, LF)   Makes 2 servings

Use fresh kale and wash and then dry it using a salad spinner or dehydrator or simply leave it on the counter for an hour.

2 cups kale, torn into chip-size pieces

1 tablespoon coconut oil

2 tablespoons coconut flour

½ teaspoon salt

1. Preheat the oven to 325°F.

2. In a bowl, combine the kale, oil, flour, and salt. Toss. Spread on a shallow baking sheet. Bake for 10 to 15 minutes, or until crispy.

Nutrition per Serving

65 calories, 10 g fat, <1 g saturated fat, 630 mg sodium, 11 g carbohydrates, 0 g sugars, 4 g fiber, 6 g protein

Kelp and Kale Chips

(V, Vg, P, GF, LF)   Makes 4 servings

Even my children love these chips. While you can buy them prepared, they
are so easy to make. Use any fresh kale or kelp. Just wash and then dry it
using a salad spinner or dehydrator or simply by leaving it on the counter for
an hour.

1 cup fresh kale, torn into chip-
size pieces

1 cup kelp

1 tablespoon coconut oil

1–2 tablespoons coconut flour

2 teaspoons pink salt or
iodized salt

1. Preheat the oven to 325°F.

2. In a bowl, combine the kale, kelp, oil, flour, and salt. Toss. Spread on a shallow baking sheet. Bake for 10 minutes, or until crispy.

Nutrition per Serving

60 calories, 5 g fat, 3.5 g saturated fat, 1,240 mg sodium, 5 g carbohydrates, <1 g
sugars, 2 g fiber, 2 g protein

Roasted Cauliflower
and Brussels Sprouts Chips

(V, Vg, P, GF, LF)   Makes 4 servings

These are better than potato chips any day.

1 medium head cauliflower

½ pound Brussels sprouts

2 tablespoons grated
Parmesan cheese or
crumbled goat cheese
(optional; omit for vegan and
lactose-free option)

1 tablespoon coconut oil or
grass-fed butter

2 teaspoons salt

1 teaspoon ground black
pepper

1 teaspoon ground red
pepper

1–2 teaspoons olive oil, for
drizzling

1. Preheat the oven to 350°F.

2. Cut the cauliflower and Brussels sprouts into thin pieces and place in a medium bowl. Add the cheese (if using), coconut oil or butter, salt, black pepper, and red pepper. Toss.

3. Spread on a baking sheet in a shallow layer. Bake for 10 to 15 minutes, or until crispy.

4. Drizzle with the olive oil.

Nutrition per Serving

130 calories, 5 g fat, 2 g saturated fat, 139 mg sodium, 13 g carbohydrates, 4 g sugars, 5 g fiber, 6 g protein

Snack Kebabs

(P, GF, LF)   Makes 4 servings for a snack, 2 servings for lunch

I usually use chicken for these kebabs, but you can use any leftovers from last night's dinner—vegetables, steak, or shrimp are always welcome additions. This power lunch or snack should keep you full for hours.

1 grilled chicken breast, cut into squares

8–10 cherry tomatoes

½ cup sliced bell peppers

8–10 olives

10 Cheddar cheese cubes (omit if lactose-free)

Thread a piece of chicken, tomato, pepper slice, olive, and cheese cube onto a skewer. Continue with the remaining ingredients and additional skewers, as desired.

Nutrition per Serving

Serving size = ¼ recipe (snack option): 240 calories, 15 g fat, 7 g saturated fat, 390 mg sodium, 4 g carbohydrates, 2 g sugars, 0 g fiber, 22 g protein

Serving size = ½ recipe (lunch option): 480 calories, 30 g fat, 14 g saturated fat, 780 mg sodium, 8 g carbohydrates, 4 g sugars, 0 g fiber, 44 g protein

Mini Roll-Ups

(P, GF, LF)   Makes 4 servings

4 gluten-free or organic corn tortillas (6" diameter) or romaine lettuce leaves

4–6 ounces sliced preservative-free turkey or chicken

¼ cup hummus

Sliced carrots, celery, and/or cucumber

Top each tortilla or lettuce leaf with turkey or chicken. Add 1 tablespoon of hummus. Layer with the carrots, celery, and/or cucumber. Roll and wrap.

Nutrition per Serving

85 calories, 3 g fat, 1 g saturated fat, 90 mg sodium, 5 g carbohydrates, 0 g sugars, 1 g fiber, 10 g protein

Hummus and Veggies

(V, Vg, P, GF, LF)   Makes 1 serving

Keep this snack handy at work or at home. Then simply dip and go!

1 cup sliced cucumber, carrots, and/or celery

3 tablespoons hummus

Dip the veggies into the hummus and enjoy!

Nutrition per Serving

160 calories, 5 g fat, 1 g saturated fat, 350 mg sodium, 25 g carbohydrates, 9 g sugars, 9 g fiber, 6 g protein

Sprouted Mung Beans

(V, Vg, P, GF, LF)   Makes 2 servings

I love mung beans, and they are great for the digestive system. These are delicious warm or cold.

2 cups mung beans

1 tablespoon coconut, olive, or safflower oil

½ teaspoon salt

1 tablespoon chopped onion

1 teaspoon ground cumin

1. In a bowl, soak the mung beans in water. I like to soak them 2 to 3 days ahead of time, so the mung beans actually sprout. Once they've sprouted, drain and dry them.

2. In a medium skillet, heat the oil over medium heat. Cook the beans, salt, onion, and cumin for 3 to 5 minutes, or until slightly browned. Delicious!

Nutrition per Serving

100 calories, 7 g fat, 6 g saturated fat, 600 mg sodium, 7 g carbohydrates, 5 g sugars, 2 g fiber, 3 g protein

MANY OF THESE RECIPES have been incorporated into your 3-Week Power Plan. With more than 50 recipes included here, you are now armed and ready to master the kitchen and nutrition and to treat food as your medicine!

CHAPTER 11

YOUR SUPER WOMAN EXERCISE RX

MUCH LIKE FOOD, exercise is everywhere. Gyms, boot camps, yoga studios, and at-home fitness solutions dot our consumer landscape. We don't have an *access* issue with exercise. We have a *time and logistics* issue—when to do it, what to do, and how often. I have watched women overexercise and overtrain and injure themselves or—on the flip side—underexercise, perhaps using light walking as their only means of exercise. Exercise and fitness, like everything else, need to be tailored to *you*.

Since I am always in a time crunch, I've learned that to keep up with any sort of exercise regimen, I need to have something available at home. Seriously—it's a 20-minute drive each way to the gym from my house and office, then 1 hour for a decent workout, then time to get cleaned up—that is a major chunk of my day! It's not often that I can spare that much time. The solution: My husband and I dedicated our last several Christmas and birthday gifts to creating a home gym that includes a reformer, a spin bike, an elliptical, exercise pads, free weights, and a full-body weight machine system. It gives me plenty of options. I can get all the cardio, strength training, and yoga I need without ever leaving the house.

I remember, years ago, pushing myself to do long, intense workouts, desperate to lose the extra weight I'd gained, but getting no results at all. I talk to patients every day who have a similar exercise history—overexercising and overtraining to lose weight, then falling fatigued on the bed and finding it difficult to make it through the rest of the day. The worst part of it, though, is when you put in all that hard work and *the scale barely budges.*

What I learned—and what I hope you take away—is that while food is the first medicine, movement and exercise follow close behind. Balance and moderation are key when it comes to exercise, and this holds true for certain Power Types more than others. We all love the high of completing a marathon, a 10K, a boot camp, or any other number of exercise goals we've had on our bucket lists. And while these sorts of events are great, they are often difficult to sustain on a day-to-day, real-life, busy super woman schedule. They can also have long-term health repercussions.

Here I'll provide three full exercise routines and many more suggestions for getting active and staying active, to reconnect you to yourself and keep your energy flowing! Next, I'll break down how exercise works best for each of the Five Power Types. You'll find tips and strategies and individualized Power Type exercise charts toward the end of this chapter to show you how to best incorporate workouts into your super woman Rx plan. Refer back to the action steps in Chapters 5 through 9 for additional exercise directions and suggestions.

YOGA

My love affair with yoga began in residency, when I needed something desperately to ease my overtaxed mind. With each breath and pose, I experienced the connection between my body and my mind and quickly came to crave a good vinyasa flow after a tough day at the hospital. I was so inspired that I actually became a certified yoga teacher, teaching classes in my late twenties and early thirties. Once I had children and my practice, I stopped teaching yoga, but that certification saved me from spending hours taking classes at a yoga studio.

You can develop your own vinyasa flow at home.

What you'll need: All you need is a yoga mat, stretchy clothing, yoga music, and your own breath.

How it works: You'll want slow music that resonates with your pace (I will often use yoga music on Pandora or a yoga CD) and a basic understanding of seven key yoga poses (see page 260). Put them together and, even on a busy morning, you should have time to do the routine once through. When you have more time, you can do cycle through all poses three or four times—you decide. *Just do it.* If you cycle through each pose one time, you'll be done in about 15 minutes. Do two cycles and you'll be at 30 minutes, and do a three-cycle vinyasa for a 45-minute routine.

Your breath: I like using the 4:7:8 breath as a starting point. Begin by inhaling slowly for 4 seconds with your eyes closed and lips closed, breathing through your nose. Hold your breath for 7 counts, extending and rounding your belly like a balloon, and then exhale through your mouth, completely blowing out all that air for 8 seconds as you bring in and flatten your belly like a pancake. Repeat this for a few cycles, and then flow into inhaling through your nose slowly for 3 to 4 seconds, and exhaling fully for 5 to 7 seconds. Focusing on extending your exhale during breathing will help you to hold any pose for a longer duration. This style of breathing is considered one of the most healing breaths and great to practice during yoga.

MOUNTAIN POSE

(This pose is static but not passive. You'll be engaging your entire body from your head to your toes, focusing on awakening and grounding it.)

Stand with your legs and feet together, toes pointing forward, your arms down by your sides with your palms facing forward. Gaze straight forward and imagine a string is attached to the top of your head, lifting you up, elongating your spine. Keeping your spine long, roll your shoulders up, back, and down—away from your ears. Distribute your weight evenly across the bottoms of both your feet. Tighten and engage your thighs and belly, and tuck your tailbone down. Inhaling deeply, steadily, and slowly through your nose, close your eyes and bring your hands together in prayer position (palms pressing into each other, your thumbs resting on your sternum) and on an inhale bring your hands to each side of your hips. Exhale completely through your mouth, feeling your feet grounded into the mat and continuing to relax your neck and shoulders. That counts as one full breath. Continue for a total of 10 full breaths.

TREE POSE

(Another centering and grounding pose, tree pose also improves balance and focus.)

From mountain pose, above, standing with your legs and feet together, hands in prayer position, gradually transfer your weight onto your left foot and leg. Once you feel stable and grounded into your left leg, begin to bend your right leg and bring the sole of your right foot up to the inside of your left leg. (If you are new to yoga, you can begin with your right foot at the inside of your left ankle; as you progress, raise your right foot to the inside of your left thigh. Always keep your foot above or below your knee, not directly on the knee joint.) Place your hands on your hips. Gently press your right foot against your left leg and hold, inhaling slowly and deeply through your nose and exhaling through your mouth. Hold this pose for a total of five breaths and then switch sides.

MORE ADVANCED: *You can press your hands together, lifting your arms up and over your head with fingertips pressed together and pointing straight up to the ceiling.*

DOWNWARD DOG

(A strengthening and calming pose, downward dog also improves circulation and bloodflow, which massages the internal abdominal organs and provides much-needed blood to your head.)

From tree pose, lower your leg and arms back down to mountain pose, with both feet on the mat and arms down by your sides. Place your palms on the mat in front of you about shoulder width apart (it's fine to bend your knees). Step your legs back one at a time, keeping your feet in line with your hands. Spread your fingers wide and press your palms down. Lift your butt up to the sky, straightening your legs and pressing the heels of your feet down. Engage your thighs, pressing back with your lower body, and stretch your arms forward (elbows straight, palms pressing into the mat—you should look like an upside-down V). Relax your head and the back of your neck. Inhale through your nose deeply and completely and exhale slowly through your mouth. Repeat for five breaths while holding the pose.

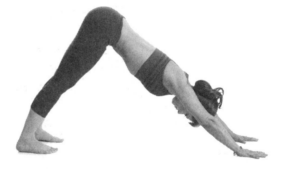

WARRIOR I

(This and Warrior II are power poses that strengthen and tone your arms and legs, firming up your belly as well.)

From downward dog pose, extend your right leg up into the air behind you, and lift your head so you can gaze slightly beyond your hands in front of you. Now, pull your right knee in toward your chest and step forward to place your right foot between your hands, directly in line with your back foot (it's okay to lift onto your fingertips to give your leg more space). If you have trouble stepping your foot all the way up between your hands, you can take a shorter step with your right foot, and then reach back and put your right hand on your right ankle and bring your right foot the rest of the way up.

With both your hands planted and your right leg bent forward with your foot between your hands, rotate your back foot out to a 45-degree angle and then press into both legs and feet. As you inhale through your nose, lift your arms up overhead, shoulder width apart and facing each other. Hips facing forward, bend your front knee to 90 degrees, and exhale. Hold this pose for a total of five breaths.

Reverse the pose by bringing both your hands back down to the mat on either side of your right foot. Step your right foot back and then repeat by stepping your left foot up and doing Warrior I on the other side. Hold for five breaths and move to the next pose.

WARRIOR II

To come out of Warrior I, lower your arms back to your mat, and step your front foot back (you are now back into downward dog pose). Swing your right leg back and up behind you as you did in the last pose and lift your head to gaze just past your fingertips. Next, bend your right knee and leg in and up toward your chest, swooping them forward to step your right foot forward between your palms in front of you. Inhale through your nose, and as you exhale through your mouth, press into your legs and feet and stand, with front leg bent at about 90 degrees. Your arms should be straight and parallel to the floor, with your right arm forward, left arm back. Palms should face up. Hold for a total of five breaths, then switch sides.

PIGEON POSE

(This hip opener increases flexibility and relieves stiffness.)

From Warrior II pose, lower your arms and place your hands back on the mat on either side of your front foot, fingertips pointing toward the front of your mat. Step your front foot back into line with your back foot. Bend your knees to come onto all fours in table pose. Slide your right knee forward, bringing your right knee to your right hand, and slide your right ankle across to your left hand. As your right leg comes forward, slide and straighten your left leg straight back until the top of your left thigh is resting on your mat, your hips facing down and forward. Your right shin should now be on your mat, crossing just in front of your wrists, and the top of your left foot should be on your mat with your left toes pointing toward the back of the mat. Inhale deeply and completely through your nose, and exhale fully through your mouth. Relax your belly and hold this pose for a total of five breaths, then switch sides and repeat.

MORE ADVANCED: *Walk your hands forward and bend your arms until your forearms are resting on the floor. Can you still go farther? Rest your chest on the floor with your arms extended in front of you.*

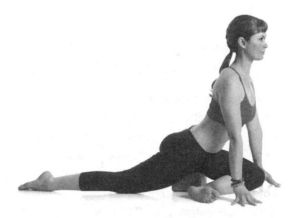

CHILD'S POSE

(Child's pose is the perfect way to finish your routine. It stretches and relaxes your back and neck and calms your whole body.)

From pigeon pose, press into your hands, bringing your back leg up and sliding your front leg back to come into table pose (on all fours). From here, bring your feet together so your big toes are touching and the soles of your feet face the ceiling. Lean back and sit onto your heels, while extending your arms and torso forward. Rest your forehead on the floor, relax your butt back and your chest forward, and hold. Take five deep breaths, inhaling through your nose and exhaling through your mouth.

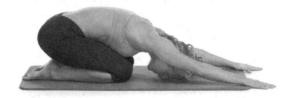

15-MINUTE MOVING MEDITATIONS
TO GROUND AND CENTER YOU

Alternatively, there are several yoga apps you can add to your smartphone, tablet, or laptop. Yoga Studio, Down Dog, Daily Yoga, and Simply Yoga are four that are highly rated. My only caveat is that if you can't be on one of these apps without being tempted into other online activity, then stay old school. If you are interested and have time for longer classes, you can find yoga studios and instructors near you at yogaalliance.org.

In addition to yoga, both tai chi and qi gong are great grounding moving meditations. These are both mentioned specifically in the Gypsy Girl and Savvy Chick chapters, pages 66 and 119, but are great for all Power Types to include.

Tai Chi

This ancient Chinese practice is used by millions of people worldwide. It is characterized by a series of slow, fluid movements that flow one into the next to create a workout that's been shown to ease anxiety, improve concentration and focus, and increase energy.

What you'll need: About 5 square feet. Do the routine barefoot, in stretchy, comfortable clothing.

How it works: Practice the following sequence as a grounding exercise each morning. Tai chi is a graceful, slow dance of movement, and you'll continue to move through all four poses fluidly for 15 minutes. Take some time to break each move down until you feel comfortable linking them together into one long sequence. You won't alternate sides like in other workouts. Don't worry about being exact—just relax and have fun. This is just a taste of tai chi. For more information on finding classes in your area, see page 266.

Stand comfortably with your feet about hip width apart, arms relaxed at your sides.

Inhale, and reach both your hands up diagonally to the right (as if you were gently picking up and petting a bird). Your right foot and leg take the weight of your body as you tap the toes of your left foot diagonally behind you.

As your inhale turns to an exhale, fluidly swoop your arms down in an arc, step your right foot next to the left one, and turn your body to face slightly left.

Continue circling your hands up until they're in front of your chin, palms facing forward. As your exhale flows into the next inhale, rotate your torso and step your right foot to the right (keep this foot flexed) so that your heel touches the floor.

As your inhale turns to an exhale, shift your weight onto your right leg (bend your knee slightly) and take your left heel up off the floor while you straighten your arms as if pressing away a heavy object. On the next inhale, step back to the beginning stance.

Repeat the sequence, moving in the same direction, for 15 minutes.

Qi Gong

Another Chinese tradition, qi gong, is also characterized by flowing movements but is often more free flowing than tai chi and has a focus on wellness. Remember that qi means "life energy"—often qi gong can include repetitions of the same move over and over to target a specifically blocked or deficient meridian. While qi gong is simple and easy to do, it's easiest to learn a few moves in a class. To find a teacher near you, call community centers and parks or karate and taekwondo schools (yep, the ones you see with cute little kids dressed in little white gi outfits). Or check adult class Web sites, Taoist temples and sanctuaries, and YMCAs.

The American Tai Chi and Qi Gong Association offers a class locator by state and city at americantaichi.net/TaiChiQigongClass.asp. You can also refer to doctortaz.com/qigong and doctortaz.com/taichi.

CARDIO

Our bodies demand that we challenge ourselves and move at a pace that raises our heart rate to at least close to double its resting rate for 10 minutes or more. Any sort of activity that challenges your lungs and your heart rate works. While all super women need this sort of challenge, the length of time and the number of times per week that you should do cardio depend on your Power Type. Some types need more aggressive and longer exercise, while others need shorter routines. (See the end of this chapter for your Power Type's specific exercise Rx.)

What you'll need: Sturdy fitness shoes appropriate for the sport you'll be participating in.

How it works: Below is a list of suggestions for a variety of cardio workouts. Although they differ, all cardio shares the goal of steadily increasing your exercise intensity and heart rate and keeping them elevated for a period of time. You'll want to start every exercise session by checking your resting heart rate, and then continue to monitor your heart rate every 10 minutes for the duration of your routine. This way, you'll be able to monitor how hard you are really working (see "How Hard Am I Working?" on page 268).

Essentials for warming up and cooling down: Next, it's important to start every workout with a few minutes of warming up, which simply means doing whatever activity you've chosen (running, for example) at a slower rate (an easy jog). This gives your body time to adjust without shocking your system. Finally, after the meat of your cardio routine—the 20 to 40 minutes where your heart rate is elevated—you'll take a few minutes to gradually slow your pace to allow your body to come back to its normal resting heart rate.

Here are a few ideas for workouts.

Walking: It doesn't get any easier than this, and walking is a great activity to do with friends, partners, and kids. Lace up your shoes and head out the door. Walk at an easy pace for the first few minutes, and then pick up your pace to a brisk walk and aim to keep within 6 to 8 on the RPE scale (see "How Hard Am I Working?" on page 268) for 20 to 40 minutes. Besides the great exercise, a wealth of research shows the many benefits of walking for boosting mood, especially of "green walks," or walking in nature (in a park, a pretty neighborhood, around a lake, at the beach). Already a regular walker? Consider switching it up. Buy some hiking or trail-friendly shoes and go off-roading. The uneven terrain and natural peaks and valleys work your body and core muscles harder than just a stroll through the park. Just plan to take it a bit slower and work up to more difficult hikes gradually.

Running: If you already run three or more times a week for at least 20 to 40 minutes, then this will be as simple as the walking workout above. Be sure to warm up with some walking and then slow jogging before you pick up your pace. While you are running, check your heart rate or do a mental RPE check to see that you are putting out an effort that is between 6 and 8 (see below). If you are not a regular runner but it's something you want to try, first check your Power Type and exercise recommendations at the end of this chapter (and in the chapter dedi-

HOW HARD AM I WORKING?

In today's world, measuring your heart rate can be done in a wide variety of ways with multiple gadgets from Fitbits to Apple Watches. Still, it's a good idea to know how to check your exercise intensity the old-school way. Here are a couple of options.

Use the target heart rate equation. Before you start your exercise, you'll need to do a little math to determine your target heart rate (65 to 85 percent of your maximum heart rate is a good range). First, in the morning before you get out of bed, check your heart rate by taking your pulse.

This is your resting heart rate (RHR) and is usually between 60 and 100 beats per minute. Next, while you are having breakfast, subtract your age from 220 for your maximum heart rate (MHR). Now subtract your RHR from your MHR to get your heart rate reserve (HRR). Multiply your HRR by 65 percent (0.65), and add your resting heart rate to this number. Now do the same for your upper target heart rate (THR). Multiply your HRR by 85 percent (0.85) and add your resting heart rate to this number.

Before you get out of bed in the morning, take your pulse
for 60 seconds = _____ (RHR)

220 minus your age = _____ (MHR)

MHR minus RHR = _____ (HRR)

HRR x 0.65 = _____ + RHR = _____ (lower THR)

HRR x 0.85 _____ + RHR = _____ (upper THR)

cated to your 3-Week Power Plan). Then ease into running gradually, beginning by doing a casual combo of walking and running. You'd warm up as in the walking exercise above, and then pick it up to a brisk walking pace for a few minutes, then jog for a few minutes, then return to walking and continue alternating. If you are just starting out, stick to 20 minutes and do intervals of walking and running, with more walking. As the weeks go by, you can gradually increase the time you run while decreasing the time you walk.

Biking: Peddling can be an especially enjoyable family outing or a great way to turn a happy hour into a happy and healthy hour. Let your friends or family know what you'd like to do ahead of time. Go easy for

Take your pulse. Before you begin your exercise, pause and take your pulse for 15 seconds by placing your left index and middle fingers between the bone and the tendon located on the thumb side of your right wrist. Multiply that number by 4 to get your pre-exercise beats per minute. Now start your routine. After you've been exercising for 10 minutes, pause and take your pulse for 15 seconds. Again multiply by 4 to check that you are within your THR. Continue checking every 10 minutes. If you're under or over your zone, adjust your exercise intensity accordingly. Over time you'll get a feel for being in your zone, which brings me to the third way you can check your output—the rating of perceived exertion (RPE).

Use the Rating of Perceived Exertion (RPE) scale. This is a simple 1 to 10 scale you can use to mentally check your level of effort (no stopping necessary). Aim to stay between 6 and 8.

0 to 1—Little to no exertion; same intensity as reading a book in bed or vegging on Netflix.

2 to 3—Slow and easy moving, such as stretching or strolling. This is your RPE during your warmups before and your cooldowns after your cardio.

4 to 5—You're starting to sweat and can feel that your breathing rate is a bit more rapid, but you can still easily carry on a conversation.

6 to 7—You're working harder, talking is becoming more difficult, but you can still speak without gasping.

8 to 9—You are close to your maximum intensity; you can only say a few words, and only with effort.

10—This is all-out intensity; you're working as hard as you can, unable to say a single word.

a few minutes, pick up your pace for 20 to 40 minutes (if you don't have a heart monitor, stick to using the RPE scale on page 269), then before you dismount, again cycle easily for a few minutes. It's a good idea to plan out your route ahead of time so you can choose a path, park, and so on that won't have a lot of traffic and will allow for steady pedaling.

Swimming: Swimming laps is fantastic exercise, and you don't have to be a great swimmer to get a great workout. Consider that water is 12 times more resistant than air, which means your body works harder in the water but stays cooler than when you take a walk (especially during hot summer months). Plus water is easy on the joints. So freestyle it up, or stick to your favorite stroke—just aim to continue moving with an RPE between 6 and 8 for 20 to 30 minutes. If you get too tired to keep going with nonstop laps, pause at one side of the pool but don't stop moving— tread water for 30 seconds to a minute, and then do another lap. You can also stand where the water is waist deep and squat, jump, and run in the water as fast as you can. Think of it as your own personal water aerobics interval class.

Using a treadmill: A treadmill can be a lifesaver when the weather turns nasty, or if you need to exercise before dawn or after sunset. Warm up on the treadmill at a slower pace of 1.5 to 2 miles per hour or so, and gradually bring your speed up after a few minutes to 3 miles per hour. Aim to keep the meat of your cardio walk between 3 and 4 miles per hour, then gradually slow the pace back to 1.5 to 2 miles per hour for a few minutes. Aim for a walk of between 20 and 40 minutes, and check your heart rate and RPE every 10 minutes.

Using an elliptical: The same guidelines suggested for the treadmill apply to the elliptical. Warm up for a few minutes at an easier pace, and then pick up the pace. Just be sure to check your heart rate and to do a mental check on your level of effort using the 1 to 10 scale. Aim to keep your effort between a 6 and an 8 for the main part of your workout (go for 20 to 40 minutes), and then cool down for a few minutes.

Taking a group class: Aerobics, kickboxing, spin class, Zumba, Jazzer-cise, water aerobics. . . . If you are someone who is motivated by being part of a social circle (hello Nightingales and Earth Mamas), you may find that you enjoy exercise classes that do double duty, offering interaction *and* exercise. Just make sure that the class you participate in has an appropriate warmup and cooldown. You'll get a decent to challenging workout that's around 45 minutes long in most of these classes, and many include a bit of strength work at the end as well. Check your local health clubs, community colleges, adult learning classes, and YMCAs.

STRENGTH TRAINING

I love strength training for myself and for all super women—as long as we ease into it gradually and don't overtrain or overstrain. Strength training helps burn body fat, build muscle, balance insulin, and prevent osteoporosis. I think two strength-training sessions per week are ideal. Pilates is a form of strength training but isometric, meaning it uses the body's own muscles to manage resistance. I've included one of the classic Pilates moves at the end of this workout, along with suggestions for finding classes and apps.

What you'll need: A yoga mat or a towel, and you can strength-train barefoot or in fitness shoes. If not otherwise noted, choose dumbbells that fatigue your muscles after 10 to 12 repetitions.

How it works: Do the following moves one or two times per week on nonconsecutive days (Monday/Thursday or Tuesday/Friday, for example). Part of getting stronger is giving your body time to recover. This is one of the coolest things about strength training—and the strength moves tear down your muscle fibers, which sends a message to your body and brain to recover, repair, and strengthen (don't worry—they'll be long, lean, sleek, and sexy muscles); you take a day or two off between workouts as your body does the work of growing stronger.

FINDING FITNESS APPS

There are tons of these, so you'll need to do a bit of research to find an app that fits your needs. Here's just a small sampling of some of the top-rated and top-grossing apps available for Androids and iPhones.

- **Cardio:** If you've always wanted to try running, Couch to 5K offers a free 8-week program. For walkers, MapMyWalk helps you record walking distances and steps. (MapMyRun is a similar app for runners.)

- **Strength training:** The 7-Minute Workout Challenge app was designed by the American College of Sports Medicine (ACSM). You'll find 12 exercises, no equipment needed. Research results from the ACSM show that this training results in a higher daily metabolism and builds strength.

- **Combo fitness:** Pear Personal Coach is an app that offers at-home workouts, cardio options and tracking, and even yoga routines.

SQUATS

(Squats strengthen and tone your entire backside and your thighs.)

Stand with your feet a little wider than hip width apart, and sit back as if you were sitting into an invisible chair. Keep your abs and back tight. Lower yourself until your legs are bent at a little less than 90 degrees. Make sure that your knees stay over your ankles. Pause and press back up. Repeat for a total of 12 repetitions. Pause for 30 seconds, then do a second set.

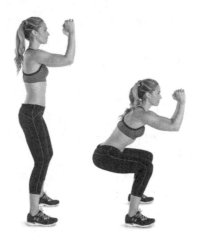

OVERHEAD SWINGS

(This exercise strengthens your hips, butt, and thighs.)

This move is traditionally done with a kettlebell (start with one weighing around 10 pounds), or you can use a dumbbell, holding it by its two ends. Stand with your feet more than hip width apart and hold the kettlebell handle with both hands, arms down, your palms facing your body. Sit back like you are sitting into a squat, then press back up just as in the last move, but instead of lowering right back into a squat as you come to the top of the move press into your heels, straighten your legs, and thrust your hips explosively upward to swing the kettlebell up to shoulder height.

Keep your wrists in line with your forearms. Your arms and shoulders should move like levers, rising and falling with the momentum and power from your hips (all the work is from your lower body, hips, and core). As the weight lowers, swinging back between your legs, sit back into your second squat. Repeat for 20 swings. Work up to 45.

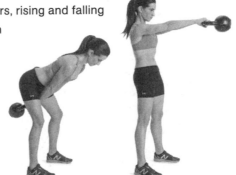

BENT-OVER ROWS

(Bent-over rows tone and tighten your upper back and the backs of your arms.)

Standing with your feet hip width apart, hold two dumbbells (8 to 15 pounds each—remember, choose a weight that gets hard to lift and lower on the 12th repetition). Bend forward from your hips about 45 degrees, gazing down but keeping your head in line with your shoulders and your neck relaxed. Circle your shoulders up, back, and down and let your arms hang straight down toward the floor, palms facing in. Contract and engage your belly and back muscles, bending your knees slightly. Keeping your arms in at your sides, bend your elbows and pull the dumbbells toward your torso until your palms are just in front of your hip bones; feel your shoulder blades draw together. Lower back to the starting position. That's 1 repetition. Do a total of 12, pause for 30 seconds, and do another set.

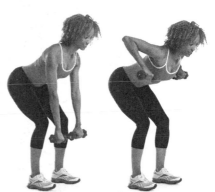

PUSHUPS

(Pushups strengthen your chest, arms, and belly and back muscles.)

Kneel on a mat or a towel. Walk your hands forward until you create a straight diagonal line from your head to your knees. Your arms should be a little wider than shoulder width apart and perpendicular to the floor, your elbows right over your wrists, and your shoulders right over your elbows. You can do modified pushups from your knees, or you can walk your feet back out so that your knees are off the floor and you are in a straight line from your head to your toes with the same arm position. Lower yourself down by bending your elbows and maintaining a straight line. Keep your abs engaged and tight, stop when your arms are bent at 90 degrees, and press back up. Continue for 12 pushups, pause, and do two more sets.

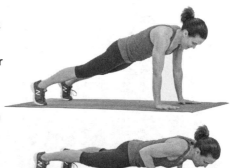

BENT- AND STRAIGHT-LEG LIFTS

(Leg lifts tone and improve your rear-end view.)

Begin on your hands and knees with your arms right under your shoulders, wrists under your elbows, and knees right under your hips, fingertips pointing forward. Contract and engage your abs and back (the goal is to stay sturdy in your middle area). Keeping your right leg bent at 90 degrees and your foot flexed, lift up your right leg until your thigh is parallel to the floor, and lower it. That is 1 bent-leg repetition. Now extend your right leg out until it is parallel to the floor and in line with your back. Engage your butt and lift your heel, then lower it. That is 1 straight-leg rep. Alternate bent-leg lifts and straight-leg lifts for a total of 12 (6 of each) without letting your back arch or sag, continuing to engage your core. Switch sides and repeat.

SKI LIFTS

(These sculpt and tone your outer thighs.)

Stand with your feet about hip width apart, behind a sturdy kitchen chair, holding the back of the chair with both hands, your knees slightly bent (not locked) and abs and back engaged. Look straight ahead. Your head should be in line with your shoulders. Holding your upper body steady, lift one leg up and out to the side. Lower and repeat on the other side. Do 12 repetitions on each side. Rest for 30 seconds, and do a second set.

You can also refer to doctortaz.com/skilifts.

THE 100

(This Pilates move is the ultimate ab toner. I highly recommend including Pilates in your routine, but it can be difficult to do on your own. Find a class at your gym or a Pilates studio, search online at pilatesteacherassociation.org/directory, or use an app like Pilates Coach.)

Lie on your back on a yoga mat. Lift and bend your legs at a 90-degree angle. Engage and contract your abs and back by sucking them in as if you were zipping up a pair of tight jeans. Inhale deeply and then exhale, reaching your arms down to the mat on either side of your torso as you lift your head and shoulders just off the mat. Pump your arms up and down in a small range of motion (keeping your arms straight) for five beats as you inhale in small puffs through your nose to match these five beats; now exhale through your nose in small puffs for five more beats. That completes 1 cycle. Do 9 more, for a total of 100 pumps.

You can also refer to doctortaz.com/thehundred.

YOUR EXERCISE RX BY POWER TYPE

For more details, turn to your Power Type's 3-Week Power Plan and review the suggestions for your specific exercise Rx.

The Gypsy Girl

Gypsy Girls need exercise but often don't do well with a daily strict regimen of adrenaline-pumping, jarring exercises such as running, spinning, kickboxing, or aggressive boot camps. They need, if you remember, grounding and adrenal repair—so yoga, Pilates, tai chi, or swimming is often a better fit. In fact, in the Gypsy Girl 3-Week Power Plan, one of the first steps in Week 1 is to include a mini session of grounding exercise first thing in the morning (see page 66). That's not to say that all weight-bearing exercises are out. Gypsy Girls are also at an increased risk for osteoporosis, so including some regular walking, and even a bit of hiking, is okay a couple times a week.

GYPSY GIRL EXERCISE RX

The focus is on grounding and stabilizing exercise, and for that reason, the cardio suggested doesn't include higher-impact activities such as running.	MONDAY*	TUESDAY*	WEDNESDAY
	Walking (see page 267)	Strength training (see routine on page 271)	Yoga (see routine on page 258)
THURSDAY	**FRIDAY**	**SATURDAY**	**SUNDAY***
Rest or walking	Strength training, yoga, or Pilates (see page 275)	Water aerobics or swimming (see page 270)	Pilates or Tai chi (page 265)

The Boss Lady

The athletic pitta element of a Boss Lady means that she needs regular exercise and movement—both as a recovery and release from mental stress, and also to satisfy her fiery personality. A mix of cardio, strength training, and yoga is often a satisfying, energizing, but not overly heating exercise Rx for a Boss Lady, with heart-pumping cardio being the preferred selection for this Power Type.

BOSS LADY EXERCISE RX

The goal is to be balanced with grounding exercise, cardio, and strength training.	MONDAY*	TUESDAY*	WEDNESDAY
	Strength training (see routine on page 271)	Cardio, kickboxing, running, spin class (see pages 267 for options)	Yoga (see routine on page 258)
THURSDAY	FRIDAY	SATURDAY	SUNDAY*
Cardio, kickboxing, running, spin class	Strength training or rest day	Yoga	Cardio, kickboxing, running, spin class

The Savvy Chick

Part Boss Lady and part Gypsy Girl, the Savvy Chick also needs a combination of adrenaline recovery work, along with a few higher-intensity adrenaline-pumping workouts. In the first week of the Savvy Chick 3-Week Power Plan, you'll see that one of the first steps is to include a mini session of grounding exercise in the morning (see page 119). The schedule I've set up below cycles from a week of grounding, lower-intensity exercise to a week of higher-intensity sessions to a final week of moderate intensity exercise. You can adjust this routine if, for example, you are feeling drained and in need of relaxing exercise on a running day, or add in a higher-intensity session if you are feeling extra energy on a tai chi day. The key is to check in with how you are feeling—physically and mentally—and adjust your workouts accordingly.

SAVVY CHICK EXERCISE RX

WEEK 1	Savvy Chicks need to cycle between more and less active exercise to match the needs of their combination Power Type.		
	MONDAY*	**TUESDAY***	**WEDNESDAY**
	Yoga (see routine on page 258)	Tai chi (see page 265)	Walking (see page 267)
THURSDAY	**FRIDAY**	**SATURDAY**	**SUNDAY***
Yoga	Qigong (see page 266)	Yoga	Rest
WEEK 2	**MONDAY***	**TUESDAY***	**WEDNESDAY**
	Walking	Running (see page 268)	Cycling (see page 269)
THURSDAY	**FRIDAY**	**SATURDAY**	**SUNDAY***
Jazzercise	Spin class	Running	Rest
WEEK 3	**MONDAY***	**TUESDAY***	**WEDNESDAY**
	Strength training (see page 271)	Walking	Yoga
THURSDAY	**FRIDAY**	**SATURDAY**	**SUNDAY***
Spin class	Walking	Strength training	Rest

The Earth Mama

Earth Mamas don't usually like exercise, but they need scheduled workouts most days of the week to increase their heart rate and burn fat, even more than the other Power Types. Why? The grounded super woman can be a little too firmly rooted to her seat, and that paired with a sluggish metabolism makes it critical for Earth Mamas to incorporate movement throughout the day. The chart below blocks out longer times for scheduled exercise and also shows how and where to interweave shorter mini-exercise breaks into the day. If longer morning exercise works better for you, then by all means do all your longer workouts in the morning. Ditto if evening offers your best exercise time—just make it happen.

EARTH MAMA EXERCISE RX

5 A.M.	Our goal is to get your heart rate up for 30 to 40 minutes most days of the week, and to also work in small bursts of activity throughout your day. An asterisk indicates a longer scheduled workout day.			
	MONDAY*	TUESDAY*	WEDNESDAY	THURSDAY
	Treadmill, 35 min (see page 270)	Spin class, 40 min (see page 270)		
	FRIDAY	SATURDAY	SUNDAY*	
			Walking for 45 min–1 hr (see page 267)	
8 A.M.	MONDAY	TUESDAY	WEDNESDAY	THURSDAY
	Park far from work for a 10-min walk	Park far from work for a 10-min walk	Park far from work for a 10-min walk	Park far from work for a 10-min walk
	FRIDAY	SATURDAY	SUNDAY	
	Park far from work for a 10-min walk	Sweep floors and vacuum, 10 min	Stand to fold/put away laundry, 10 min	

10:30 A.M.	MONDAY	TUESDAY	WEDNESDAY	THURSDAY
		Walk around your office building or block, 10 min	Walk around your office building or block, 10 min	Walk around your office building or block, 10 min
	FRIDAY	**SATURDAY**	**SUNDAY**	
	Walk around your office building or block, 10 min	Hike for 1 hr (see page 267)	Jog around the block, 10 min	

12:30 P.M.	MONDAY	TUESDAY	WEDNESDAY	THURSDAY
	Walk for 10 min during lunch break		Walk for 10 min during lunch break	Do some yoga poses for 10 min after lunch
	FRIDAY	**SATURDAY**	**SUNDAY**	
	Walk for 10 min during lunch break	Sweep off front and back porch, 10 min	Walk to library, museum, or park, 10 min	

2:30 P.M.	MONDAY	TUESDAY	WEDNESDAY	THURSDAY
	Walk around your office building or block, 10 min	Walk around your office building or block, 10 min	Do some yoga poses, 10 min	
	FRIDAY	**SATURDAY**	**SUNDAY**	
		Play catch with the kids or fetch with the pooch, 10 min	Treadmill or outdoor run/walk, 35 min, or rest	

5 or 6 P.M.	MONDAY	TUESDAY	WEDNESDAY	THURSDAY
	Walk the dog, 10 min		Zumba, 45 min	After-dinner walk, 40 min (see page 267)
	FRIDAY	**SATURDAY**	**SUNDAY**	
		Walk the dog, 10 min	Walk, 10 min	

7 or 8 P.M.	MONDAY	TUESDAY	WEDNESDAY	THURSDAY
		Walk around the block or ride a stationary bike, 10 min		Walk the dog, 10 min
	FRIDAY	SATURDAY	SUNDAY	
	Walk around the block or on the treadmill, 10 min			

The Nightingale

The Nightingale needs restful and energizing exercise that involves movement but not stress. That means that high-intensity exercise often backfires for this Power Type—depleting the immune system and sidelining her for long periods of time. Instead, to get regular, energizing, and immunity-boosting exercise, Nightingales get their best results from walking in nature and participating in regular and gentle yoga, tai chi, or qi gong.

NIGHTINGALE EXERCISE RX

Energy level Low	This chart schedules your exercise in weekly chunks based on your energy level (low or moderate). If you find your energy fluctuating, customize your workouts accordingly.		
	MONDAY*	TUESDAY*	WEDNESDAY
	Yoga (page 258), 20–40 min	Tai chi (page 265), 20–40 min	Rest
	THURSDAY	FRIDAY	SATURDAY	SUNDAY*
	Easy nature walk in park, 20–30 min	Tai chi, 20–40 min	Yoga, 20–40 min	Swimming or walking, moderate intensity (page 270)

Energy level Moderate	MONDAY	TUESDAY	WEDNESDAY
	Brisk walking, 40 min, and 10-min bursts of activity (see "Earth Mama Exercise Rx" on page 279)	Rest	Tai chi, 40 min, and 10-min bursts of activity
THURSDAY	**FRIDAY**	**SATURDAY**	**SUNDAY**
Brisk walking, 40 min, and 10-min bursts of activity	Yoga, 30 min, and 10-min bursts of activity	Brisk walking, 40 min, and 10-min bursts of activity	Rest

WRAP-UP AND WHAT'S NEXT

We are making progress! You know your Power Type, your nutritional needs, and now, your exercise strategy. But wait—there's more! We have a few more ingredients to mix together to create the best version of *you*. Up next—the super woman mind and body recharge!

CHAPTER 12

BUILD YOUR
FORTRESS OF SOLITUDE

CREATING YOUR FORTRESS of Solitude is about designing a sanctuary in your physical, mental, emotional, and spiritual world that nurtures and nourishes the Wonder Woman in you.

In 2004, I got married (*a journey that's a book in itself*). One of the many happy things we did early on was our 3-week honeymoon to Hawaii. Three weeks! That was the first time since probably before high school that I'd had any sort of a real, carefree, non-business-related vacation, and 21 days was the longest amount of time I'd had to relax in at least 14 years. While I'd already addressed some of my health issues, I'd just scratched the surface of my nutritional deficiencies, my hair was still shedding, and I was certainly stressed from wedding planning and frazzled from work. Hawaii was a break from all of it—the emergency room night shifts and family wedding drama—and a chance to return to a normal sleep cycle. I was forced to unplug and truly relax. Six weeks after returning from that trip, my hair came back—all of it. Suddenly, I had the hair of my childhood—thick, coarse, and luxuriant. What the?! After all I had been through—it took Hawaii? Vik? Not only had I completely stopped shedding, I also felt absolutely renewed, refreshed, and reenergized—inside and out! It took me a while to recognize that those precious few weeks of complete rest had reset my entire body and my nervous system. I realized how truly powerful it was to have a complete break from stress and to have uninterrupted sleep, and that loads of quiet time were just as important as getting food, supplements, and exercise right.

That was the first of many aha moments, the realization of how critical it is to nourish my whole self—mind, body, and soul. Since that time, I try really hard to take physical and mental health breaks (vacations and retreats), and I incorporate mindfulness practices like journaling, meditation, and breath work as a part of my super power soul-feeding regimen. And I prescribe these things to all my patients. In fact, my treatment plans include an entire section that every patient receives with guidelines for creating her own Fortress of Solitude.

While I rarely get to enjoy honeymoon-length vacations these days (maybe when I reach retirement?), I do have strategies that keep my mind and spirit balanced even when my schedule isn't. This chapter will show you how even the busiest super women can use deliberate mindfulness and spiritual tools to replenish their energy.

CREATE YOUR PERSONAL PARADISE

Batman had the Bat Cave, Superman had the Fortress of Solitude, and Wonder Woman had Paradise Island. It's up to you to create your own personal super woman haven where you can go to replenish and restore. In this section, we'll explore how to make your living spaces—personal and community—devoid of kryptonite energy drains and full of tranquility and rejuvenating relaxation. Color can be thought of as a form of visual energy, while textures in the fabrics of your furniture or the blankets on your bed can be described as holding a kind of tactile energy. Even scents carry an aromatic energy (for more on aroma therapy, see "Aroma or Essential Oil Therapy" on page 312 and "The *Essential* Essential Oils" on page 312). Our senses absorb and interpret everything we come into contact with through a myriad of complex channels. Knowing how each affects and influences you will help you to get the most out of each room in your home.

All throughout your house, your goal will be to nurture a healthy and balanced mind and body. With that in mind, you'll want some rooms to stimulate and energize, and others to relax and soothe. I've broken down the house by rooms and spaces; for each, I'll discuss best colors, textures, aromas, and other elements. Let's get started.

Your Bedroom: Make It a Haven

It's important to have multiple things you love to see, feel, and smell in and about your bedroom, but you'll want to limit this space to only three activities: intimacy, sleep, and relaxation. Use the following tips to get the most from your bedroom.

- **Think tranquility.** Ambiance-wise, this means bringing in gentle blues and subtle greens because they are soothing to the eyes and mind. Add some artwork you love, or a picture with a favorite quote or reading on it. Positive words and messages can boost positive feelings, according to Yale researchers.
- **Namaste your nightstand.** Put a prayer, meditation, or dream journal next to your bed. Add some lavender-colored and -scented candles and essential oils such as bergamot and vanilla for soothing aromatherapy and colors.
- **Go screen free.** It took some loving persuasion to convince my husband that we needed to ditch the TV in our room (and by "loving persuasion" I mean a big ole FIGHT). Many of my patients insist that a television in the bedroom is a great way to unwind at night, and I get it, but no—it's not. It might be a way to turn your brain off, but being mindLESS isn't the same as being mindFULL or rested. Watching a show might feel like being transported to another space or reality (Calgon, Take Me Away), but that's an illusion—videos can't and won't replenish your soul. Studies actually show that watching TV results in a mildly agitated reaction (the light from the screen isn't your friend; see the next tip), especially if you close out the day with the news (talk about a horror show).
- **Black out.** I'm not talking about popping Xanax or installing a Jägermeister shot machine in your boudoir. What I'm referring to is the way that even the smallest light from a digital clock or a charging smartphone can disrupt the natural sleep hormones that your brain pumps out at night. Replenishing through sleep is one of the most important ways you can recharge your super powers— especially your willpower—so when you are hitting the hay, pull down the light-canceling curtains, put black tape over any little lights on chargers, and put a scarf over digital clocks. And while we're on the topic of shutting things out, that goes for sound too. While you might not be able to fully soundproof your bedroom, you might find it helpful to have a white noise machine to dampen the sounds of kids or neighbors.
- **Create a serenity space.** This can simply be your side of the bed, but if

you have the room, go for the addition of a comfy chair, a meditation cushion, even a little mantel on which to put items that speak to your soul: a Buddha, a cross, pictures of loved ones, a few candles, an aromatherapy diffuser, whatever nourishes your spirit. Keep your journal in this space.

- **Make yoga part of your bedtime ritual.** Bring in your yoga mat for a few stretches before bed, or for when you wake up in the morning. See page 258 for a simple routine.
- **Invest in the best bed.** That goes for your mattress, pillows, sheets, and blankets. Your bed should make you feel like you're in a Four Seasons honeymoon deluxe suite. This is one area where you don't want to scrimp.
- **Keep the crumbs out**—of bed, that is. Save eating for your kitchen or dining room. 'Nuff said.
- **Light up your libido.** Deep, dark maroon colors may be too heat inducing and stimulating for 24/7 display in your boudoir, but pull out a luscious burgundy velvet throw or comforter and hello! Ditto for wine-colored candles and natural scents including cinnamon, bergamot, cedarwood, chocolate, rose, and patchouli. Just watch your libido light up. You can add some matching lingerie for a hard-to-miss red-hot signal to your spouse or mate that says you are in the mood.

The Bathroom

Many of the same rules apply as for your bedroom. Your bathroom can be a fantastic sanctuary, but it also needs to do double duty. At the end of your day, you can use your bathing area as your own personal spa, equipped with aromatherapy, bath salts, and facial masks (beauty treatments are covered in the next chapter).

- **Add ambiance.** Don't forget the violet and pink candles and some soothing scents and music to calm and cheer your mind.
- **Optimize your walls.** Research shows that words or quotes with positive meanings or messages can help you feel more optimistic. So look for or create a simple framed picture that says "Enthusiastic," or "Loving," or "Creative," and watch your day brighten up.
- Soft shades of blues and greens are healing and balancing.

The Kitchen

This is probably the number one hangout for most families and get-togethers. Why does everyone always gravitate toward the kitchen? It can be home base to many members of the family for cooking, chores, homework, and dining. Social colors such as aqua, yellows, and pinks can be cheery and inviting. Clear the clutter from counters, and organize your kitchen for eating well. Your refrigerator should be well stocked and your pantry organized with the right grains, oils, snacks, and beans or lentils. (See "The Super Powered Kitchen," page 190.)

Other Community Spaces

We've covered the main spaces in the home, but redoing other community areas can be a great family project. Take the time to think about what each room of the house represents. Every house is unique, as is every family and Power Type. Optimize energy in all areas, from your living room, den, dining room, backyard, home gym, music room, craft room, entryways and mudrooms to even the laundry area (okay, maybe laundry won't be spiritual, but it can be welcoming).

Nature is the ultimate healer. Backyards, porches, and decks can be especially nurturing spaces for bolstering your serenity and tranquility. If you have the outdoor space, consider creating a specific meditation or contemplation area in your yard.

At Work

You've heard the saying "A cluttered desk means a cluttered mind." Whether it's a home office, a cubicle, or a private corner suite, the space you work in needs to be organized, energized, and calm all at once. Not a tall order at all! Order and flow serve all three. If you have a choice in color, keep in mind that yellow hues stimulate and increase feelings of confidence.

USE THESE TOOLS TO SUPER CHARGE YOUR MENTAL AND EMOTIONAL POWERS

Now that you've made a good start on your physical space, it's time to head into an area that may be scarier than your junkiest junk drawer—your *head*. Fortunately, your biggest battle can be fought and won with a few simple strategies. The only caveat? That you put them to good practice on a daily basis. Within each of the 3-Week Power Plans, you've learned about mental strategies that serve your Power Type best. Below, you'll find specific instructions for how to incorporate all of the mindful tools. If you didn't see one mentioned for your specific Power Type, it's not because it wouldn't be helpful. All of the following super charging tools work if you bring an open mind and a willing heart.

Recharging for mental health is essential to regaining your super powers. You can be uber-disciplined with your diet, supplements, and exercise, but if you don't dedicate the same commitment to mental healing, your efforts will often be in vain. I see it most in myself. When I've worked too many hours, or I have too many deadlines, and I haven't carved out enough downtime, my patience wears thin, my ability to connect weakens, and I am not myself.

Meditation

Meditation helps train your mind and focus your brain. The mental buzzing, all the thought-noise—it's so hard to turn it off. I recall first trying to meditate after experiencing a few stressful events, and I could not make it past a minute! My mind could not focus, my thoughts kept racing—it was just too hard. But after a week or two of forced sitting, it got better: First, I could get to 2 minutes, then 5 minutes, and then 10 and more.

Meditation actually gives you *back* time in your day. The downtime you give your brain by *not* thinking gives it time to recharge and replenish in a way no other activity can. Think about it: Even when you sleep, your dreams take over—slumber isn't necessarily rest time for your mind as it goes hopping off on who knows what crazy adventure or nightmare. But when you meditate by simply focusing all your attention on one thing, usually your breath, you shut off all that mental static. *Ahhh.* What a release that is. Just a few minutes can do wonders for getting through a stressful and overwhelming day.

Below is a meditation from one of my early mentors, and his practice still stays with me today.

How to meditate: Sit somewhere quiet and set your phone timer or a kitchen timer for 3 minutes. Take a deep breath, and blow it all out. Close your eyes. Inhale again, focusing entirely on that inhale: Feel the air go all the way in and your belly expand, and then exhale, blowing all the air slowly out of your mouth, feeling your belly contract. Continue, focusing all your mental energy on each inhale and each exhale. When your mind wanders—and it will because that is the nature of your mind—simply bring your focus back, again and again, to your breath. Let your thoughts drive quietly by in your mind, like cars zipping down a road: As soon as one thought pops up, let it drive on by, and let the next one drive on through, and so on. Continue until your timer goes off. It doesn't matter if you spend all but one breath wandering around in your mental landscape—the effort to meditate counts even if you are terrible at it. Over time, you will get better. Each day, take a few minutes to quiet your mind, center your breath, close your eyes, and just focus on one breath at a time!

There are also lots of great apps for meditating, such as the Insight Timer, Mindfulness App, Meditation Studio, Headspace, and more. Search on your smartphone or tablet, read descriptions, and find one that works for you.

Breathing

Air may be the most important ingredient for good health. When stressed, we hold our breath, take shallow breaths, and feel like we cannot breathe. Taking a few moments to breathe slows you down and makes you focus on relaxation. Slow belly breathing lowers blood pressure and heart rate, easing anxiety and improving restful sleep. One of my favorite breaths—the 4:7:8 breath—is an easy, quick way to learn to breathe for relaxation and healing (see page 259 in Chapter 11 for full directions).

Affirmations

I am a huge believer in affirmations. I do think they really reprogram your brain's pathways over time to shift away from habitual negative thinking to a positive mind-set. Research indicates that using these sorts of conscious and purposeful inner directions can rewire your neural pathways to be more powerful. Affirmations can come from anywhere—books, prayers, quotes that speak to you, or your favorite yoga class. If you search online for "affirmations" plus "courage," "serenity," "optimism," "energy," and so on, you'll find hundreds for every circumstance and situation. Here are a few classics you can use.

"I am getting better, healthier, and happier every day in every way."

"I am beautiful just as I am right in this moment."

"I am grateful for all the abundance in my life."

"I am awake and aware of the wisdom and healing abilities of my body."

"I honor and respect myself and my body and mind."

You can also design your own affirmations. There are just a few basic rules for coming up with effective phrases. What do you notice about the five I offered above? First, they are in the present tense. You might not have a lot of abundance in your life right now, but by saying the affirmation as if it already is true—acting "as if"—your brain believes it to be so. So it's "I am" and "I have," not "I am going to have" or "I will have." Second, avoid negative words such as "don't," "not," or "shouldn't." Affirmations work best if kept on the glass-half-full side of the equation. Finally, the affirmation can't be something you completely reject. You can't say "I am the perfect weight" if you are firmly convinced that you are not, but you can say "I see the beauty inside myself right now."

Journaling, Drawing, and Coloring

Coloring books, journaling, doodling, painting—any sort of hand-to-paper activity that taps creativity—will move cluttered thoughts out of your brain and physical body to calm the nervous system and declutter your mind. One of my favorite books is *The Artist's Way*, and I believe that practicing its ritual exercise of morning pages (more on this below) tapped my own creativity and led me down my road to integrative medicine. I often recommend this book to my patients, along with other artistic endeavors. Try the following:

1. **Scribble a stream of consciousness.** Julia Cameron, author of *The Artist's Way*, has made somewhat famous her exercise of "morning pages," writing three pages freely, first thing in the morning, as soon as you open your eyes. The thought is that this opens the channel to your inner world and literally dumps the junk thoughts. The reality is that I don't have time most mornings to grab my journal and write, but I do try to check in through pen and paper on a daily basis. Here's my adapted

version: I try to write a bit during the first half of my day (first thing in the morning isn't always possible with my family's schedule), so whenever I have about 15 minutes or so to myself, I grab my notebook and pen and start writing. This is often a mishmash of to-do lists, random thoughts, and whatever else is rolling around in my head. Don't overthink it! I know that when I write I feel better, so I've made it a habit. I know writing regularly will make you feel better too. So do it. The rules are that no editor or teacher is allowed in or invited to my writing sessions, plus I don't check spelling, punctuation, or grammar—I simply set a timer and write. If I can't think of what to write, then I write, "I can't think of anything to write," until I think of something else to put down. You'd be surprised what comes out. Give it a try and see.

2. **Sketch and color your mind beautiful.** If you are completely resistant to writing, you can still benefit from a sort of visual journaling to relax your mind. Sketching, painting, or even using the adult coloring books that are so popular these days is a great way to tap into your creative side and helps you to take your mind off stressors of the day. Go to an art store and treat yourself to a good sketch pad and some colored pencils. Set aside 15 to 30 minutes per day to color or sketch—it's not just for kids.

Spirituality and Prayer

This includes your personal definition of spirituality, finding a faith or belief system that works for you, and sharing your spirituality with others. If we look back to our ancient healers, they truly believed all disease was the result of *spiritual disconnection*. My own spirituality is eclectic. I have Bibles, Korans, the Bhagavad Gita, and books by Joel Osteen and Marianne Williamson around my house, and I use them all. I can start off with some morning yoga while listening to a Hindu chant, read a Bible passage before I head into the office, and close out my evening with a Muslim prayer. You may be drawn to a certain faith, or to multiple faiths. Follow what speaks to you—the universe is there to guide you! I encourage you to find your own spiritual home and community. It may be a church, a mosque, a community center, a meditation group, or the living room of a lovely friend—we all need connection with others and a sense of belonging to be our best selves.

Therapy

I have met many women who end up far too deep into the tunnel of despair—where it's too late for a few simple at-home tools (breathing techniques and meditation alone won't cut it). Anxiety and depression are two of the most common mental health issues I see in the women I treat. According to the Anxiety and Depression Association of America, anxiety and depression affect more than 40 million Americans and often present together. Women are more than twice as likely to be affected as men. Women have a different brain chemistry than men, and this in part may account for some of the differences in how they are able to deal with the stressors of life. Research has shown that the fight-or-flight response system in the brain is more readily active in women and stays triggered longer than in men—this is thought to be due to imbalances in estrogen and progesterone. Also, studies show that serotonin in women is processed more slowly than in the male brain, and recent research shows women are more sensitive to a hormone that regulates the stress response, making them twice as vulnerable as men to stress-related disorders (see "A Word about Antidepressants, on the opposite page).

If you feel that even a simple, basic task (making a phone call) is overwhelming, or that you are so fatigued that you can't even get dressed or take a shower—you just want to hide—you may need some extra help. I encourage you to talk with your primary care doctor and discuss a referral for therapy, or you can directly call a therapist in your area. The American Psychological Association offers resources at http://locator.apa.org. Just plug in your city and state and you should get a list of therapists, along with summaries about how they work. Please see below for resources for psychotherapy and hypnotherapy, both of which I have witnessed helping many of my patients.

◆ **Psychotherapy:** I often recommend that my super women who are severely depressed or anxious talk to a therapist. Psychotherapy, often referred to as "talk therapy," is defined as the treatment of mental issues using psychological rather than medical means. Research suggests that women suffering mood disorders do benefit from going to both group and individual therapy. Participating in, and learning from therapy is another way to bring balance and strength to your mind and your life, to help you create an even stronger Fortress of Solitude and sense of serenity. There are several types of therapy, and many therapists use a blended approach. According to the National Association of Cognitive-Behavior Therapists, cognitive behavioral therapy (CBT) emphasizes the role of thinking patterns, their effect on your feelings and actions, and how you can work to identify and discard defeating and negative thinking and thought patterns. CBT teaches you how to replace them with effective, empowering, and positive thoughts and actions. CBT is known for being shorter term than some other therapies, and is particularly helpful in treating anxiety- and depression-related issues. It is highly instructive and comes with a lot of homework and active participation, and can be received as one-on-one therapy or in a group setting. CBT works to improve your focus and concentration, while managing your emotional response. To find a certified cognitive behavioral therapist in your area, visit www.nacbt.org/find-a-therapist/.

◆ **Hypnotherapy:** Hypnosis is an empowered state of awareness, perception, or consciousness that heightens inner absorption, concentration, and focused attention. Hypnotherapy is used by licensed and trained health practitioners to treat psychological or physical issues

A WORD ABOUT ANTIDEPRESSANTS

In a Canadian study, researchers found that between 2007 and 2011 antidepressants were prescribed more than twice as often to women as to men (9.3 percent versus 4.2 percent in adults ages 25 to 44, and 17.2 percent versus 8.2 percent in those ages 45 to 64). More than 10 percent of women take antidepressants, and 23 percent—nearly a quarter—of women in their forties and fifties take one. While medications are not my first choice for treating depression or anxiety, if I have a patient who is suffering from severe depression, who has tried and failed to use other methods to relieve her symptoms, or who just doesn't have the energy to connect the dots or get to the root of her issues—she needs a solution *now*. If this is the scenario, I will prescribe an antidepressant and collaborate with psychiatrists I trust. That said, I am cautious with antidepressants. The cavalier go-to attitude of prescribing these medications appears to be an international epidemic, as they are often used before trying the more natural and organic steps suggested in this book.

such as anxiety, phobias, alcoholism, chronic pain, and for smoking cessation and weight loss. I often recommend hypnosis to help patients learn how to tap into a state of relaxation. I remember one patient in my early years of practice who could not stop coughing, but we couldn't find any physical cause for her symptoms. I suggested hypnotherapy, and after she had a few sessions and learned a few self-hypnosis tricks, her unexplained constant coughing stopped! While you can learn self-hypnosis, it is often helpful to start off with a few sessions with a licensed hypnotherapist. For more information, check out the American Society of Clinical Hypnosis locator page at asch.net/Public/MemberReferralSearch.aspx.

BUILD YOUR BODY'S FORCE FIELD WITH BODYWORK

Many different types of bodywork, from acupuncture to reiki, are available. The certifying bodies vary widely, as do the origins of each. Here's a look at the methods that can help you to fortify and heal your body. Be sure to check out the spa treatments listed by Power Type in the next chapter as well!

Acupuncture

Studies show that acupuncture can alleviate the side effects of chemotherapy and works to balance the nervous system to minimize stress and inflammation. Additionally, acupuncture actually lowers levels of cortisol, the stress hormone that is the root cause of many illnesses today. Lowering cortisol reduces inflammation and anxiety, improves sleep, and promotes healthy eating. I've personally experienced tremendous healing from acupuncture and still use it as an essential part of my self-care and wellness. I've recommended it, and continue to, because I see *great results* for my patients who suffer from migraines, hormonal imbalances, gastrointestinal issues, and many other pain-related issues. To find a board-certified acupuncturist, visit mx.nccaom.org/Find-APractitioner.aspx, the National Certification Commission for Acupuncture and Oriental Medicine's find-a-practitioner page. You can also search for a practitioner at medicalacupuncture.org, the site of the American Academy of Medical Acupuncture.

Massage Therapy

There is a vast body of research that shows the benefits of massage in relieving stress and reducing neck pain and muscle tension. Massage can also lower anxiety, improve mood, and decrease arthritis pain, symptoms of carpal tunnel syndrome, and migraines. I recommend a weekly massage to most of my super women! To find a licensed massage therapist, visit the American Massage Therapy Association at amtamassage.org.

Reiki

Like many other energy systems of medicine, reiki focuses on the transfer of energy from practitioner to patient. The hands of a reiki practitioner pass healing energy into the patient's body to restore balance and calm. Many of my patients use energy healing and find it beneficial. While I have tried to access this energy in my own work with patients, I find that I am not as gifted in this particular skill, and leave it to the amazing practitioners I often meet. You can find a reiki practitioner at the International Association of Reiki Professionals at iarp.org.

Craniosacral Therapy

This technique involves gentle hand pressure and manipulations of the skull and base of the spinal column, resulting in pain and tension relief. The technique works to harmonize the natural rhythm of cerebrospinal fluid in the central nervous system. It is known to relieve migraines, improve sleep, and ease asthma. Additional benefits include reduced neck pain and pain from TMJ (temporomandibular joint) syndrome, ear infections, and sinus infections. Visit the American CranioSacral Therapy Association's Web site at acsta.org to find a qualified therapist.

A WELL-ROUNDED AND HAPPY HABITAT

By empowering, protecting, and enhancing the areas discussed in this chapter—your personal spaces, your mind and mental state, your spirit and your body—you'll create a force field around your life that will keep you happy and healthy, helping you to recharge your super powers for the roller-coaster ride that is life.

Next up? Let's get beautiful!

CHAPTER 13

SUPER BEAUTY

WHAT IS DEEMED beautiful is influenced by your culture, and even by the generation in which you were raised. While Western theories of beauty are finally relaxing their hold on the super skinny, Marilyn Monroe would still probably be told to shave her size 12 body down to a size 4 to meet today's super model standards! Every culture has its own standards of beauty, but besides facial symmetry, few other ideals are universal. Almost everyone everywhere resonates with thick, lustrous hair, clear skin, and *radiance*—that ultimate determinant of beauty.

I think of beauty as being almost identical to health—women can run around buying a million products (or procedures) to be "beautiful," but *real* inner radiance—true beauty—comes from a secret sauce of body and mind balance, health, and happiness. Beauty is *not* only skin deep—it's exactly the opposite. How you look on the outside is a true reflection of how healthy you are on the inside, and vice versa. I see a true shift in my patients when they stop buying the next magic-bullet beauty fix and they start giving their unique Power Type the ingredients it needs, inside and out, to be glowing and gorgeous. As you follow your Power Plan you'll see this relationship between your health and your beauty, and your glow, *your radiance,* will grow brighter.

I can always spot it. I'll see a patient at a follow-up appointment a few months after the first time we met, and it's like someone turned the lights back on. It's one of the top reasons I love doing what I do, and I'm thrilled to show you how you can shine brighter than ever before.

With so many beauty products and regimens to choose from, it can be difficult to figure out what is best for you. Knowing your Power Type unlocks that door and allows you to identify your key beauty needs.

Ready?

Each Power Type, as you've learned, has unique characteristics: If you are a Gypsy Girl, you live in that creative space. A Boss Lady? You are comfortable commanding and leading. Savvy Chicks are the visionaries, Earth Mamas nurture, and Nightingales serve. And just as your medical conditions, nutritional needs, and exercise requirements are unique, so are your beauty needs. One size does not fit all and that includes beauty regimens and treatments!

One of the biggest challenges in the beauty industry is finding products that are not only unique and address your skin type but also are free of chemicals, dyes, and other additives that impact your health. The Environmental Working Group (EWG) is a nonprofit, nonpartisan organization that works to educate the public about all the ingredients in our products, including all beauty, body, and hair products. A recent report by the EWG found that the United States allows more than 1,000 chemicals in cosmetics and body care products that are not allowed by the European Union. Your skin is one of the largest organs on your body,

BEWARE OF BEASTLY BEAUTY INGREDIENTS

You might eat organic and local, keep pesticides out of your garden, and use only toxin-free cleaners, but it's important to know what's in your beauty products as well. According to the Environmental Working Group (EWG), the average woman uses 12 products containing 168 ingredients every day. And your teen and tween super women are far from immune: Adolescent girls' bodies are contaminated with 16 potentially toxic chemicals commonly found in beauty products, according to a recent study. Plus, a recent EWG survey found that the average teen used 40 percent more products than adults! Teens are more sensitive to chemical exposure and have more to lose, since many of these products can affect a developing body and reproductive system.

The products you put on your skin and hair are absorbed into your skin and scalp's inner layers. This includes all hair products, gels, foams, sprays, makeup, body lotions, and cleansers. Thankfully the EWG provides information about what you should look for and avoid. They even have a database of more than 62,000 products you can search to find out what's in your makeup bag, bathroom, and shower, at ewg.org/skindeep/.

and both your skin and your scalp are readily accessible and vulnerable to absorption of all things—good or bad. The health implications of some of these chemicals are disturbing and profound. Many of them are endocrine disruptors, meaning they throw off and damage the very thing we have spent a lot of time talking about balancing in this book—your hormones.

So while we talk beauty and making sure you look as good on the outside as I know you are feeling on the inside, we need to keep in mind that caring for our skin and hair should not add to our toxic load. (See "Beware of Beastly Beauty Ingredients," page 297.)

In the last section of this chapter, I'll walk you through each of the Power Types and my best and healthiest recommendations for your skin and hair care. First, since a complete beauty regimen tends to include cleansing, toning, and moisturizing for your face and body and shampooing and conditioning for your hair, I want to get you familiarized with several DIY beauty ingredients and recipes. I'm a fan of making your own moisturizers, facial masks, hair conditioners, and more because it allows you to reduce chemicals and increase the purity of your beauty products even more. Don't worry, though, if you are too busy to make your own products—simply look for products with the ingredients recommended for your Power Type.

Finally, I have included spa treatments for your Power Type. These treats are a prescription, not just a suggestion, for all super women. You *must* gift yourself spa treatments regularly to maximize your super powers—and that's a doctor's order! You can find day spas at either spafinder.com or yelp.com. When I'm traveling, I like to check both. I'll see what's nearby on spafinder, and then I'll check Yelp to see what the reviews say. If both check out, I'll call and see what a spa offers. I'll discuss what's best for each Power Type later in this chapter, but treating yourself to extra-special beautifying times is not a luxury—it's a requirement. And day spas are the perfect way to do it.

THE BASICS

All women need to follow three basic steps in their beauty regimen.

Cleanse your face, skin, and hair to remove makeup, impurities, and toxins. Some women do not cleanse at all, while others overcleanse and dry out their skin and hair.

Tone your skin to help balance your skin's pH and remove trace remnants of makeup. (See page 303 for more information on balancing the acidity and alkalinity of your skin.)

Moisturize your skin to help restore its natural moisture without clogging your pores. When it comes to your hair, conditioning helps to prevent it from breaking, drying, or being brittle.

See Resources (page 316) for online ordering suggestions for all beauty ingredients in this chapter.

And that's where the one-size-fits-all conversation about the beauty routine stops. It's important to understand the unique needs of your skin and hair type so you can create the beauty recipes that best fit your specific super woman Power Type. Commercial products for both skin and hair are often loaded with chemicals that irritate and harm the skin, so let's get started learning about stocking your super beauty pantry.

Let's take a look at the beauty needs of each Power Type.

GYPSY GIRLS: REPLENISH AND MOISTURIZE

When we think of the Gypsy Girl and her nutritional need for protein and fat, it's easy to see the connection to her most frequent beauty concerns: dry hair, brittle nails, and premature wrinkling. With this dryness in mind, the Gypsy Girl Power Type must focus on hydration and building collagen, the protein matrix that makes up your skin's connective tissue and keeps your skin and your hair plump, shiny, and healthy.

The Gypsy Girl 3-Week Power Plan addressed many of the "inside job" factors of your beauty equation through food, exercise, rest, and supplements. (Trust me! Those B vitamins are working on your hair and nails right now.) But you need a matching outer beauty regimen. Here are my recommendations for your best skin and hair.

Cleanse

Gypsy Girl cleansers should be free from harsh chemicals and abrasive or drying agents because they are too damaging to your skin. Instead, look for gentle, simple, and moisturizing skin products. If you are going to buy a cleanser, choose one that hydrates and is cream or oil based, but without waxes or other pore-clogging ingredients. Look for the ingredients listed below in your cleansers. However, I suggest making your own face and skin cleanser and shampoo. It's so simple and affordable—and good for you! Just mix one of the natural oils below with some castile soap (like Dr. Bronner's Unscented Mild Castile Liquid Soap), which will clean your face and hair without stripping them.

- Olive oil
- Coconut oil
- Jojoba oil
- Argan oil
- Rose oil

DIY face cleanser: Mix 1 teaspoon of any two of the above ingredients together (choosing organic products is best) with 1 teaspoon of castile soap. Gently apply a thin layer to your face with your fingertips. Use warm water and a washcloth to gently remove (no harsh or vigorous scrubbing).

DIY hair wash: You can simply use castile soap with 10 to 20 drops of oil (I like jojoba, argan, or rose oil). Wash and rinse as you normally would. Wash your hair every 2 to 3 days. Washing more often will dry out hair that is already susceptible to drying.

Don't want to make your own? Pick a shampoo with the fewest ingredients and chemicals; go to doctortaz.com/shampoo.

Tone

I like to tone with essential oils rather than astringents, which are loaded with drying and skin-stripping alcohol. Using a few drops of any of the following essential oils will tone and tighten your skin without drying your face. You can use clean fingers to gently apply a small amount of one of the essential oils listed below. You can wipe off gently with a cotton ball if you feel any excess oil. If you have time, incorporate a quick facial massage, which Chinese medical practitioners have long thought stimulated circulation and built collagen (possibly the secret behind so many Chinese people's flawless skin?). Not sure of the technique? Check it out on doctortaz.com/facialmassage.

- Lemon oil
- Lemongrass oil
- Rose oil

DIY facial massage: Massage a few drops of one of the above oils into your skin, for 1 to 3 minutes a day.

Moisturize

The great news is that many of the ingredients you need to cleanse with can also double as moisturizers and conditioners. Nothing relaxes a Gypsy Girl like warming up any of the oils listed and massaging it into the scalp before bed—just this alone can ground your vata, or air, energy and promise you a good night's sleep! You can lather some on your face as well, mixed with relaxing herbs like lavender or sandalwood, for an extra-deep slumber.

DIY face moisturizers: *In the morning:* Combine 1 teaspoon olive oil with 3 to 5 drops lavender oil or rose oil and apply lightly to your face. *In the evening:* Massage 1 teaspoon argan oil nightly into your scalp and/or face.

DIY conditioner: I love to use coconut oil in my hair. It doesn't get any simpler, and it smells great. Simply massage a tablespoon or so into your hair (more if your hair is long and thick, less if it's short). Let it sit for a couple minutes and then rinse. Add a little castile soap to your rinse if your hair feels too oily.

For a deep hair treat: Once a week, add a quarter-size dollop of coconut oil to your hair, comb it, and twist it into a loose bun (if long). Place a soft towel over your pillow, or sleep in a shower cap. In the morning, use castile soap or a nontoxic shampoo to wash it out.

Spa Treatments for Gypsy Girls

There are three special treats I like to recommend to the Gypsy Girl because they help to ground and calm her mind and body.

Craniosacral massage: In this technique, the cranial bones are manipulated by a licensed practitioner, relaxing the nervous system but also leaving you glowing! You can find a therapist at the American Cranio-Sacral Therapy Association's Web site at acsta.org.

Shirodhara: This is one of my favorite Ayurvedic treatments—the gentle, slow drip of oil on the forehead brings instant relaxation to those classic 11 worry lines on the forehead.

Microcurrent therapy: This is a treatment that uses extremely small pulses of electricity to strengthen facial muscles and to keep skin from premature wrinkling. It has been shown to improve production of collagen and elastin.

BOSS LADIES: BE CALM AND COOL

The Boss Ladies, if you remember, "run hot." They generate a lot of heat since all that commanding and directing can tax the digestive system. In many Boss Ladies, you can literally feel that heat emanating from their scalps; in fact, if you are a Boss Lady, close your eyes and lift your left or right arm (it doesn't matter which) so your hand hovers a few inches above your head, palm down. Focus for 30 seconds, and I bet under that hand you can feel that warm sensation of heat! For this reason, a lot of the beauty recommendations for Boss Ladies include ingredients that cool the skin and scalp or just help combat inflammation.

Cleanse

With a tendency toward oily skin or skin that breaks out frequently, Boss Ladies need a cleanser that is pH balanced—that won't strip the skin of its natural oils but also won't add pore-clogging or aggravating ingredients to the surface of the skin. Many commercial cleansers for the hair and scalp are actually too alkaline—the skin is at its best when the pH is right around 5.5, or slightly acidic. Try not to buy cleansers or shampoos that are too alkaline, as they won't help the skin maintain this lower pH, which is necessary for preventing bacterial overgrowth, fine lines, and wrinkles. Better yet, make your own with natural ingredients like apple cider vinegar, lemon juice, and yogurt. The lactic acid in yogurt and milk makes them excellent cleansers for Boss Ladies. Here is the complete list of natural ingredients for this Power Type.

- **Organic raw apple cider vinegar:** made from fermented apples to preserve enzymes and nutrients not found in white vinegar; good for skin and hair; reduces age spots, removes dead skin and toxins, fights acne, balances pH (so your skin won't become too dry or too oily), and minimizes the appearance of wrinkles
- **Lemon juice:** has healing and toning properties, is antibacterial, and can help stop breakouts
- **Yogurt and milk:** reduce fine lines, and the lactic acid in dairy helps to dissolve dead skin and to tighten your pores
- **Chickpea flour:** reduces dryness and removes impurities without being overly drying
- **Bentonite clay:** has minerals including iron, sodium, calcium, potassium, and magnesium that cleanse and heal skin

- **Aloe vera:** contains emollients that provide wound healing and reduce skin inflammation
- **Fuller's earth:** unclogs pores and reduces excess oil secretion, making it a great treatment for acne-prone skin

DIY cleanser: Mix 1 teaspoon apple cider vinegar in 8 teaspoons water and 1 teaspoon yogurt and apply to skin. You can allow this to sit on the skin for 10 to 15 minutes. Rinse and pat dry.

DIY hair wash: Mix as above but in a larger volume to cleanse the scalp. Use as you would a shampoo, and then follow with castile soap.

DIY face mask: My sisters and I used to make this one at home all the time, and this recipe is handed down straight from my mom.

2 teaspoons chickpea flour, organic

1 teaspoon lemon juice, organic and local (if possible)

1 teaspoon plain yogurt, organic

Mix all the ingredients together, apply on the face for 10 to 15 minutes, and then wash off.

For additional suggested cleansers/shampoos, see doctortaz.com/beauty.

Tone

One of the things I love about using natural ingredients is that many can be used for multiple purposes. Try using any of the following ingredients to correct your pH, which really is the goal of skin care for a Boss Lady. Just apply a few drops or dab your face after cleansing with your fingertips. You can either wipe these off with a cotton ball or leave them on your skin. Some, such as apple cider vinegar and rose oil, double as cleansers and moisturizers.

- Raw apple cider vinegar
- Lemon juice
- Frankincense oil
- Lavender oil
- Sandalwood oil
- Rosemary oil
- Basil oil

- Peppermint oil
- Tea tree oil (especially helpful if you are acne prone)
- Calendula
- Comfrey
- Indian gooseberry or amla: This one is also great used as a scalp toner.

DIY hair toner mix: 1 teaspoon of amla juice into your shampoo or just let the juice soak into your scalp for 20 minutes and rinse it out. This fruit is incredibly cooling to the body and scalp.

Moisturize

Moving on to moisturizing, the best moisturizers for Boss Ladies are those that maintain pH but still provide an additional layer of nongreasy moisture to the skin. While a Gypsy Lady needs a thicker-consistency moisturizer, Boss Ladies need moisturizers that moisturize but don't add to the oiliness that they may already have on the face or scalp. Many essential oils are great moisturizers as they serve exactly that purpose.

DIY face moisturizer: Try adding a few drops of frankincense, rose, or lavender oil to a teaspoon of olive or jojoba oil and applying a very thin layer to your face. You can also add to your favorite nontoxic moisturizer.

DIY hair conditioner: Any of the essential oils mentioned earlier in your Boss Lady list also makes for a great conditioner. You can massage 6 to 8 drops of bergamot, lavender, lemon, or sandalwood oil into the ends of your hair. (Leave in or rinse out.)

Spa Treatments for Boss Ladies

Sticking with the theme of "cooling," spa treatments that dissipate heat or regulate inflammation are excellent treatments for Boss Ladies. Think about heat in your body, scalp, or face as a low-level fire that needs the right ingredients to blow it out completely.

Scalp/TMJ massage: A weekly must for a Boss Lady, this type of massage lowers mental tension and relaxes the tight muscles of the scalp and jaw that are often held contracted due to stress. Search for an experienced massage therapist at the American Massage Therapy Association, amtamassage.org.

Exfoliation: Facial treatments that exfoliate the surface layer of the skin may be helpful for Boss Ladies since their skin can sometimes have a rougher texture due to clogged pores, excess sebum, and oil. Ask at your local spa what sort of exfoliation treatments they offer. Lactic and glycolic acid peels and microdermabrasion can help to refine skin texture. Pumpkin enzymes also help to exfoliate. No time for the spa? Try this natural exfoliator: Mix 1 to 2 tablespoons of any of the following into some olive or jojoba oil to make a paste. Massage into your face gently in circular motions, and then wash off.

- Sugar
- Sea salt
- Ground oatmeal
- Baking soda
- Ground almonds

SAVVY CHICKS: BALANCE HOT AND COLD

Alternating between Gypsy Girl and Boss Lady traits, Savvy Chicks have combination needs when it comes to skin and hair—they need moisture like a Gypsy Girl but simultaneously have too much of it, thanks to their Boss Lady side with its tendency toward heat. Given this duality, the beauty regimen of a Savvy Chick can be a bit complex—but not impossible. The key? Always remember to order products for both sides of your skin's and hair's characteristics, so you'll be ready to pivot toward products for dry or moist hair and skin as they fluctuate from dry to oily, rough to smooth—and back again.

Cleanse

One of the greatest cleansing challenges for a Savvy Chick is keeping her pores clean since they are often enlarged by the fluctuation of skin moisture levels. This can create a cycle, with pores enlarging, then getting more easily clogged because they are larger. Most Savvy Chicks notice this the most in the area of the T-Zone, where oil glands are more plentiful. Harsh chemicals in cleansers often worsen this type of combination skin since they strip moisture in the places that need it most. The best cleansers for combination skin would include a mix of the ingredients for Gypsy Girls and Boss Ladies. I like oil cleansing for Savvy Chicks, followed by a gentle wash—this way there is no overstripping and no greasy residue. For hair, I find that what works best is to precondition the hair the night before with any of the oils listed below, followed the next day with shampooing and then regular conditioning.

DIY face cleanser:

Step 1—Cleanse with any one of the following facial or scalp oils or use the Gypsy Girl cleanser list. This will remove dirt and impurities but maintain the pH of the skin.

- Olive oil
- Coconut oil
- Jojoba oil

- Argan oil
- Avocado oil
- Macadamia oil

Step 2—Wash with apple cider vinegar, lemon juice, or yogurt afterward to reduce topical oil and set the right skin pH. You can also mix all of these ingredients together.

DIY hair wash: Follow the recommendations for Boss Ladies on page 303, or try a mixture of ¼ cup organic coconut milk (found in the dairy aisle), ¾ cup castile soap, and 10 drops of lavender or rose oil. Combine all these ingredients in a jar and shake well. Store in your fridge. Shake again before you use the mixture or put it in a foaming dispenser. You'll need a tablespoon or so—use as you would a regular shampoo.

Tone

The role of scalp or facial toners for Savvy Chicks is similar to that for Boss Ladies—to maintain a slightly acidic pH and prepare the skin for moisturizing. Following cleansing, simply use a cotton ball to dab on any one of the following:

- Aloe vera gel, juice, or essential oil

- Lemon oil
- Hazel oil

DIY hair toner: A few drops of the above oils can be added to any shampoo or massaged into the scalp the night before shampooing, not just to tone the scalp, but also to get a great night's sleep.

Moisturize

I think Savvy Chicks need to have two moisturizers—one for oilier days and one for dryer days. Or they can change moisturizers by the season. An easier trick is to keep a base moisturizer on hand but add ingredients to it as needed. For example, your base moisturizer could be water based or a nonclogging oil like olive oil or jojoba. For oiler days, add a few drops of frankincense or lavender to the base—pH balancers that also tackle inflammation. On drier days, add coconut oil, shea butter, or avocado or macadamia oil—thicker ingredients with more moisturizing tendencies. You can do the same with your shampoo as well.

DIY hair treatments: When it comes to a Savvy Chick's scalp and hair, follow the recommendations given for Boss Ladies on page 303. You can also use plain whole milk yogurt or sour cream once a week as a hair treatment. Add a dollop of either, massage it in, and let sit for 20 minutes, then rinse. Both will strip away oils and are moisturizing at the same time.

Spa Treatments for Savvy Chicks

Savvy Chicks need the spa. But, as with their beauty regimen, they'll need different treatments depending on which super woman is dominating—Gypsy or Boss. When there is too much heat and commanding, the Rx is a soothing massage, scalp massage, and the more cooling treatments such as a cooling stone facial massage, a cucumber facial, or a soak in a peppermint-infused tub. At other times, grounding may be more of the issue, so adding in Ayurvedic treatments like shirodhara (see page 44) may be a better option to calm an excitable nervous system.

Exfoliation: Exfoliation and collagen building are Savvy Chick issues as well. When the skin or scalp starts to feel rough, dry, or flaky, weekly facial or scalp exfoliation with some of the DIY exfoliators mentioned for Boss Ladies is helpful (see page 304).

Microcurrent, microneedling, and cosmetic acupuncture: On the other hand, if you have premature wrinkling, microcurrent therapy (page 301) and microneedling (for more information on acupuncture, turn to Chapter 12) are treatments that can help the skin build collagen. Another personal favorite for me is cosmetic acupuncture—it's not as harsh as microneedling (which I also love) but a beauty treatment that applies the principles of Chinese medicine to the face. Each point on the face

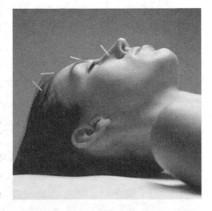

also corresponds with a meridian and, by needling that point, the muscle underneath relaxes, collagen builds up, and the meridian becomes unblocked.

EARTH MAMAS: BALANCE FOR BEAUTY

Out of all the Power Types, Earth Mamas, when in balance, win the prize for their hair and skin. They typically have thick, shiny, lustrous hair and skin that glows—no, *radiates*—seemingly without effort. They are less prone to wrinkling but can battle oily skin and hair when out of balance.

Cleanse

Balancing cleansers are usually best for Earth Mamas. With their thicker skin texture, Earth Mamas need cleansers that work with their skin, rather than stripping it or leaving it sticky or greasy. Since Earth Mamas can at times have oilier skin, moisturizing cleansers are often unnecessary. Here are a few good cleansers for Earth Mama skin and hair.

- Olive oil
- Honey
- Lemon juice
- Milk
- Rosemary oil
- Peppermint oil
- Geranium oil
- Citrus oil (lemon and orange)

DIY face cleanser: Mix 1 teaspoon of honey with 2 teaspoons of lemon juice. Apply a few drops of this mixture to your face, massaging it in gently. Then wash off. Store the remainder in an airtight jar so you can reuse it. Alternatively, you can use any of the oils with the lemon in place of the honey, especially if your skin is feeling dry.

DIY hair wash: For your hair, simply add a few drops of any of the above to your favorite shampoo or castile soap.

Tone

Toning for Earth Mamas is a step to help them maintain their skin moisture without triggering breakouts. Any of the essential oils listed below are good natural toners for Earth Mama skin.

- Rosemary oil
- Peppermint oil
- Geranium oil
- Citrus oil

- Rose oil
- Cypress oil
- Patchouli oil

DIY face toner: Simply massage a few drops of any of these oils into the skin. This step can also double as a moisturizing step, since Earth Mamas don't need a lot of thick, heavy moisturizers. Leave the oil on your skin.

If you don't want to use an oil-based toner, try the following alcohol-free ingredients to gently tone your skin.

- Witch hazel
- Aloe vera gel
- Green tea extract
- Cucumber juice or water (make the juice by blending up some peeled cucumber and then pressing it through a paper towel in a strainer set above a container; make the water by putting cucumber slices in a cup of water and storing in the fridge for 24 hours)

Moisturize

As we mentioned, Earth Mamas do well using the right essential oils as moisturizers or using lightweight moisturizers that balance the skin and hair without necessarily adding more moisture. The most helpful ingredients include many of the essential oils that we have already listed for Earth Mamas or the following:

- Olive oil
- Grapeseed oil
- Hyaluronic acid

- Niacinamide
- Glycerin
- L-carnitine

Look for moisturizers and conditioners with these ingredients—or add them to your favorite existing products.

DIY face moisturizer: A few drops of any of these oils applied to your face will do.

DIY hair conditioner: Mix 1 tablespoon olive oil with ¼ teaspoon jojoba oil, and dilute with ½ cup of warm water. Shake well and apply. Let sit for a minute and then rinse.

Spa Treatments for Earth Mamas

With a slight tendency toward being stagnant, Earth Mama spa treatments should be focused on movement and balance—improving circulation through the face, scalp, and body. Here are some suggested spa treatments for Earth Mamas.

Facials: A monthly facial peel may help to manage excess facial oil and breakouts. Peels that include pumpkin enzyme or glycolic or lactic acid improve skin texture and can resolve breakouts.

Lymphatic massage: Bodywork is always a treat, but Earth Mamas respond particularly well to lymphatic massage. This massage technique improves the flow of lymph and blood through the body, since almost 70 percent of the body's lymphatic vessels lie under the surface of the skin. Gentle strokes returning lymph flow to the heart can help the Earth Mama!

Thai massage: With deep compressions and gentle stretching and pulling, Thai massage, sometimes called "lazy man's yoga," can be another invigorating massage for Earth Mamas, improving circulation and drainage. While this massage can be practiced on a massage table, it was traditionally offered on a mat on the floor. Search for a massage therapist who offers this type of therapy in your area at amtamassage.org.

Acupuncture: One of my favorites, acupuncture is great for Earth Mamas, moving energy through the body and improving circulation (more information on page 41).

NIGHTINGALES: FORTIFY AND MAINTAIN

Nightingales can have the most challenging skin, and building and maintaining collagen seems to be their biggest issue. Both skin and hair can lose moisture and feel dry and rough to the touch. Premature wrinkling can be a concern, and hair may be brittle, with hair loss a common complaint. But a Nightingale can maintain skin and hair texture once she is back in balance. Here are helpful ingredients to maintain Nightingale skin and hair.

Cleanse

Thicker oil- or cream-based cleansers are best for Nightingale skin. Many of the cleansers we recommended for Gypsy Girls are also good fits for Nightingales. These cleansers return moisture to the skin and protect the delicate skin barrier.

- Avocado oil
- Macadamia oil
- Coconut oil
- Rose oil

DIY cleanser: Mix 1 tablespoon olive oil with 2 or 3 drops of rose oil. Rub the mixture into your face and wipe off with a warm washcloth.

DIY hair treatment: Lather the above combination into your scalp and shampoo it out the next day to moisturize without a greasy look.

Tone

I think the best toner for Nightingale skin and hair is lemon juice or any other citrus fruit since the vitamin C can help boost collagen. Additional toners include:

- Rose water
- Liquid vitamin E
- Cucumber juice or water (see page 309 for details on making)

DIY face toner: Try dipping a cotton ball in lemon juice and dabbing it on your skin, or use citrus juice to wash your hair.

Moisturize

Moisturizing is key for Nightingale skin—and an essential step. Nightingale skin needs a barrier to protect it from the elements. The oils we have mentioned double as not just cleansers but moisturizers as well. Other ingredients to look for in a great Nightingale moisturizer include:

- Glycerin
- Hyaluronic acid
- Evening Primrose oil
- Grapeseed oil
- Baobab oil
- Ceramides

DIY face moisturizer and hair conditioner: Apply a thin layer in the morning prior to putting on your makeup, and at night add a thicker layer to your skin, after you've cleansed. You can also add them to your hair at night to rejuvenate it.

AROMA OR ESSENTIAL OIL THERAPY

According to the National Association for Holistic Aromatherapy, aroma-therapy is "the art and science of using naturally extracted aromas from plants to balance, harmonize, and promote the health of body, mind, and spirit." Within this chapter you've heard me talk a lot about using essential oils as topical cleansers, toners, and moisturizers, but here I'm talking about using essential oils for their aroma, not applying them directly to the skin. In this way you can use essential oils to help calm or balance your emotional moods. The essential oils used in aromatherapy are natural oils that have been obtained from a plant, fruit, seed, or herb via a distillation process using steam, water, or steam and water, or have been cold pressed (as with citrus peel oils). Please find the most common essential oils below.

The Essential Essential Oils

I've discussed many of these oils for use on the skin in various recipes. Here is a list of how to use essential oils in an aroma diffuser to achieve the following effects.

ESSENTIAL OIL	WHAT IT DOES
Peppermint	Invigorates, energizes, relieves nausea and migraines
Citrus peel—lemon, mandarin, and orange	Uplifts, calms, and detoxifies
Lemongrass	Cleanses, relieves headaches
Rosemary	Invigorates, stimulates, and energizes
Eucalyptus	Invigorates
Tea tree	Has antibacterial, antifungal, antiviral properties; good acne treatment
Lavender	Relaxes, calms, and soothes
Roman chamomile	Relaxes, soothes, and sedates
Clary sage	Acts as an aphrodisiac, cleanses, and relaxes
Frankincense	Eases congestion, boosts mood, relaxes
Geranium	Balances
Bergamot	Relaxes, boosts mood, refreshes
Sandalwood	Enhances mental clarity, calms, boosts libido
Patchouli	Boosts mood and relaxes
Clove	Relieves stress and headaches
Ylang ylang	Acts as an aphrodisiac
Ginger	Emotionally warms

Spa Treatments for Nightingales

With their service-minded outlook, Nightingales need the spa to rest, recover, and rejuvenate. Specific spa treatments can also help Nightingales restore collagen and improve the hair and skin barrier. Aggressive treatments, including microdermabrasion, cosmetic acupuncture, and microneedling, may not be a good fit until the skin barrier becomes stronger and more intact. Instead, consider any of the following:

- Vitamin C masks/peels: Vitamin C, or L-ascorbic acid, is known to repair the skin and increase collagen.
- Moisturizing masks containing hyaluronic acid, evening primrose oil, or niacinamide: All are known to repair the skin barrier.
- Oxygen facials: These help to restore vibrancy to dull skin or skin exposed to harsh chemicals, wind, dry weather, or UV light.
- Algae therapy: The trace minerals in algae help to repair the skin surface, rebuilding the skin and hair barrier and repairing collagen.

With a little TLC, Nightingales can restore and beautify their skin and hair! They just need to take the time to nurture and pamper themselves.

YOUR BEAUTY POWERS ARE ACTIVATED

Your beauty regimen, just like your Power Plan, needs to be tailored and individualized to you! Now you have all the tools in this chapter to connect your health to your beauty regimen—leaving you feeling—*and looking*—amazing! From the inside to the outside, you'll be glowing and, most importantly, you will be radiant.

Parting Thoughts

IT IS MY deepest hope that *Super Woman Rx*—the ultimate biohack of your health—will have you feeling, looking, and being your *BEST*. I know that once your health and your chemistry are in balance, amazing things will unfold and you'll be able to live the life you were meant to live!

Remember that when your chemistry and health are off the mark, not only do *you* suffer—sometimes silently, sometimes loudly—but everyone whose life you touch bears the weight as well. This ripple effect—you feel lousy, irritable, and agitated so you yell at your partner, spouse, mom, colleagues, kids, friends—has a way of throwing everyone you come into contact with off balance as well.

No more! Now you have the tools to prevent this. If you feel yourself slipping off balance—and let's face it, life happens—you now you have the Super Woman Rx in your back pocket to get you back on track. Plus, you'll begin to see Power Types in all the people around you—maybe you already have. You'll catch yourself thinking about your friend, "Wow, I thought *I* was a Boss Lady, but *she's* a bigger Boss Lady than I am!" And it works for guys too—granted, not too many men are going to want to be called a Gypsy Girl, but if you know a flighty, artistic, creative guy who has a certain style about him (his clothes always look great), you may have just met, or long known, a Gypsy *Guy*. Men and women ask me all the time, "Hey, when are you going to write a book for guys (or kids or parents)?" Stay tuned. There's more to come on the Power Type front. Until then, it's still a helpful habit, and for me, a bit of a fun game to play. Look around and become aware of the various Power Types in the people around you. It can change your communication, deepen your understanding, and shift your interactions with the people in your life from adversarial to cooperative and encouraging. Are you surrounded by Earth Mamas or Savvy Chicks? Is your mom a Nightingale, your daughter an Earth Mama, or your sister a Gypsy Girl? You'll begin to see a positive ripple effect as you interact with and actually influence your colleagues, partners, children, and neighbors—even the cashier at your grocery store. This book will help you to better understand all the people in your life.

Many of my super women patients use my plans to build a better super tribe of women and cut loose those people who are destructive, energy-sucking vampires. You will, too. I've only been able to touch on one one-hundredth of the stories of super women and super men who support and nourish me every day to be—well—me!

EVEN SUPER WOMEN HAVE A BAD DAY

At the end of your 21-day Power Plan, you'll notice the changes in your health, especially in the benchmarks—as I call them—of energy, mood, sleep, and cognition. I am hoping that I sparked the flame of motivation and desire to get on this journey back to *you*. Still, every super woman has a bad day—or days—or sometimes even a bad month or year. As a woman, you will ebb and flow, wax and wane, and change with the circumstances and demands of your life and your age. One moment you might be single, at another, married. You may be in the thick of raising children and nurturing your family or maybe you're a new empty nester. You might be a high-powered corporate executive, or maybe you suddenly find yourself starting your own small business.

Change keeps us alive, charged, and vibrant. Change helps us reinvent, avoid stagnation, and find super powers in ourselves that we did not know we had. All of this is the journey, the triumphs and tragedies of being *you*. Just remember, every super woman has a bad day.

As you walk through your life, remember that you will evolve and use the Super Woman Rx to revisit your needs. An Earth Mama today may be a Savvy Chick tomorrow, and her health needs—like her life—will change. Every medical and scientific aspect of your health is just like life—changeable, plastic, dynamic, and on a continuum.

It is my deepest hope and prayer that this book will guide you in your darkest moments and propel you forward to your happiest ones. I know that you are amazing, powerful, and brilliant—but we all get a bit lost sometimes. Use this book as a road map to reconnect with yourself at any stage of your life—*no matter your age, role, or circumstances*. Find your super powers, be a super woman, and let your light join that of millions of other women to change our world.

Blessings, peace, and hope to all
Dr. Taz

Resources

THESE DAYS THERE are so many great products and resources available online and on the shelves! Here's a list of the brands and some tools that I personally love using and frequently recommend. You can find many of these online at doctortaz.com or centrespringmd.com or you can find them on your favorite Web site or at a local shop.

ALOE VERA JUICE

Lily of the Desert
   (lilyofthedesert.com)

Nature's Way (naturesway.com)

BEAUTY RESOURCES

Beauty Counter (beautycounter.com)

EWG (ewg.org/skindeep)
Check the beauty/skin products you
   utilize here to ensure they're safe
   (lower chemical load).

DIGESTIVE ENZYMES

DigestGold
EnzyMedica (enzymedica.com)

GFCF
Integrative Therapeutics
   (integrativepro.com)

Orthodigestizyme
OrthoMolecular
   (orthomolecularproducts.com)

ESSENTIAL OILS

Doterra (doterra.com)

GLUTAMINE

Glutagenics
Metagenics (metagenics.com)

GlutaShield
Orthomolecular
   (orthomolecularproducts.com)

HERBS

Ashwagandha
Banyan Botanicals
   (banyanbotanicals.com)

Astragalus
Gaia Herbs (gaiaherbs.com)

Slippery Elm
Gaia Herbs (gaiaherbs.com)

PROTEIN POWDER, GUT HEALING SHAKES

Chocolate protein powder
Vega (myvega.com)

Dr. Taz's Protein Powder
EastWest by Dr. Taz MD
   (doctortaz.com)

Ultra Clear and Ultra Meal
Metagenics (metagenics.com)

Vanilla protein powder
Garden of Life (gardenoflife.com)

OTHER VITAMINS, MINERALS, AMINO ACIDS, AND BLENDS

Amalaki
Banyan Botanicals
   (banyanbotanicals.com)

BOOST (vitamin B/energy blend)
EastWest by Dr. Taz MD
   (doctortaz.com)

Epsom salt
Dr. Teal's
   (drteals.pdcbrandsusa.com)

Ghee
Banyan Botanicals
   (banyanbotanicals.com)

Hormone Helper (balance)
EastWest by Dr. Taz MD
   (doctortaz.com)

Liquid iron
Integrative Therapeutics
   (integrativepro.com)

L-Theanine
Integrative Therapeutics
   (integrativepro.com)

Lush Locks (hair support)
EastWest by Dr. Taz MD
   (doctortaz.com)

Magnesium
Metagenics (metagenics.com)

Natural Calm (magnesium drink)
Natural Vitality (naturalvitality.com
   /natural-calm/)

Omega-3
Nordic Naturals
   (nordicnaturals.com)

Sleep Savior (aiding in sleep)
EastWest by Dr. Taz MD
   (doctortaz.com)

Vitamin D
OrthoMolecular
   (orthomolecularproducts.com)

KITCHEN TOOLS (ALL AVAILABLE ON AMAZON.COM)

Blender

NutriBullet (nutribullet.com)

Ninja (ninjakitchen.com)

Vitamix (vitamix.com)

Food processor

Hamilton Beach
   (hamiltonbeach.com)

Cuisinart (cuisinart.com)

Frother

PowerLix Milk Frother
   (amazon.com)

Elementi original Premier Milk Frother
   (amazon.com)

Immersion blender

KitchenAid (kitchenaid.com)

Hamilton Beach
   (hamiltonbeach.com)

Mason jars

Golden Spoon (at Walmart or
   amazon.com)

Ball Mason (at Walmart or
   amazon.com)

Pressure cooker

Instant Pot (instantpot.com)

Presto (gopresto.com)

Spiralizer

Zestkit (amazon.com)

Spiralife (amazon.com)

References

Chapter 1: The Super Woman Syndrome

American Psychological Association. 2010. "Gender and Stress." Accessed February 16, 2017 apa.org/news/press/releases/stress/2010/gender-stress.aspx. stressinamericaorg.

American Society for Aesthetic Plastic Surgery. 2017. "American Society for Aesthetic Plastic Surgery Reports More Than $15 Billion Spent for the First Time Ever." News release, March 15. Accessed April 8, 2017. surgery.org/media/news-releases/americans -spend-more-than-15-billion-on-aesthetic-procedures-for-the-first-time-ever.

Anxiety and Depression Association of America. 2017. "Facts: Anxiety and Depression." Accessed February 16, 2017. adaa.org/living-with-anxiety/women/facts.

Bureau of Labor Statistics. US Department of Labor. 2016. "American Time Use Survey—2015 Results." News release, June 24. Accessed February 16, 2017. bls.gov/news.release /pdf/atus.pdf.

Chandra, A., C. E. Copen, and E. H. Stephen. 2013. "Infertility and Impaired Fecundity in the United States, 1982–2010: Data from the National Survey of Family Growth." *National Health Statistics Reports* 67 (August 14): 1–18. cdc.gov/nchs/data/nhsr /nhsr067.pdf.

Duke University Libraries. "Miss America Protests: Women's Liberation Movement Print Culture." Accessed February 16, 2017. library.duke.edu/digitalcollections/wlmpc /Series/Miss%20America%20Protests.

———. "Women's Liberation Movement Print Culture." Accessed February 16, 2017. library.duke.edu/digitalcollections/wlmpc/

Fryar, Cheryl D., Cynthia L. Ogden, and Gu M.D. Giuping. 2012. "Anthropometric Refer- ence Data for Children and Adults: United States, 2007–2010." *Vital and Health Statistics*, 11th ser., no. 252 (October). cdc.gov/nchs/data/series/sr_11/sr11_252.pdf.

Gladstone, Leslie W. 2001. "American Women: The Long Road to Equality: What Women Won from the ERA Ratification Effort." Library of Congress. Accessed February 16, 2017. memory.loc.gov/ammem/awhhtml/aw03e/aw03e.html.

Heart Foundation. 2015. "Heart Disease Scope and Impact." Accessed February 16, 2017. theheartfoundation.org/heart-disease-facts/heart-disease-statistics/.

History, Art & Archives. United States House of Representatives. "The Women's Rights Movement, 1848–1920." Accessed February 16, 2017. history.house.gov/Exhibitions -and-Publications/WIC/Historical-Essays/No-Lady/Womens-Rights/.

Library of Congress. 2010. "Rosie the Riveter Transcript (Journeys and Crossings, Library of Congress Digital Reference Section)." Accessed April 10, 2017. loc.gov/rr/program /journey/rosie-transcript.html.

———. "Women in the Civil Rights Movement—Civil Rights History Project." Accessed February 16, 2017. loc.gov/collections/civil-rights-history-project/articles-and -essays/women-in-the-civil-rights-movement/.

Migraine Research Foundation. "Migraine Is a Women's Health Issue." Accessed February 16, 2017. migraineresearchfoundation.org/about-migraine/migraine-in-women/.

National Alliance on Mental Illness. 2009. "Women and Depression Fact Sheet." (October 30). Accessed February 16, 2017. nami.org.

National Bureau of Economic Research. 2009. "Women and Post-WWII Wages." Accessed April 10, 2017. nber.org/digest/nov02/w9013.html.

Office on Women's Health. 2014. "Chronic Fatigue Syndrome." (September 4). Accessed February 16, 2017. womenshealth.gov/publications/our-publications/fact-sheet/chronic-fatigue-syndrome.html#.PBS, *American Experience*. 2001. "People & Events: Mrs. America: Women's Roles in the 1950s." Accessed February 16, 2017. pbs.org/wgbh/amex/pill/peopleevents/p_mrs.html.

Patten, S. B., J. L. Wang, J. V. Williams, S. Currie, C. A. Beck, C. J. Maxwell, and N. El-Guebaly. 2006. "Descriptive Epidemiology of Major Depression in Canada." *Canadian Journal of Psychiatry* 51 (2): 4–90.

PCOS Foundation. 1999. "What Is PCOS?" Accessed February 16, 2017. pcosfoundation.org/what-is-pcos.

Petitti, Diana. 2005. "Four Decades of Research on Hormonal Contraception." *The Permanente Journal* 9 (1): 29–34.

Statista.com. "Revenue of the Cosmetic/Beauty Industry in the United States from 2002 to 2016." Accessed February 16, 2017. statista.com/statistics/243742/revenue-of-the-cosmetic-industry-in-the-us/.

Stroke.org. 2016. "Women and Stroke." (January 26). Accessed February 16, 2017. stroke.org/understand-stroke/impact-stroke/women-and-stroke.

Tyrer, Louise. 1999. "Introduction of the Pill and Its Impact." *Contraception* 59 (1).

US Census Bureau Public Information Office. 2012. "Facts for Features: Women's History Month: March 2012—Facts for Features & Special Editions—Newsroom—US Census Bureau." (February 22). Accessed February 16, 2017. census.gov/newsroom/releases/archives/facts_for_features_special_editions/cb12-ff05.html.

Wolfe, Molly. 2015. "This Day in History: National Organization for Women Was Founded." The White House (June 30). Accessed February 16, 2017. obamawhitehouse.archives.gov/blog/2015/06/30/day-history-national-organization-women-was-founded.

Women's International Center. 1995. "WIC—Women's History in America." Accessed February 16, 2017. wic.org/misc/history.htm.

Chapter 4: Super Tools for Super Women

Clarke, Tainya C, L. I. Black, B. J. Stussman, P. M. Barnes, and R. L. Nahin. 2015. "Trends in the Use of Complementary Health Approaches among Adults: United States, 2002–2012." *National Health Statistics Report* 79. Hyattsville, MD: US Department of Health and Human Services, Centers for Disease Control and Prevention, National Center for Health Statistics. cdc.gov/nchs/data/nhsr/nhsr079.pdf.

Tai-Seale, M., T. G. McGuire, and W. Zhang. 2007. "Physician and Patient Behavior: Time Allocation in Primary Care Office Visits." *Health Services Research* 45 (5) (October): 1871–94.

Chapter 5: The Gypsy Girl's 3-Week Rx

Hirschfield, Robert M. A. 2001. "The Comorbidity of Major Depression and Anxiety Disorders." *The Primary Care Companion to the Journal of Clinical Psychiatry* 3 (6) (December 1): 244–54.

Kessler, Ronald C., Sergio Aguilar-Gaxiola, Jordi Alonso, Somnath Chatterji, Sing Lee, Johan Ormel, T. Bedirhan Üstün, and Philip S. Wang. 2009. "The Global Burden of Mental Disorders: An Update from the WHO World Mental Health (WMH) Surveys." *Epidemiologia e Psichiatria Sociale* 18 (1): 23–33.

Meng, Hongdao, Lauren Hale, and Fred Friedberg. 2010. "Prevalence and Predictors of Fatigue In Middle-Aged And Older Adults: Evidence from the Health and Retirement Study." *Journal of the American Geriatrics Society* 58 (10): 2033–34.

Remes, Olivia, Carol Brayne, Rianne Van Der Linde, and Louise Lafortune. 2016. "A Systematic Review of Reviews on the Prevalence of Anxiety Disorders in Adult Populations." *Brain and Behavior* 6 (7) (June 5).

World Health Organization. 2016. "Investing in Treatment for Depression and Anxiety Leads to Fourfold Return." News release, April 13. Accessed February 17, 2017. who.int/mediacentre/news/releases/2016/depression-anxiety-treatment/en/.

"2005 Sleep in America Poll—Adult Sleep Habits and Styles." 2005. *Sleep Health* 1 (2) (March).

Chapter 6: The Boss Lady's 3-Week Rx

Beaufrere, A. M., N. Neveux, P. Patureau Mirand, C. Buffiere, G. Marceau, V. Sapin, L. Cynober, and Dominique Meynial-Denis. 2014. "Long-Term Intermittent Glutamine Supplementation Repairs Intestinal Damage (Structure and Functional Mass) with Advanced Age: Assessment with Plasma Citrulline in a Rodent Model." *Journal of Nutrition, Health & Aging* 18 (9) (November 5).

Grundmann, Oliver, and Saunjoo L. Yoon. 2010. "Irritable Bowel Syndrome: Epidemiology, Diagnosis and Treatment: An Update for Health-Care Practitioners." *Journal of Gastroenterology and Hepatology* 25 (4) (January 13): 691–99.

International Foundation for Functional Gastrointestinal Disorders. 2016. "Facts about IBS." November 24.. Accessed February 21, 2017. aboutibs.org/what-is-ibs/facts -about-ibs-2.html.

Lee, Sun-Young, Jeong Hwan Kim, In-Kyung Sung, Hyung-Seok Park, Choon-Jo Jin, Won Hyeok Choe, So Young Kwon, Chang Hong Lee, and Kyoo Wan Choi. 2007. "Irritable Bowel Syndrome Is More Common in Women Regardless of the Menstrual Phase: A Rome II-based Survey." *Journal of Korean Medical Science* 22 (5) (October 31): 851.

Tanghetti, E. A., A. K. Kawata, S. R. Daniels, K. Yeomans, C. T. Burk, and V. D. Callender. 2014. "Acne in the Adult Female Patient: A Practical Approach." *Journal of Clinical and Aesthetic Dermatology* 7 (21) (February).

Chapter 8: The Earth Mama's 3-Week Rx

Centers for Disease Control and Prevention. 2016. "Childhood Obesity Facts." December 22. Accessed February 21, 2017. cdc.gov/obesity/data/childhood.html.

Vahratian, Anjel. 2008. "Prevalence of Overweight and Obesity among Women of Childbearing Age: Results from the 2002 National Survey of Family Growth." *Maternal and Child Health Journal* 13 (2) (April 16): 268–73.

Vesely, J. M., and L. G. DeMattia. 2014. "Obesity: Dietary and Lifestyle Management." *Family Physician Essentials* 425 (October): 11–15.

Chapter 10: The Nightingale's 3-Week Rx

Arranz, Lorena, Noelia Guayerbas, León Siboni, and Mónica De La Fuente. 2007. "Effect of Acupuncture Treatment on the Immune Function Impairment Found in Anxious Women." *American Journal of Chinese Medicine* 35 (1): 35–51. Accessed February 21, 2017.

Chacko, Sabu M., Priya T. Thambi, Ramadasan Kuttan, and Ikuo Nishigaki. 2010. "Beneficial Effects of Green Tea: A Literature Review." *Chinese Medicine* 5 (1) (April 6): 13.

Chattopadhyay, Chandan, Mitali Chatterjee, Kajari Sarkar, Nandini Chakrabarti, Sonali Mukherjee, and Aroy Chaudhuri. 2012. "Black Tea (Camellia sinensis) Decoction Shows Immunomodulatory Properties on an Experimental Animal Model and in Human Peripheral Mononuclear Cells." *Pharmacognosy Research* 4 (1) (January): 15–21.

Kim, Sun Kwang, and Hyunsu Bae. 2010. "Acupuncture and Immune Modulation." *Autonomic Neuroscience* 157 (1–2) (October 28): 38–41.

National Cancer Institute. 2012. "Cruciferous Vegetables and Cancer Prevention." June 7. Accessed February 21, 2017. cancer.gov/about-cancer/causes-prevention/risk /diet/cruciferous-vegetables-fact-sheet.

Patil, Vaishali M., Sukanya Das, and Krishnan Balasubramanian. 2016. "Quantum Chemical and Docking Insights into Bioavailability Enhancement of Curcumin by Piperine in Pepper." *Journal of Physical Chemistry A* 120 (20) (May 26): 3643–53.

Chapter 10: Super Sustaining Nutrition

Environmental Working Group. 2017. "Clean Fifteen: EWG's 2017 Shopper's Guide to Pesticides in Produce." Accessed February 21, 2017. Accessed February 21, 2017. ewg.org/foodnews/clean_fifteen_list.php.

———. 2017. "Dirty Dozen: EWG's 2017 Shopper's Guide to Pesticides in Produce." Accessed February 21, 2017. ewg.org/foodnews/dirty_dozen_list.php.

Chapter 11: Power-Packed Exercise

Abbott, Ryan, and Helen Lavretsky. 2013. "Tai Chi and Qigong for the Treatment and Prevention of Mental Disorders." *Psychiatric Clinics of North America* 36 (1) (March 1): 109–19. doi:10.1016/j.psc.2013.01.011.

American Heart Association. 2016. "Target Heart Rates." October. Accessed February 21, 2017. heart.org/HEARTORG/HealthyLiving/PhysicalActivity/FitnessBasics /Target-Heart-Rates_UCM_434341_Article.jsp#.WKxR2BiZPAJ.

Centers for Disease Control and Prevention. 2015. "Target Heart Rate and Estimated Maximum Heart Rate." August 10. Accessed February 21, 2017. cdc.gov/physicalactivity /basics/measuring/heartrate.htm.

National Center for Complementary and Integrative Health. 2016. "Yoga: In Depth." September 26. Accessed February 21, 2017. nccih.nih.gov/health/yoga/introduction .htm.

Pearson, David G., and Tony Craig. 2014. "The Great Outdoors? Exploring the Mental Health Benefits of Natural Environments." *Frontiers in Psychology* 5 (October 21).

Chapter 12: Build Your Fortress of Solitude

Albert, Paul. 2015. "Why Is Depression More Prevalent in Women?" *Journal of Psychiatry & Neuroscience* 40 (4) (July 1): 219–21.

American Massage Therapy Association. 2005. "25 Reasons to Get a Massage." March 2. Accessed February 21, 2017. amtamassage.org/articles/1/News/detail/3124.

Anxiety and Depression Association of America. 2016. "Facts & Statistics." August. Accessed February 21, 2017. adaa.org/about-adaa/press-room/facts-statistics.

———. 2016. "Live and Thrive—Women: Facts." Accessed February 21, 2017. adaa.org /living-with-anxiety/women/facts.

Blanchfield, Anthony, James Hardy, and Samuele Marcora. 2014. "Non-conscious Visual Cues Related to Affect and Action Alter Perception of Effort and Endurance Performance." *Frontiers in Human Neuroscience* 8 (December 11).

Cameron, Julia. 2016. *The Artist's Way: A Spiritual Path to Higher Creativity.* London: Macmillan.

Elliot, A. J., and M. A. Maier. 2014. "Color Psychology: Effects of Perceiving Color on Psychological Functioning in Humans." *Annual Review of Psychology* 65 (1) (January 3): 95–120.

Harvard Health Publications. 2011. "Women and Depression." May 1. Accessed February 21, 2017. health.harvard.edu/womens-health/women-and-depression.

———. 2015. "Relaxation Techniques: Breath Control Helps Quell Errant Stress Response." January 26. Accessed February 21, 2017. health.harvard.edu/mind-and -mood/relaxation-techniques-breath-control-helps-quell-errant-stress-response.

Kim, Mi Kyoung, and Sung Don Kang. 2013. "Effects of Art Therapy Using Color on Purpose in Life in Patients with Stroke and Their Caregivers." *Yonsei Medical Journal* 54 (1) (January 1): 15–20.

Leach, Liana S., Helen Christensen, Andrew J. Mackinnon, Timothy D. Windsor, and Peter Butterworth. 2008. "Gender Differences in Depression and Anxiety Across the Adult Lifespan: The Role of Psychosocial Mediators." *Social Psychiatry and Psychiatric Epidemiology* 43 (12): 983–98.

Levy, Becca R., Corey Pilver, Pil H. Chung, and Martin D. Slade. 2014. "Subliminal Strengthening: Improving Elders' Physical Function over Time through an Implicit-Age-Stereotype Intervention." *Psychological Science* 25 (12) (December 25): 2127–35.

Li, Qian-Qian, Guang-Xia Shi, Qian Xu, Jing Wang, Cun-Zhi Liu, and Lin-Peng Wang. 2013. "Acupuncture Effect and Central Autonomic Regulation." *Evidence-Based Complementary and Alternative Medicine* (May 26): 1–6.

National Center for Complementary and Integrative Health. 2016. "Meditation: In Depth." April. Accessed February 21, 2017. nccih.nih.gov/health/meditation/overview .htm#hed3.

Pratt, L. A., D. J. Brody, and G. Qiuping. 2011. "Antidepressant Use in Persons Aged 12 and Over: United States, 2005–2008." Centers for Disease Control and Prevention. October 19. Accessed February 21, 2017. cdc.gov/nchs/data/databriefs/db76.htm.

Sharma, Pulkit, Ruby Charak, and Vibha Sharma. 2009. "Contemporary Perspectives on Spirituality and Mental Health." *Indian Journal of Psychological Medicine* 31 (1) (January): 16–23.

Stuckey, Heather L., and Jeremy Nobel. 2010. "The Connection Between Art, Healing, and Public Health: A Review of Current Literature." *American Journal of Public Health* 100 (2) (February): 254–63.

Chapter 13: Super Beauty

Eisenhardt, Stefan, Benno Runnebaum, Klausdieter Bauer, and Ingrid Gerhard. 2001. "Nitromusk Compounds in Women with Gynecological and Endocrine Dysfunction." *Environmental Research* 87 (3): 123–30.

Environmental Working Group. 2001. "National Academy of Sciences: Formaldehyde Causes Cancer." April 8. Accessed February 21, 2017. ewg.org/news/news -releases/2011/04/08/national-academy-sciences-formaldehyde-causes-cancer.

———. 2008. "Teen Girls' Body Burden of Hormone-Altering Cosmetics Chemicals." September 24. Accessed February 21, 2017. ewg.org/research/teen-girls-body-burden -hormone-altering-cosmetics-chemicals.

———. 2017. "Myths on Cosmetics Safety" Accessed February 21, 2017. ewg.org /skindeep/myths-on-cosmetics-safety/.

Hutter, H.-P., P. Wallner, H. Moshammer, W. Hartl, R. Sattelberger, G. Lorbeer, and M. Kundi. 2005. "Blood Concentrations of Polycyclic Musks in Healthy Young Adults." *Chemosphere* 59 (4): 487–92.

Integrative, PDQ, Alternative, and Complementary Therapies Editorial Board. 2005. "Aromatherapy and Essential Oils (PDQ®)." National Center for Biotechnology Information. October 24. Accessed February 21, 2017. ncbi.nlm.nih.gov/pubmedhealth /PMH0032645/.

National Association for Holistic Aromatherapy. "What Are Essential Oils?" Accessed February 21, 2017. naha.org/index.php/explore-aromatherapy/about-aromatherapy /what-are-essential-oils/.

Pan, Shawn, Chaoshen Yuan, Abderrahmane Tagmount, Ruthann A. Rudel, Janet M. Ackerman, Paul Yaswen, Chris D. Vulpe, and Dale C. Leitman. 2016. "Parabens and Human Epidermal Growth Factor Receptor Ligand Cross-Talk in Breast Cancer Cells." *Environmental Health Perspectives* 124 (5) (May): 563–69.

Rimkus, Gerhard G., and Manfred Wolf. 1996. "Polycyclic Musk Fragrances in Human Adipose Tissue and Human Milk." *Chemosphere* 33 (10): 2033–43

Acknowledgments

This book is for every woman—the women who cry in my exam rooms feeling defeated by the world, the women who hold it together every day, and the women around the world trying to protect their families and build better communities—even in the face of violence, misogyny, and persecution. Every woman I have ever met delays her care until everyone else around her is taken care of. It is my hope that this book is your guide, as well as a home, a place to return to every few months to check in to protect and guard your health. Without it, none of us can do what we were meant to do.

To Mom. Crossing an ocean, entering a new country, raising children, trying to find your voice and community and purpose, navigating that space of what you were told was a woman's role and what you wanted—always modeling a work ethic that we, your girls, still to this day cannot emulate (and I work hard!!!!).

To my sister, Shireen Haque, whose recipes are scattered throughout this book. Thanks for sharing your culinary talent with my readers. Watch out! They may want more. And to my hubby, Vik, and my son, Kubby—we would not be super women without super men and super boys like you!!!

To my amazing team—Jessica, Lindsay, Marianne, Margot—you guys rock! You kept me on track and made this come alive.

And to my team at Centrespring MD—the work we do matters. Thank you for your dedication.

Dr. Taz

Index

Underscored page references indicate boxed text. **Boldface** references indicate photographs or illustrations.

A

abhyanga therapy, 44
acne/breakouts, 40, 86
acupuncture, 41, 106, 172, 294, 307
ACV (apple cider vinegar) tonic, 94, 150
ADHD, 57
adrenal adaptogens, 125
adrenal glands, 50, 62, 73–74, 115, 124–25, 175
adrenaline, 105, 179
affirmations, 289–90
Alba, Jessica, 111
alcohol, 47
algae therapy, 313
allergies, 165
allopathic medicine, 35
aloe vera juice, 95
amenorrhea, 113
American Academy of Medical Acupuncture, 294
American CranioSacral Therapy Association, 295
American Massage Therapy Association, 295
amla, 106
amylase, 48, 99
ANA (antinuclear antibodies), 141
androgenetic alopecia (hair loss), 60
anorexia, 57–58
anovulatory (missed) cycles, 60
antidepressants, 293
anti-inflammatory diet, 46–47
antinuclear antibodies (ANA), 141
anxiety, 3, 56–57, 112, 166, 292
apple cider vinegar (ACV) tonic, 94, 150
aromatherapy, 79, 105, 312
artificial sweeteners, 47
ashwagandha, 74, 125
aspartame, 47

asthma, 165
astragalus root, 125, 171
Ayurvedic Medicine
abhyanga, 44
chakras, 43–44
cooling foods, 104
defined, 16
doshas, 42, 61–62, 115, 140, 167
overlap with TCM, 43
overview, 41–42
pittas, 88–89
shirodhara, 44
typing, 43–44

B

balancing hormones
Boss Ladies' 3-Week Power Plan, 175–78
Gypsy Girls' 3-Week Power Plan, 73–76
Savvy Chicks' 3-Week Power Plan, 123–27
Barrett's esophagus, 165
bathroom, personalizing, 286
beauty routines, 296–313
aromatherapy, 312
basics, 298–99
Boss Ladies' 3-Week Power Plan, 105, 302–5
Earth Mamas' 3-Week Power Plan, 158, 308–10
essential oil therapy, 312
Gypsy Girls' 3-Week Power Plan, 79, 299–301
Nightingales, 310–13
overview, 296–98
Savvy Chicks' 3-Week Power Plan, 305–8

W

Y